Shoulder Instability in the Athlete

Editor

STEPHEN R. THOMPSON

CLINICS IN SPORTS MEDICINE

www.sportsmed.theclinics.com

Consulting Editor
MARK D. MILLER

October 2013 • Volume 32 • Number 4

ELSEVIER

1600 John F. Kennedy Boulevard ● Suite 1800 ● Philadelphia, Pennsylvania, 19103-2899

http://www.theclinics.com

CLINICS IN SPORTS MEDICINE Volume 32, Number 4
October 2013 ISSN 0278-5919, ISBN-13: 978-0-323-26412-9

Editor: Jennifer Flynn-Briggs
Developmental Editor: Donald Mumford

Clinics in Sports Medicine (ISSN 0278-5919) is published quarterly by Elsevier Inc., 360 Park Avenue South, New York, NY 10010-1710. Months of issue are January, April, July, and October. Business and Editorial Offices: 1600 John F. Kennedy Blvd., Ste. 1800, Philadelphia, PA 19103-2899. Customer Service Office: 3251 Riverport Lane, Maryland Heights, MO 63043. Periodicals postage paid at New York, NY and additional mailing offices. Subscription prices are $324.00 per year (US individuals), $523.00 per year (US institutions), $159.00 per year (US students), $367.00 per year (Canadian individuals), $631.00 per year (Canadian institutions), $222.00 (Canadian students), $446.00 per year (foreign individuals), $631.00 per year (foreign institutions), and $222.00 per year (foreign students). Foreign air speed delivery is included in all *Clinics* subscription prices. All prices are subject to change without notice. **POSTMASTER:** Send address changes to *Clinics in Sports Medicine*, Elsevier Health Sciences Division, Subscription Customer Service, 3251 Riverport Lane, Maryland Heights, MO 63043. Customer Service (orders, claims, online, change of address): Elsevier Health Sciences Division, Subscription Customer Service, 3251 Riverport Lane, Maryland Heights, MO 63043. Tel: 1-800-654-2452 (U.S. and Canada); 314-447-8871 (outside U.S. and Canada). Fax: 314-447-8029. E-mail: journalscustomerservice-usa@elsevier.com (for print support); journalsonlinesupport-usa@elsevier.com (for online support).

Reprints. For copies of 100 or more of articles in this publication, please contact the Commercial Reprints Department, Elsevier Inc., 360 Park Avenue South, New York, NY 10010-1710. Tel.: 212-633-3874; Fax: 212-633-3820; E-mail: reprints@elsevier.com.

Clinics in Sports Medicine is covered in *MEDLINE/PubMed (Index Medicus) Current Contents/Clinical Medicine, Excerpta Medica,* and *ISI/Biomed.*

Printed and bound by CPI Group (UK) Ltd, Croydon, CR0 4YY

Transferred to digital print 2012

Contributors

CONSULTING EDITOR

MARK D. MILLER, MD
S. Ward Casscells Professor of Orthopaedic Surgery, University of Virginia; Team
Physician, James Madison University, Charlottesville, Virginia

EDITOR

STEPHEN R. THOMPSON, MD, MEd, FRCSC
Private Practice, Sports Medicine and Arthroscopic Surgery, Orthopaedic Surgery of
Maine, Eastern Maine Medical Center, Bangor, Maine; Division of Orthopedic Surgery,
Western University, London, Ontario, Canada

AUTHORS

DAVID W. ALTCHEK, MD
Attending Surgeons, Hospital for Special Surgery, New York, New York

GEORGE S. ATHWAL, MD, FRCSC
Division of Orthopedic Surgery, Western University; Bioengineering Research Laboratory,
Hand and Upper Limb Centre, St. Joseph's Health Centre, London, Ontario, Canada

JEAN-CHRISTIAN BALESTRO, MD
Sydney Shoulder Specialists, St Leonards, Sydney, New South Wales, Australia

RYAN T. BICKNELL, MD, MSc, FRCS(C)
Associate Professor, Division of Orthopaedic Surgery, Department of Surgery, Kingston
General Hospital—Nickle 3, Queen's University, Kingston, Ontario, Canada

ROBERT BLEAKNEY, MD, FRCPC
Radiologist, Department of Medical Imaging, Mount Sinai Hospital, Toronto, Ontario,
Canada

AARON J. BOIS, MD, MSc, FRCSC
Clinical Lecturer, Section of Orthopaedic Surgery, Department of Surgery, University of
Calgary, Calgary, Alberta, Canada

JAMES P. BRADLEY, MD
Clinical Professor of Orthopaedics, Head Team Physician, Pittsburgh Steelers, Burke
and Bradley Orthopaedics, University of Pittsburgh Medical Center, Pittsburgh,
Pennsylvania

STEPHEN F. BROCKMEIER, MD
Assistant Professor, Department of Orthopaedic Surgery, University of Virginia,
Charlottesville, Virginia

ROBERT H. BROPHY, MD
Associate Professor, Department of Orthopaedic Surgery, Washington University School of Medicine, St Louis, Missouri

LAUCHLAN CHAMBERS, MD, MPH
Fellow in Sports Medicine and Shoulder Surgery, Hospital for Special Surgery, New York, New York

RYAN M. DEGEN, MD
Division of Orthopedic Surgery, Western University, London, Ontario, Canada

JOSHUA S. DINES, MD
Attending Surgeon, Department of Sports Medicine and Shoulder Surgery, Hospital for Special Surgery, New York, New York

TIM DWYER, MBBS, FRACS, FRCSC
Orthopaedic Surgeon, Department of Surgery, Women's College Hospital, University of Toronto Orthopaedic Sports Medicine, Toronto, Ontario, Canada

JOSHUA W. GILES, BESc
Bioengineering Research Laboratory, Hand and Upper Limb Centre, St. Joseph's Health Centre, London, Ontario, Canada

EWAN B. GOUDIE, BMedSci (Hons), MRCSEd
Specialty Registrar, Department of Trauma and Orthopaedics, Royal Infirmary of Edinburgh, Edinburgh, United Kingdom

JUSTIN W. GRIFFIN, MD
Resident Physician, Department of Orthopaedic Surgery, University of Virginia, Charlottesville, Virginia

F. WINSTON GWATHMEY Jr, MD
Fellow, Orthopaedic Sports Medicine, Massachusetts General Hospital, Boston, Massachusetts

JOSHUA D. HARRIS, MD
The Methodist Center for Sports Medicine, Division of Sports Medicine, Department of Orthopaedic Surgery, Houston, Texas

THOMAS C. HARRIS, MS
Senior Medical Physicist, Department of Radiation Oncology, Massachusetts General Hospital, Boston, Massachusetts

MITHUN A. JOSHI, MBBS
Sydney Shoulder Specialists, St Leonards, Sydney, New South Wales, Australia

RICHARD W. KANG, MS, MD
Orthopaedic Surgery Fellow, Department of Sports Medicine and Shoulder Surgery, Hospital for Special Surgery, New York, New York

W. BEN KIBLER, MD
Shoulder Center of Kentucky, Lexington Clinic, Lexington, Kentucky

PRADEEP KODALI, MD
Assistant Professor, Department of Orthopaedic Surgery, Ironman Sports Medicine Institute, University of Texas Health Sciences Center at Houston, Houston, Texas

ROBERT B. LITCHFIELD, MD, FRCSC
Division of Orthopedic Surgery, Western University, London, Ontario, Canada

LEONARD C. MACRINA, MSPT, SCS, CSCS
Physical Therapist, Champion Sports Medicine, A Physiotherapy Associates Clinic; American Sports Medicine Institute, Birmingham, Alabama

GREGORY T. MAHONY, BA
Research Assistant, Department of Sports Medicine and Shoulder Surgery, Hospital for Special Surgery, New York, New York

MATTHEW D. MILEWSKI, MD
Elite Sports Medicine, Connecticut Children's Medical Center; Professor of Orthopaedics, University of Connecticut School of Medicine, Farmington, Connecticut

ANTHONY MINIACI, MD, FRCSC
Professor, Department of Orthopaedic Surgery, Orthopaedic and Rheumatologic Institute; Department of Biomedical Engineering, Lerner Research Institute, Cleveland Clinic, Cleveland, Ohio

IAIN R. MURRAY, BMedSci (Hons), MRCSEd, Dip SEM
Clinical Lecturer, Department of Trauma and Orthopaedic Surgery, The University of Edinburgh, Edinburgh, United Kingdom

CARL W. NISSEN, MD
Elite Sports Medicine, Connecticut Children's Medical Center; Assistant Professor of Orthopaedics, University of Connecticut School of Medicine, Farmington, Connecticut

MASSIMO PETRERA, MD
Orthopaedic Surgeon, Department of Surgery, Women's College Hospital, University of Toronto Orthopaedic Sports Medicine, Toronto, Ontario, Canada

FRANK A. PETRIGLIANO, MD
Assistant Professor-in-Residence and Attending Surgeon, Department of Orthopaedic Surgery, David Geffen School of Medicine at UCLA, California

HAIFENG REN, MD, FRCS(C)
Division of Orthopaedic Surgery, Department of Surgery, Kingston General Hospital—Nickle 3, Queen's University, Kingston, Ontario, Canada

C. MICHAEL ROBINSON, BMedSci (Hons), FRCSEd
Consultant Orthopaedic Surgeon, Department of Trauma and Orthopaedics, Royal Infirmary of Edinburgh, Edinburgh, United Kingdom

ANTHONY A. ROMEO, MD
Program Director, Shoulder and Elbow Fellowship, Section Head, Shoulder and Elbow Surgery, Professor, Division of Sports Medicine, Department of Orthopedic Surgery, Midwest Orthopaedics at Rush, Rush Medical College, Rush University Medical Center, Rush University, Chicago, Illinois; Co-Team Physician, Chicago White Sox; Co-Team Physician, Chicago Bulls

AARON SCIASCIA, MS, ATC, PES
Shoulder Center of Kentucky, Lexington Clinic, Lexington, Kentucky

JON K. SEKIYA, MD
Larry S. Matthews Collegiate Professor of Orthopaedic Surgery, Professor, MedSport, University of Michigan, Ann Arbor, Michigan

ERIC P. TANNENBAUM, MD
House Officer, Department of Orthopaedic Surgery, University of Michigan, Ann Arbor, Michigan

JOHN S. THEODOROPOULOS, MD, MSc, FRCSC
Orthopaedic Surgeon, Department of Surgery, Women's College Hospital, University of Toronto Orthopaedic Sports Medicine; Mount Sinai Hospital, Toronto, Ontario, Canada

STEPHEN R. THOMPSON, MD, MEd, FRCSC
Private Practice, Sports Medicine and Arthroscopic Surgery, Orthopaedic Surgery of Maine, Eastern Maine Medical Center, Bangor, Maine; Division of Orthopedic Surgery, Western University, London, Ontario, Canada

GILLES WALCH, MD
Centre Orthopédique Santy, Lyon, France

RICHARD E.A. WALKER, MD, FRCPC
Clinical Assistant Professor, Department of Radiology, Faculty of Medicine, University of Calgary, Foothills Medical Centre, Calgary, AB, Canada

JAMES P. WARD, MD
Fellow in Sports Medicine, University of Pittsburgh Medical Center, Pittsburgh, Pennsylvania

JON J.P. WARNER, MD
Chief, The MGH Shoulder Service, Co-Director, The Boston Shoulder Institute, Massachusetts General Hospital, Professor of Orthopaedic Surgery, Harvard Medical School, Boston, Massachusetts

KEVIN E. WILK, PT, DPT, FAPTA
Champion Sports Medicine, A Physiotherapy Associates Clinic, Birmingham, Alabama; Rehabilitation Consultant, Tampa Bay Rays Baseball Team, Tampa Bay, Florida; American Sports Medicine Institute, Birmingham, Alabama

TREVOR WILKES, MD
Shoulder Center of Kentucky, Lexington Clinic, Lexington, Kentucky

ALLAN A. YOUNG, MBBS, MSpMed, PhD, FRACS (Orth)
Sydney Shoulder Specialists, St Leonards, Sydney, New South Wales, Australia

Contents

> The glenohumeral joint provides greater freedom of motion than any other joint in the body at the expense of decreased stability. Shoulder instability can occur in overhead throwing athletes (chronic, overuse injuries) but more commonly occurs in contact athletes (acute traumatic dislocations). Our understanding of the anatomy and pathologic entities has evolved significantly since initial descriptions of shoulder instability and this has facilitated an evolving repertoire of treatment options. This article reviews the functional anatomy and biomechanics of shoulder stability and outlines the bony and soft tissue lesions associated with shoulder instability in the athlete.

> Surgical management of recurrent shoulder instability can be complicated in the setting of associated osseous defects of the glenoid, humeral head, or both. A wide variety of surgical options exist for the management of complex shoulder instability. Interventions for addressing glenoid and humeral head bone defects, and their biomechanical effects, are reviewed. Further studies are required to delineate critical defect values and develop validated treatment algorithms.

> The overhead throwing or serving motion requires the coordinated activation of all of the bony segments in a kinetic and kinematic chain to generate and regulate the forces and motions to accomplish the task. Proper mechanics create the optimum forces and motions. Pathomechanics are frequently associated with alterations in performance and injury risk or injury. Knowledge of normal mechanics and possible pathomechanics can help in the evaluation of athletes with shoulder pain. The evaluation should be comprehensive, including the presence of pathomechanics, the anatomic and physiologic reasons for the pathomechanics, and evaluation of all elements in the kinetic chain.

bone loss. Athletes with recurrent instability and associated bone loss have high failure rates when treated with a soft tissue reconstruction procedure. Therefore it is preferred to manage recurrent instability in contact athletes with the Latarjet-Patte procedure. In this article, the authors describe their technique. They have found this procedure to be safe and effective, with very low recurrence and early return to sport. A meticulous surgical technique is important to avoid intraoperative and postoperative complications.

Thorough evaluation of the athlete with persistent shoulder instability and appropriate use of imaging modalities, such as 3-dimensional computed tomography, can help quantify the severity of bony deficiency. Based on obtained imaging and examination, surgical and nonsurgical methods can be considered. In many situations both the humeral- and glenoid-sided bone loss must be addressed. Depending on the extent of bone loss, athletic demands, and surgeon experience, arthroscopic or open surgical options can provide shoulder stability and return athletes to their prior level of activity.

Glenohumeral instability in pediatric and adolescent patients covers a wide range of disease, from traumatic anterior instability to multidirectional instability. The rates of recurrent instability are high. Conservative and operative treatment options have shown variable success. Given the high risk of recurrent instability, young, active patients who seek to return to competitive contact sports should consider arthroscopic stabilization after a first-time instability event. Multidirectional instability should be treated initially with conservative rehabilitation. Patients who fail extensive conservative treatment may benefit from surgical stabilization. Arthroscopic techniques may approach the results of traditional open capsular shift procedures.

Athletes participating in contact sports often subject their shoulders to intense activity and high-energy forces. When one or more of the posterior stabilizing structures is damaged, posterior shoulder instability often ensues. Orthopedists must know how to perform the specific physical examination maneuvers to determine posterior shoulder instability and what imaging tests are necessary. Initial management traditionally includes 6 months of conservative nonoperative rehabilitation. If the athlete's shoulder instability persists after conservative treatment, surgery is directed at repairing any soft or bony lesions. Depending on the surgery performed, athletes may expect to gradually return to play between 5 and 8 months.

a systematic approach to the diagnosis and treatment. The surgeon must develop a clear understanding of the etiology of the failure and take the necessary steps during the management algorithm to prevent a subsequent recurrence. When planning revision surgical stabilization, the surgeon must analyze and address risk factors for recurrence, which include younger age, contact/collision sports, higher level of competition, capsular laxity, glenoid bone loss, and engaging Hill-Sachs deformities. The surgeon must provide the athlete with the surgery that provides the best chance to return to sport and the lowest risk of recurrent instability. While revision arthroscopic Bankart repair may be appropriate in some cases in which there is minimal glenoid bone loss and robust labral and capsular tissue is available, an open procedure such as a Latarjet may be indicated for athletes at high risk for recurrence.

Kevin E. Wilk and Leonard C. Macrina

There exists a wide range of shoulder instabilities, from subtle subluxations (as seen in overhead athletes) to gross instability. An appropriate rehabilitation program plays a vital role in the successful outcome following an episode of shoulder instability. Nonoperative rehabilitation is often implemented for patients diagnosed with various shoulder instabilities. Based on the classification system of glenohumeral instability and several key factors, a nonoperative rehabilitation program may be developed. This article discusses these factors, and the nonoperative rehabilitation and postoperative programs designed to return patients to their previous level of function. In addition, a rehabilitation program that focuses on restoring strength, improved posture, scapula stability, neuromuscular control and proprioception will be emphasized.

CLINICS IN SPORTS MEDICINE

Foreword

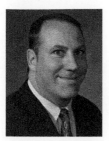

Mark D. Miller, MD
Consulting Editor

Although shoulder instability is a common problem in sports medicine, it has been some time since we focused on this problem in an issue of *Clinics in Sports Medicine*. I invited a rising star in orthopedic sports medicine, Dr Stephen Thompson, to guest edit this issue. He has put together a very ambitious issue that covers the whole gambit of shoulder instability. Like most good reviews, the issue begins with anatomy and biomechanics, focuses on examination and imaging, addresses surgical timing, and then covers a variety of conditions. Internal impingement, multidirectional instability, bone loss, revision surgery, posterior instability, and a variety of other clinical conditions are thoroughly addressed. There are also articles dedicated to both contact and noncontact athletes, instability in pediatric patients, and rehabilitation.

This is a comprehensive treatise on shoulder instability and Dr Thompson has assembled an all-star cast. He has done a masterful job, and this will be an issue that you will want to study carefully.

Mark D. Miller, MD
University of Virginia
James Madison University
400 Ray C. Hunt Drive, Suite 330
Charlottesville, VA 22908-0159, USA

E-mail address:
mdm3p@virginia.edu

Clin Sports Med 32 (2013) xiii
http://dx.doi.org/10.1016/j.csm.2013.08.001

Preface

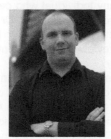

Stephen R. Thompson, MD, MEd, FRCSC
Editor

*It deserves to be known how a shoulder which is subject to frequent dislocations
should be treated.*

—*Hippocrates*

The diagnosis and management of shoulder instability remains a challenging topic. Despite being one of the first orthopedic conditions recognized in the medical literature, the optimal methods of diagnosis and management continue to be defined. Athletes, whether their sport involves contact or not, typically rely a great deal on their shoulders for successful performance. When the careful balance between motion and stability is tipped to one direction, performance can suffer greatly. As such, athletes with shoulder instability are a particularly challenging group of individuals to treat. Their often competing desires for motion, strength, and stability can result in serious angst among even the most seasoned orthopedic surgeons.

This issue of *Clinics in Sports Medicine* is designed to both introduce the novice surgeon to the treatment of shoulder instability in the athlete and provide an update to the experienced surgeon on the pathoanatomy, diagnosis, and management of this common condition. It is my distinct pleasure to have had the opportunity to assemble this collection of articles written by some of the world's foremost experts. Authors from Canada, the United States, Australia, United Kingdom, and France provide an international view on how athletes with shoulder instability are treated.

Drs Murray, Goudie, Petrigliano, and Robinson from the Shoulder Injury Clinic of the Edinburgh Orthopaedic Trauma Unit provide the basis for the entire volume through their discussion on functional anatomy and biomechanics of shoulder stability. The discussion of biomechanics as it relates to complex shoulder instability is furthered by Drs Degen, Giles, Thompson, Litchfield, and Athwal from the University of Western Ontario. The athlete involved in overhead activities represents a unique subset and

Clin Sports Med 32 (2013) xv–xvii
http://dx.doi.org/10.1016/j.csm.2013.07.018
0278-5919/13/$ – see front matter © 2013 Published by Elsevier Inc.

sportsmed.theclinics.com

Drs Kibler and Wilkes along with Mr Sciascia from the Shoulder Clinic of Kentucky provide an outstanding and unique perspective on the mechanics and pathome-chanics of the throwing motion that should be read by any individual who cares for the overhead athlete. Drs Bois and Walker from the University of Calgary, Dr Kodali from the University of Texas Health Sciences Center at Houston, and Dr Miniaci from the Cleveland Clinic provide a beautifully illustrated review of the different imag-ing modalities used in the diagnosis of shoulder instability.

Dr Bradley, drawing on his many years of experience as team physician of the Pittsburgh Steelers, provides his advice along with his colleague, Dr Ward, on how to manage the in-season athlete with shoulder instability. Drs Chambers and Altchek from the Hospital for Special Surgery review the subtle distinctions between microinst-ability and internal impingement in the overhead athlete. Transitioning into manage-ment, Drs Harris and Romeo of Rush University provide an excellent review of how best to manage the contact athlete with instability in an arthroscopic fashion. Drs Joshi, Young, and Balestro from Sydney, Australia then collaborate with Dr Walch from Lyon, France to provide their technique for managing a contact athlete with insta-bility in an open fashion using the Latarjet-Patte procedure. The difficult problem of dealing with an athlete who has bone loss is nicely reviewed by Drs Griffin and Brock-meier from the University of Virginia.

As with most of orthopedics, the pediatric patient presents its own unique chal-lenges and Dr Milewski and Nissen from the Connecticut Children's Medical Center use their dual sports medicine and pediatric training to provide an outstanding review of how to deal with pediatric and adolescent shoulder instability. Drs Tannenbaum and Sekiya from the University of Michigan nicely introduce instability in the posterior direction.

Moving into specific and difficult clinical scenarios, Dr Kang, Mr Mahoney, Mr Harris, and Dr Dines provide an outstanding review of posterior instability that occurs in base-ball players that has been termed "Batter's Shoulder." Drs Dwyer, Petrea, Bleakney, and Theodoropoulos from the University of Toronto rely on their experience with National Hockey League players to describe the findings and management of shoulder instability in ice-hockey players. Drs Ren and Bicknell from Queen's University review the especially difficult concepts of the unstable painful shoulder and microinstability in the young athlete.

Rather than provide detailed results in each section, Dr Brophy from Washington University provides an outstanding summary of the results of shoulder stabilization surgery in athletes. Drs Gwathmey and Warner from Harvard then review the chal-lenging problem of failed surgery and provide expert commentary on how best to manage these scenarios. Last, Dr Wilk and Mr Macrina from the American Sports Medicine Institute in Birmingham, Alabama provide a guide for the nonoperative reha-bilitation of glenohumeral instability using their years of experience in dealing with the highest levels of professional athletes.

I sincerely hope that readers find this issue of Clinics in Sports Medicine particularly useful and relevant to their practice. I could not have assembled this issue without the assistance of a great number of individuals. First and foremost, I sincerely thank each author who graciously gave of their time to provide their insight so that others may learn. I also thank the editorial staff at Elsevier, and Jennifer Flynn-Briggs and David Parsons, who expertly guided this issue into production. It almost goes without saying that I thank my friend and mentor, Dr Mark Miller, for asking me to edit this issue. Of course, I must thank my lovely wife, Shannon, for continuing to allow me to work on these projects. Thank-you also to my son, Harper, for sleeping just long enough each day for me to get some work done. Last, I would like to thank my dear friend,

Kim Murphy, who has been instrumental in so many projects I have worked on that I wouldn't be where I am today without her.

Stephen R. Thompson, MD, MEd, FRCSC
Sports Medicine and Arthroscopic Surgery
Orthopaedic Surgery of Maine
Eastern Maine Medical Center
Bangor, Maine

E-mail address:
theskip@gmail.com

Functional Anatomy and Biomechanics of Shoulder Stability in the Athlete

Iain R. Murray, MRCSEd, Dip SEM[a],*, Ewan B. Goudie, MRCSEd[b],
Frank A. Petrigliano, MD[c], C. Michael Robinson, FRCSEd[b]

KEYWORDS

- Instability • Anterior • Posterior • Multidirectional

KEY POINTS

- The large range of motion afforded by the glenohumeral joint results in a propensity for instability.
- The constitutional trait of laxity facilitates extensive motion in multiple planes and may be essential to athletic performance.
- Range of motion and joint distractibility are increased in hyperlaxity, which is considered as instability when associated with loss of function.
- Strength and stability of the joint are highly dependent on both static and dynamic restraints.
- Soft tissue lesions associated with anterior instability include the Bankart lesion, superior labrum anterior and posterior detachment tear, humeral avulsion of the glenohumeral ligaments (HAGL), anterior labroligamentous periosteal sleeve avulsion, and defects of the rotator interval.
- Bony lesions associated with traumatic anterior instability include bony Bankart lesions and Hill-Sachs impression fractures.
- Soft tissue lesions associated with posterior instability include reverse Bankart lesions, plastic deformation of the capsule, Kim lesions, posterior labrocapsular periosteal sleeve avulsion lesions, Bennett lesions, and posterior HAGL.
- Posterior glenoid bone defects and reverse Hill-Sachs impression fractures have been associated with posterior instability.
- Atraumatic instability is most commonly associated with underlying ligamentous laxity or overuse injury but can also be associated with traumatic injury bringing subacute injury to clinical attention.

[a] Department of Trauma and Orthopaedic Surgery, The University of Edinburgh, EH16 4SA, UK;
[b] Department of Trauma and Orthopaedics, Royal Infirmary of Edinburgh, EH16 4SA, UK;
[c] Department of Orthopaedic Surgery, David Geffen School of Medicine at UCLA, California, CA 90095, USA
* Corresponding author.
E-mail address: iain.murray@ed.ac.uk

Clin Sports Med 32 (2013) 607–624
http://dx.doi.org/10.1016/j.csm.2013.07.001
0278-5919/13/$ – see front matter © 2013 Elsevier Inc. All rights reserved.

INTRODUCTION

The glenohumeral joint provides greater freedom of motion than any other joint in the body at the expense of decreased stability. Glenohumeral joint movements include flexion-extension, abduction-adduction, circumduction, and rotation. Shoulder instability can occur in overhead throwing athletes (chronic overuse injuries) but more commonly occurs in contact athletes (acute traumatic dislocations). It can be conceptually regarded as a continuum of pathology with possible contributions from many of the bony and soft tissue intra-articular shoulder structures. Our understanding of the anatomy and pathologic entities has evolved significantly since initial descriptions of shoulder instability and this has facilitated an evolving repertoire of treatment options. This article reviews the functional anatomy and biomechanics of shoulder stability and outlines the bony and soft tissue lesions associated with shoulder instability in the athlete.

WHAT IS INSTABILITY?

The constitutional trait of hyperlaxity and the pathologic condition of instability represent distinct clinical entities.[1] Laxity is the asymptomatic passive translation of the humeral head on the glenoid and may be essential to athletic performance. In hyperlaxity, this range of joint motion and joint distractibility are increased without loss of function. Glenohumeral instability is defined as excessive translation of the humeral head on the glenoid associated with a functional deficit.[1] These abnormal translations of the humeral head can occur actively or passively and are classically accompanied by symptoms of pain and apprehension. In athletes, instability can present as frank dislocation, subluxation events, or more subtly as microinstability. Symptomatic instability and hyperlaxity both exhibit a spectrum of clinical diversity, and there is no single diagnostic test for the presence of either condition. Although they generally occur independently,[2] instability and hyperlaxity may coexist, particularly in elite athletes who are often hyperlax and prone to injury through sport. In the compensated athlete, static soft tissue and bony deficiency are often counteracted by advanced neuromuscular control. Symptomatic instability results from acute or chronic deterioration in the compensatory dynamic stabilizers of the glenohumeral joint or a frank traumatic event.

NORMAL SHOULDER STABILITY

The balance between stability and mobility within the shoulder is achieved through complex interactions involving static and dynamic restraints.[1] The bony static stabilizers include the glenoid, humeral head, and proximal humerus. The soft tissue passive stabilizers include the glenoid labrum, negative intra-articular pressure, articular cartilage surface, the glenohumeral ligaments, and the glenohumeral joint capsule. Soft tissue dynamic stabilizers are tendon-muscle complexes that provide both function and stability to the shoulder. The joint reaction force is primarily maintained by the rotator cuff muscles, long head of biceps, and the deltoid. However, all muscles that cross the glenohumeral joint, including pectoralis major and latissimus dorsi, can act as dynamic stabilizers.

Static Bony Stabilizers

- *Articular conformity*: The glenoid surface is pear-shaped; the inferior aspect of the glenoid takes the shape of a true circle and the superior aspect of the glenoid is 20% narrower.[3] The sphere-shaped humeral head has 3-fold the surface area of the glenoid, with only 25% to 30% of the humeral head in contact with the glenoid surface in any one position.[4] This serves to highlight the importance of the soft tissues and muscles surrounding the joint in providing stability during shoulder function. The dimensional relationship between the humeral head and the glenoid can be expressed as the maximum diameter of the glenoid divided by the maximum diameter of the humeral head (glenohumeral ratio) (**Fig. 1**). This ratio is about 0.75 in the sagittal plane and 0.6 in the transverse plane.[5] The area of contact between the humeral head and glenoid moves superiorly with abduction.[5] The balance stability angle is the maximum angle that the humeral joint reaction force can make with the glenoid center line before dislocation results.[6] The effective glenoid arc is the arc of the glenoid (including the increased depth afforded by the labrum) able to support the net humeral joint reaction force. The shape of the underlying bone, cartilage, and labrum all influence the balance stability angle and the effective glenoid arc.[6]

- *Glenoid version*: Mean retroversion of the glenoid (see **Fig. 1**) has been reported as 1.23° (range 9.5° of anteversion to 10.5° of retroversion).[7] Excessive retroversion or anteversion can be associated with reduced stability. Average glenoid inclination has been reported to be 4.2° of superior inclination (range −7° to 15.8°).[7]
- *Coracoacromial arch*: The coracoacromial arch, composed of the coracoid, coracoacromial ligament, and acromion, acts to prevent anterosuperior migration of the humeral head.

Static Soft Tissue Stabilizers

- *Capsuloligamentous structures*: Different portions of the glenohumeral ligament and capsule are responsible for maintaining stability in each anatomic plane; cadaveric[8] and clinical studies[9] have confirmed the varying contributions of

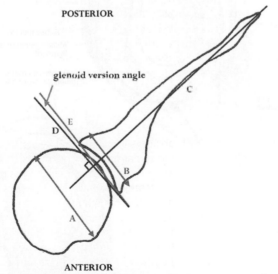

POSTERIOR

glenoid version angle

ANTERIOR

Fig. 1. Static bony stabilizers. The dimensional relationship between the humeral head and the glenoid can be expressed as the maximum diameter of the glenoid (*B*) divided by the maximum diameter of the humeral head (*A*). A method for measuring the glenoid version angle is also shown. Line *C* represents the plane of the body of the scapula and line *E* represents the plane of the osseous glenoid. The angle between line *E* and line *D* (line *D* is drawn perpendicular to line *C*) represents the glenoid version angle.

each structure with different shoulder positions (**Fig. 2**). The complex anatomy of each structure accommodates their role as a primary stabilizer as well as a secondary stabilizer in a position-dependent manner. The anterior and posterior bands of the inferior glenohumeral ligament form a slinglike structure that cradles the humeral head in position. As the shoulder is brought into abduction and external rotation, the anteroinferior aspect of the capsule and the anterior band of the inferior glenohumeral ligament are the most important static constraints to anterior translation of the humeral head. Conversely, with the arm positioned in adduction, flexion, and internal rotation, the posterior band of the inferior glenohumeral ligament and the posterior aspect of the capsule provide the major constraints against posterior instability. With the shoulder in adduction and neutral rotation, the rotator interval complex (comprising the superior glenohumeral ligament, the rotator interval capsule, and the coracohumeral ligament) and the inferior glenohumeral ligament complex resist inferior subluxation.[10] The middle glenohumeral ligament functions to limit both anterior and posterior translation of the arm at 45° of abduction and 45° of external rotation.[11] The functional

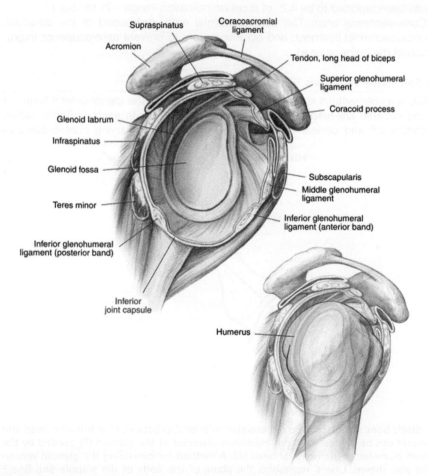

Fig. 2. Static soft tissue stabilizers. (*From* Miller MD. Orthopaedic surgical approaches. Philadelphia: Elsevier Saunders, 2008; with permission.)

interaction between stabilizers on opposite sides of the joint has been described as the "circle concept of ligamentous stability."[12]

- *The glenoid labrum:* The glenoid labrum is a triangular rim of fibrocartilaginous tissue that functions as an extension of the bony glenoid, increasing the depth and surface area of the glenohumeral articulation and contributing around 10% to glenohumeral stability.[13,14] The capsular attachments of the labrum provide further stability with contraction of the rotator cuff. Superiorly, the long head of the biceps tendon shares its origin with labral tissue and the supraglenoid tubercle.

- *The rotator interval:* The rotator interval is a triangular space within the glenohumeral joint capsule that comprises the coracohumeral ligament, the superior and middle glenohumeral ligaments, the long head of the biceps, and a thin layer of capsule. The coracohumeral ligament and associated lateral aspect of the subscapularis are important to maintain stability of the long head of the biceps tendon in the bicipital groove. It is bordered by the coracoid at its base, and the supraspinatis and subscapularis muscles, which converge to an apex laterally. The coracoid separates the subscapularis from the supraspinatus medial to the joint. These muscles insert laterally converging over the intertubercular sulcus.

- *Negative intra-articular pressure:* A degree of stabilization occurs through the vacuumlike effect produced within the closed shoulder compartment and the adhesion-cohesion effect produced by the synovial viscous fluid.[15]

Dynamic Stabilizers

- *Concavity compression:* The rotator cuff, deltoid, and long head of biceps work synergistically to compress the humeral head to the glenoid (concavity compression). The contribution of each depends on the conditioning and strength of the individual structures.[14] The neuromuscular presetting action of the rotator cuff provides the concavity compression required for stability before movement.[16] With their strong influence on shoulder stability, the muscles may contribute not only to stabilization of the shoulder joint but also instability.[17,18]

- *Rotator cuff:* Direct attachments to the capsule allow the rotator cuff muscles to contribute to stability by increasing articular tension; joint compression of the muscular structures provides additional support. In addition, rotator cuff muscles serve to depress the humeral head within the glenoid cavity, and a proprioceptive muscular reflex response counters capsular stretch and shoulder motion detected by sense receptors. Together with the coracoacromial arch, the supraspinatus guards the joint superiorly, the infraspinatus and teres minor stabilize it posteriorly, and the subscapularis protects the shoulder anteriorly.

- *Long head of biceps:* This tendinous structure serves to depress the humeral head while preventing excessive torsion of the glenohumeral joint in rotation with a flexing elbow.

- *Scapular rotators:* Trapezius, rhomboids, latissimus dorsi, serratus anterior, and levator scapulae ensure that the humerus and scapula move synchronously to maintain normal joint articulation throughout the range of motion.

CLASSIFICATION OF SHOULDER INSTABILITY

The cause of shoulder instability is complex and multifactorial, and although several classification systems have been suggested, there is no all-encompassing system that adequately serves as a guide to treatment, predicts outcome, or facilitates communication between clinicians. Instability has been described in terms of direction (anterior, posterior, inferior, or multidirectional), degree of instability (dislocation, sub-luxation, or microinstability), chronology (acute, chronic, or acute on chronic), and whether instability is under voluntary control.[19,20]

Two typical groups of individuals who develop glenohumeral instability have been described based on the cardinal features of their condition.[21] The acronym TUBS describes patients with traumatic instability, who characteristically have unidirectional instability (traumatic, unilateral, with a Bankart lesion generally requiring surgical treatment). The acronym AMBRI describes instability that is typically atraumatic, multidirectional, and bilateral, responds to rehabilitation, and occasionally requires an inferior capsular shift. These patients classically have underlying ligamentous laxity and develop instability insidiously. It is now recognized that this system is oversimplistic; these 2 groups represent extremes in a spectrum of pathologic conditions, with many patients exhibiting overlapping traits (**Fig. 3**). Many patients with hyperlaxity who report instability without a traumatic precipitant have predominantly unidirectional or bidirectional instability.[2] Similarly, traumatic unidirectional instability occurs bilaterally in a quarter of patients with excessive capsular elastin also noted in many of these patients, implying an element of inherited predisposition.[22]

More recently, the FEDS classification (**Fig. 4**) which is based on the 4 cardinal features of instability used most frequently in existing classifications (frequency, etiology, direction, and severity) has been demonstrated to have high intra-observer and inter-observer agreement.[23]

Many patients are able to voluntarily dislocate their shoulder. Although this can occur in those with anterior instability, it typically occurs in patients with posterior instability. Voluntary instability may be associated with an underlying psychological condition and outcomes from surgical treatment are rarely good unless the underlying emotional condition is addressed.[24]

The concept of instability being caused by a combination of structural (traumatic and atraumatic) and neurologic system disturbances has led to a classification of instability as a continuum of pathologies that can be displayed graphically as a triangle (the Stanmore classification) (**Fig. 5**).[25] The polar pathologies are labeled type I (traumatic instability), type II (atraumatic instability), and type III (neurologic dysfunctional or muscle patterning). Polar groups I and II and the axis I-II representing the spectrum

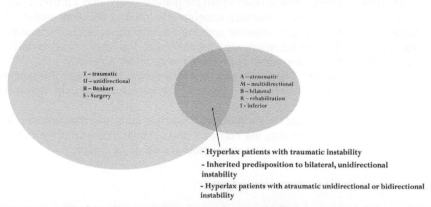

- Hyperlax patients with traumatic instability
- Inherited predisposition to bilateral, unidirectional instability
- Hyperlax patients with atraumatic unidirectional or bidirectional instability

Fig. 3. The traditional dichotomy between TUBS and AMBRI patients is now recognized as being oversimplistic; many patients exhibit overlapping traits. Examples include hyperlax patients with traumatic unidirectional instability and ligamentously lax patients with traumatic injuries.

FREQUENCY–The patient is asked, *"How many episodes have you had in the last year?"*

> Solitary – *'1 Episode'*
> Occasional- *'2 -5 Episodes'*
> Frequent – *'>5 Episodes'*

ETIOLOGY – The patient is asked, *'Did you have an injury to cause this?'*

> Traumatic – *' Yes'*
> Atraumatic – *' No'*

DIRECTION – The patient is asked, *' What direction does the shoulder go out most of the time?'*

> Anterior- *'Out the Front'*
> Inferior- *' Out the Bottom'*
> Posterior- *'Out the Back'*
> The direction is confirmed at the time of the physical examination using provocative tests. During translation testing, the physician asks, which one of the following directions most closely reproduces your symptoms, and then translates anterior, inferior, and posterior. To confirm, the physician may ask which one of these tests most closely reproduces your symptoms: and the anterior apprehension test, the sulcus test, and the posterior jerk test is performed. With the history and physical examination using provocative tests, the patient should be able to distinguish and identify the *primary direction* of his or her instability.

SEVERITY–The patient is asked,*'Have you ever needed help getting the shoulder back in joint?'*

> Subluxation– *'No'*
> Dislocation – *'Yes'*

Fig. 4. The FEDS classification of shoulder instability. (*From* Kuhn JE. A new classification system for shoulder instability. Br J Sports Med 2010;44(5):341–6; with permission.)

of injuries between them correspond to the TUBS-AMBRI classification. The direction of instability is not considered in the Stanmore classification, with the investigators arguing that it is less relevant to effective management whether the instability is structural, nonstructural, or both.[26]

Without an all-encompassing classification, we advocate an individual or algorithmic approach to diagnosis where the clinical manifestation of instability (chronicity, direction, presence of trauma, degree of instability, and volitional control) is combined with the underlying pathologic attributes on an injury (considering soft tissue and bony injuries).[1] In considering the most appropriate treatment, these features should be

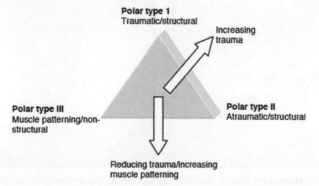

Polar type 1
Traumatic/structural

Increasing trauma

Polar type III
Muscle patterning/nonstructural

Polar type II
Atraumatic/structural

Reducing trauma/increasing muscle patterning

Fig. 5. Stanmore classification of shoulder instability. (*From* Jaggi A, Lambert S. Rehabilitation for shoulder instability. Br J Sports Med 2010;44(5):333–40; with permission.)

combined with a consideration of the athletic needs of an individual and the timing within the athletic calendar.

PATHOGENESIS OF INSTABILITY IN THE ATHLETE

Three broad etiologic categories have been implicated in instability of the shoulder: repetitive microtrauma to the shoulder, acute traumatic events, and purely atraumatic causes. It is crucial to identify the correct pathogenesis of instability so that treatment can be appropriately tailored to the patient's needs.

PATHOANATOMY OF TRAUMATIC ANTERIOR INSTABILITY

Traumatic anterior shoulder instability in the athlete usually occurs with a posteriorly directed force applied to the anterior aspect of an abducted, externally rotated arm. A direct blow (from posterior) can also cause a traumatic anterior dislocation. The humeral head is driven forward, producing a spectrum of soft tissue and bony lesions that are implicated in the pathogenesis of recurrent instability.

Soft Tissue Lesions

Bankart lesion
The Bankart lesion, with detachment of the anteroinferior labrum with its attached inferior glenohumeral ligament complex (IGHLC), was traditionally described as the "essential lesion" of anterior traumatic dislocation of the shoulder occurring in 90% of cases of anterior instability (**Fig. 6**). Although the Bankart lesion is almost always present in patients with traumatic instability,[27,28] it does not produce instability in isolation. The underlying cause is multifactorial, with plastic deformation of the IGHLC regarded central to development of recurrent anterior instability.[29]

Plastic deformation of the IGHLC
Plastic deformation of the IGHLC occurs during the initial dislocation before detachment of the labrum and becomes progressively more severe with recurrent episodes of instability.[30] In a cadaveric study, IGHLC specimens were loaded in tension to failure and 3 modes of failure were observed: at the site of the glenoid insertion (40%), in the mid-substance of the ligament (35%), and at the site of the humeral insertion (25%). Even when failure occurred at the site of the glenoid insertion, it occurred

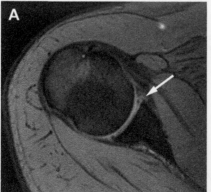
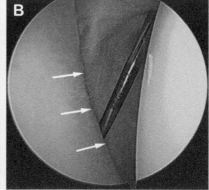

Fig. 6. Magnetic resonance image showing disruption of the anteroinferior glenoid labrum (*arrow, A*). Arthroscopic image confirming discontinuity of the glenoid surface and redundant anterior labrum (*arrows, B*).

only after significant elongation of the IGHLC.[31] Clinical studies have reinforced that capsular stretching can occur simultaneously with a Bankart lesion during an anterior dislocation, with an abnormal capsular redundancy reported in up to 28% of patients with recurrent anterior instability.[32]

Variations in anterior capsulolabral pathoanatomy
Various other patterns of capsulolabral injury have been described.

- Superior labrum anterior and posterior detachment (SLAP) (**Fig. 7**). This may occur in continuity with Bankart lesions and defects of the rotator interval. It is more common in throwing athletes perhaps because of the eccentric loads on the biceps anchor during the deceleration phase of throwing.[33,34] A cadaveric study demonstrated a significant effect on anteroposterior and superoinferior translation with complete lesions.[35]
- Humeral avulsion of the glenohumeral ligaments (HAGL) (**Fig. 8**). This lesion is typically recognized after first-time dislocations and probably represents a variant from the normal pattern of anterior capsular stretching or rupture.[36] It may occur in isolation or in conjunction with a Bankart lesion.
- Anterior labroligamentous periosteal sleeve avulsion (ALPSA) (**Fig. 9**). This is similar to the Bankart lesion, however, the anterior scapular periosteum does not rupture and the IGHLC, labrum, and periosteum are stripped and displaced in a sleeve-type fashion medial on the glenoid neck.[37]

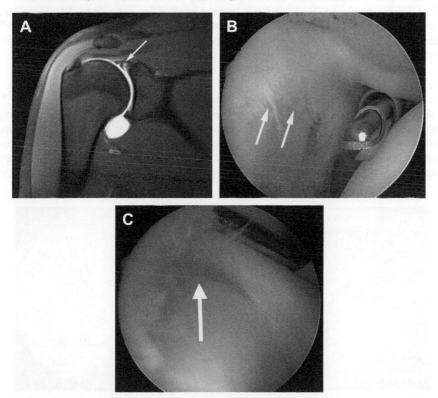

Fig. 7. Coronal magnetic resonance image demonstrating disruption of the superior labrum in keeping with an SLAP tear (*arrow, A*). On arthroscopic examination, the superior labrum can be seen to be detached from its attachment to the superior glenoid (*arrows, B* and *C*).

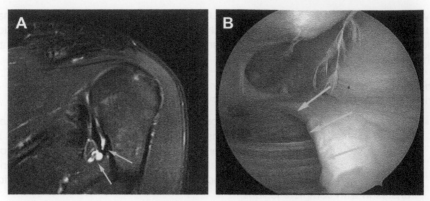

Fig. 8. Magnetic resonance image showing avulsion of the glenohumeral ligaments on from their proximal humeral insertion (HAGL lesion) (*arrows, A*). Arthroscopic appearance of an HAGL lesion (*arrows, B*).

Defects of the rotator interval

There is wide physiologic variability in the rotator interval capsule between individuals, from a small opening to a wide gap. It is therefore difficult to define what is abnormal and contributing to pathologic instability. Although open closure of isolated rotator interval defects has been described, it is not uncommon for patients to develop recurrent instability into a large, inferior pouch after this type of limited surgical repair.[38,39] There may be a role for arthroscopic rotator interval closure as an adjunct to other techniques to reduce failure rates.[40]

Disruption of neuromuscular control

Neuromuscular control plays an important role in the regulation of shoulder stability.[41] One study showed that proprioception of the affected shoulder was altered in patients with glenohumeral instability compared with the asymptomatic extremity.[42] This was eliminated after shoulder reconstruction, suggesting that surgery restores some of the proprioceptive characteristics. An arthroscopic study demonstrated a direct afferent neurologic pathway between the proprioceptive receptors in the joint capsule and

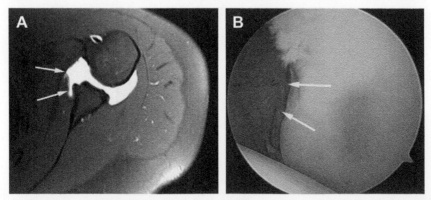

Fig. 9. Magnetic resonance (*A*) and arthroscopic (*B*) appearance of an ALPSA lesion. In this lesion the IGHLC, labrum and periosteum are stripped and displaced in a sleeve-type fashion medial on the glenoid neck (*arrows*).

the cerebral cortex.[43] More research is necessary to further our understanding of the role of proprioception in the unstable shoulder.

Bony Lesions

Bony Bankart lesion

As the humeral head dislocates anteriorly, it may produce a bony Bankart lesion (**Fig. 10**) a compression fracture, or wear of the glenoid rim (**Fig. 11**). Anterior glenoid defects result in loss of glenoid concavity and compromise the static shoulder restraints predisposing to instability.[44] Biomechanical studies demonstrate an inverse relationship between the size of the glenoid defect and joint stability.[45] Cadaveric studies report that glenoid lesions measuring more than half of the glenoid length reduced dislocation resistance by more than 30%; defects wider than 20% glenoid length predispose to recurrence despite Bankart repair.[19,45]

Hill-Sachs impression fracture

When the humeral head impacts on the anterior glenoid, a Hill-Sachs impression fracture is created on the posterolateral aspect of the humeral head. Most lesions are small to moderate in size and do not influence shoulder stability.[1] Hill-Sachs lesions can be classified according to their size as mild (2 cm × 0.3 cm), moderately severe (4 cm × 0.5 cm), and severe (4 cm × 1 cm or greater).[46] A Hill-Sachs lesion that extends into the zone of contact between the humeral head and glenoid during abduction, external rotation, and horizontal extension (glenoid track) has a risk of engagement, resulting in glenohumeral dislocation.[47] Because of the contribution of Hill-Sachs lesions to recurrent instability, the defect should be addressed in patients with severe defects or defects larger than 60% of the humeral head radius, and in those who engage in 90° of abduction and 90° of external rotation (the 90/90 position).[48,49]

PATHOANATOMY OF TRAUMATIC POSTERIOR INSTABILITY

The most frequent cause of recurrent posterior shoulder instability in the athlete is repetitive microtrauma to the posterior shoulder complex. In contrast to anterior instability, acute dislocation is usually not the most common initial presentation of posterior instability.[50] A spectrum of soft tissue and bony pathologies is encountered, the nature of which depends on the cause of the instability.

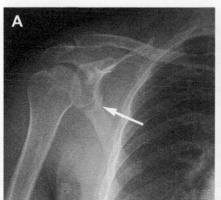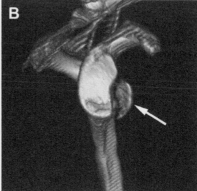

Fig. 10. Plain radiograph (*A*) and magnetic resonance image (*B*) illustrating an acute bony Bankart lesion with a large visible bony fragment (*arrows*).

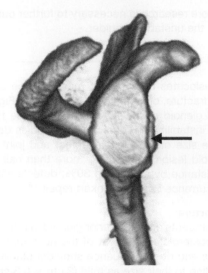

Fig. 11. Three-dimensional computed tomography reconstruction demonstrating anteroinferior glenoid bone loss (*arrow*).

Soft Tissue Lesions

Repetitive bench press lifting, overhead weight lifting, rowing, swimming, or other activities that involve repetitive loading of the shoulder in front of the body can be sources of repetitive microtrauma.[50] In these activities, the shoulder is repetitively placed in a flexed and internally rotated position. The resulting posterior load causes lesions of the posterior labrum, frequently accompanied by stretching of the posteroinferior aspect of the capsule.[51–53]

Reverse Bankart lesion

Tears of the posteroinferior aspect of the capsulolabral complex (reverse Bankart lesion) involving the posterior band of the inferior glenohumeral ligament are more common when there has been a discrete injury to the shoulder (**Fig. 12**).[54–57] They may be degenerative in origin, caused by recurrent episodes of instability.[52,58,59]

Plastic deformation of the capsule

With recurrent subluxation, the capsule undergoes plastic deformation, producing a patulous posteroinferior capsular pouch and increased joint volume. This excessive capsular laxity and large capsular recess can be a cause of posterior instability.[52,57,60]

Variations in posterior capsulolabral pathoanatomy

Several variations from the typical pattern of capsulolabral pathoanatomy have been described.

- Kim lesion. This incomplete and concealed avulsion of the posteroinferior aspect of the labrum may be associated with unidirectional or posteroinferior instability.[61]
- Posterior labrocapsular periosteal sleeve avulsion (POLPSA). In this lesion, the posterior labrum and the intact posterior scapular periosteum are stripped from the glenoid, producing a redundant recess that communicates with the joint space.[62]

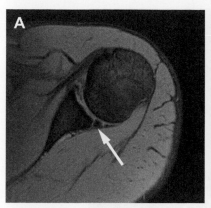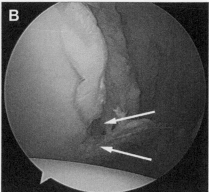

Fig. 12. Magnetic resonance image showing disruption of the posteroinferior glenoid labrum (*arrow, A*). Arthroscopic image confirming discontinuity of the glenoid surface and the posterior labrum (*arrows, B*).

- Bennett lesion. This is an extra-articular curvilinear calcification along the posteroinferior glenoid near the attachment of the posterior band of the inferior glenohumeral ligament.[63] It has been hypothesized that POLPSA may represent the acute stage of a Bennett lesion.[62]
- Posterior humeral avulsion of the glenohumeral ligament. This lesion represents an avulsion of the posterior band of the inferior glenohumeral ligament from its attachment on the humerus.[64]

Bony Lesions

Instability may theoretically occur through increased glenoid retroversion, posterior glenoid erosion, engaging anterior humeral head defects, localized posterioinferior glenoid hypoplasia, or increased humeral head retroversion. No clear association has been demonstrated between posterior instability and the latter 2 conditions.[53]

Glenoid retroversion
Glenoid version varies widely in the normal population and is often documented in patients with instability.[7,65] Studies of the degree of association between glenoid retroversion and posterior instability have produced conflicting results.[66–68] It is probable that excessive glenoid retroversion is rarely a primary cause of instability but should be considered a contributory factor.[53]

Posterior glenoid bone defects
Damaged posterior stabilizers may present as posterior rim fractures (reverse bony Bankart lesions) after an acute traumatic dislocation or erosions as a result of localized glenoid hypoplasia or repeated subluxations (**Fig. 13**).[52,69,70] There is a relationship between the extent of glenoid erosion seen on computed tomography and recurrent instability.[71]

Reverse Hill-Sachs impression fracture
Posterior dislocation often results in an osteochondral fracture of the anterior humeral head medial to the lesser tuberosity, in the region of the anatomic neck from impaction on the posterior glenoid rim (a reverse Hill-Sachs lesion). This may extend into the zone of contact between the humeral head and the glenoid during flexion, adduction, and internal rotation, producing subsequent engagement and subjective instability or dislocation.[72]

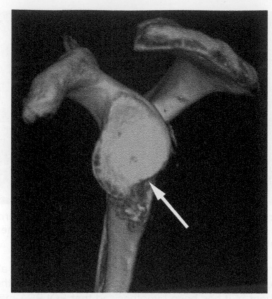

Fig. 13. Computed tomography reconstruction demonstrating posteroinferior glenoid bone loss (*arrow*).

PATHOANATOMY OF ATRAUMATIC INSTABILITY

It is challenging to define atraumatic instability because activities of daily living and improper shoulder mechanics may lead to damage at a molecular level. Many athletes with evidence of constitutional ligamentous laxity develop unilateral instability only after a discrete injury; whilst some degree of inherited predisposition to traumatic instability is implied by its occurrence bilaterally in a quarter of patients.[73] Atraumatic instability includes the diagnosis of multidirectional instability (MDI). Studies have shown an excessive elastin component in capsular tissue and skin of patients with MDI.[74] Patients with MDI tend to have a generalized increase in joint volume with posterior, inferior, and anterior capsular redundancy.[2] Bony abnormalities are not generally present, however pathologic findings may be present when a traumatic dislocation is superimposed in the setting of MDI. Muscle imbalance, especially rotator cuff weakness can lead to dependency on the capsule as the primary restraint to translational forces, which may ultimately result in fatigue failure beyond the visco-elastic material properties of the capsule. This ultimately leads to capsular stretching that may progress to symptoms of instability.[75]

SUMMARY

Glenohumeral joint motion results from a complex interplay between static and dynamic stabilizers that require intricate balance and synchronicity. Instability of the shoulder is a commonly encountered problem in active populations, especially young athletes. The underlying pathoanatomy predisposing to further episodes and the needs of individual athletes must be considered in determining the most appropriate treatment.

REFERENCES

1. Murray IR, Ahmed I, White NJ, et al. Traumatic anterior shoulder instability in the athlete. Scand J Med Sci Sports 2013;23(4):387–405.

2. Johnson SM, Robinson CM. Shoulder instability in patients with joint hyperlaxity. J Bone Joint Surg Am 2010;92(6):1545–57.
3. Huysmans PE, Haen PS, Kidd M, et al. The shape of the inferior part of the glenoid: a cadaveric study. J Shoulder Elbow Surg 2006;15(6):759–63.
4. Codman E. The shoulder. Boston: Thomas Todd; 1934.
5. Saha AK. Dynamic stability of the glenohumeral joint. Acta Orthop Scand 1971; 42(6):491–505.
6. Lee T. Clinical anatomy and biomechanics of the glenohumeral joint (including stabilizers). In: Romeo A, Provencher MT, editors. Shoulder instability: a comprehensive approach. Philadelphia: Saunders; 2012. p. 3–19.
7. Churchill RS, Brems JJ, Kotschi H. Glenoid size, inclination, and version: an anatomic study. J Shoulder Elbow Surg 2001;10(4):327–32.
8. Gerber C, Werner CM, Macy JC, et al. Effect of selective capsulorrhaphy on the passive range of motion of the glenohumeral joint. J Bone Joint Surg Am 2003; 85-A(1):48–55.
9. Lippitt SB, Harris SL, Harryman DT 2nd, et al. In vivo quantification of the laxity of normal and unstable glenohumeral joints. J Shoulder Elbow Surg 1994;3(4): 215–23.
10. Jost B, Koch PP, Gerber C. Anatomy and functional aspects of the rotator interval. J Shoulder Elbow Surg 2000;9(4):336–41.
11. Burkart AC, Debski RE. Anatomy and function of the glenohumeral ligaments in anterior shoulder instability. Clin Orthop Relat Res 2002;(400):32–9.
12. Curl LA, Warren RF. Glenohumeral joint stability. Selective cutting studies on the static capsular restraints. Clin Orthop Relat Res 1996;(330):54–65.
13. Howell SM, Galinat BJ. The glenoid-labral socket. A constrained articular surface. Clin Orthop Relat Res 1989;(243):122–5.
14. Halder AM, Kuhl SG, Zobitz ME, et al. Effects of the glenoid labrum and glenohumeral abduction on stability of the shoulder joint through concavity-compression: an in vitro study. J Bone Joint Surg Am 2001;83-A(7):1062–9.
15. Miller SJ. Shoulder anatomy and biomechanics. In: Miller SJ, editor. Sports medicine - core knowledge in orthopaedics. Philadelphia: Mosby Elsevier; 2006. p. 239–51.
16. Labriola JE, Lee TQ, Debski RE, et al. Stability and instability of the glenohumeral joint: the role of shoulder muscles. J Shoulder Elbow Surg 2005;14(1 Suppl S): 32S–8S.
17. Mihata T, Gates J, McGarry MH, et al. Effect of rotator cuff muscle imbalance on forceful internal impingement and peel-back of the superior labrum: a cadaveric study. Am J Sports Med 2009;37(11):2222–7.
18. Sciaroni LN, McMahon PJ, Cheung TG, et al. Open surgical repair restores joint forces that resist glenohumeral dislocation. Clin Orthop Relat Res 2002;(400): 58–64.
19. Gerber C, Nyffeler RW. Classification of glenohumeral joint instability. Clin Orthop Relat Res 2002;(400):65–76.
20. Allen A. Clinical evaluation of the unstable shoulder. In: Warren RF, Craig EV, Altchek DW, editors. The unstable shoulder. Philadelphia: Lippincott-Raven; 1999. p. 93–106.
21. Thomas SC, Matsen FA 3rd. An approach to the repair of avulsion of the glenohumeral ligaments in the management of traumatic anterior glenohumeral instability. J Bone Joint Surg Am 1989;71(4):506–13.
22. Dowdy PA, O'Driscoll SW. Shoulder instability. An analysis of family history. J Bone Joint Surg Br 1993;75(5):782–4.

23. Kuhn JE. A new classification system for shoulder instability. Br J Sports Med 2010;44(5):341–6.
24. Rowe CR, Pierce DS, Clark JG. Voluntary dislocation of the shoulder. A preliminary report on a clinical, electromyographic, and psychiatric study of twenty-six patients. J Bone Joint Surg Am 1973;55(3):445–60.
25. Lewis A, Kitamura T, Bayley JI. Mini symposium: shoulder instability (ii). The classification of shoulder instability: new light through old windows! Curr Orthop 2004;10:758–67.
26. Jaggi A, Lambert S. Rehabilitation for shoulder instability. Br J Sports Med 2010; 44(5):333–40.
27. Baker CL, Uribe JW, Whitman C. Arthroscopic evaluation of acute initial anterior shoulder dislocations. Am J Sports Med 1990;18(1):25–8.
28. Taylor DC, Arciero RA. Pathologic changes associated with shoulder dislocations. Arthroscopic and physical examination findings in first-time, traumatic anterior dislocations. Am J Sports Med 1997;25(3):306–11.
29. Speer KP, Deng X, Borrero S, et al. Biomechanical evaluation of a simulated Bankart lesion. J Bone Joint Surg Am 1994;76(12):1819–26.
30. Robinson CM, Dobson RJ. Anterior instability of the shoulder after trauma. J Bone Joint Surg Br 2004;86(4):469–79.
31. Bigliani LU, Pollock RG, Soslowsky LJ, et al. Tensile properties of the inferior glenohumeral ligament. J Orthop Res 1992;10(2):187–97.
32. Rowe CR, Patel D, Southmayd WW. The Bankart procedure: a long-term end-result study. J Bone Joint Surg Am 1978;60(1):1–16.
33. Digiovine NM, Jobe FW, Pink M, et al. An electromyographic analysis of the upper extremity in pitching. J Shoulder Elbow Surg 1992;1(1):15–25.
34. Glousman R, Jobe F, Tibone J, et al. Dynamic electromyographic analysis of the throwing shoulder with glenohumeral instability. J Bone Joint Surg Am 1988; 70(2):220–6.
35. Pagnani MJ, Deng XH, Warren RF, et al. Effect of lesions of the superior portion of the glenoid labrum on glenohumeral translation. J Bone Joint Surg Am 1995; 77(7):1003–10.
36. Wolf EM, Cheng JC, Dickson K. Humeral avulsion of glenohumeral ligaments as a cause of anterior shoulder instability. Arthroscopy 1995;11(5):600–7.
37. Neviaser TJ. The anterior labroligamentous periosteal sleeve avulsion lesion: a cause of anterior instability of the shoulder. Arthroscopy 1993;9(1):17–21.
38. Field LD, Warren RF, O'Brien SJ, et al. Isolated closure of rotator interval defects for shoulder instability. Am J Sports Med 1995;23(5):557–63.
39. Levine WN, Arroyo JS, Pollock RG, et al. Open revision stabilization surgery for recurrent anterior glenohumeral instability. Am J Sports Med 2000;28(2):156–60.
40. Treacy SH, Field LD, Savoie FH. Rotator interval capsule closure: an arthroscopic technique. Arthroscopy 1997;13(1):103–6.
41. Levine WN, Flatow EL. The pathophysiology of shoulder instability. Am J Sports Med 2000;28(6):910–7.
42. Lephart SM, Warner JJ, Borsa PA, et al. Proprioception of the shoulder joint in healthy, unstable, and surgically repaired shoulders. J Shoulder Elbow Surg 1994;3(6):371–80.
43. Tibone JE, Fechter J, Kao JT. Evaluation of a proprioception pathway in patients with stable and unstable shoulders with somatosensory cortical evoked potentials. J Shoulder Elbow Surg 1997;6(5):440–3.
44. Boileau P, Villalba M, Hery JY, et al. Risk factors for recurrence of shoulder instability after arthroscopic Bankart repair. J Bone Joint Surg Am 2006;88(8):1755–63.

45. Itoi E, Lee SB, Berglund LJ, et al. The effect of a glenoid defect on anteroinferior stability of the shoulder after Bankart repair: a cadaveric study. J Bone Joint Surg Am 2000;82(1):35–46.
46. Rowe CR, Zarins B, Ciullo JV. Recurrent anterior dislocation of the shoulder after surgical repair. Apparent causes of failure and treatment. J Bone Joint Surg Am 1984;66(2):159–68.
47. Yamamoto N, Itoi E, Abe H, et al. Contact between the glenoid and the humeral head in abduction, external rotation, and horizontal extension: a new concept of glenoid track. J Shoulder Elbow Surg 2007;16(5):649–56.
48. Kaar SG, Fening SD, Jones MH, et al. Effect of humeral head defect size on glenohumeral stability: a cadaveric study of simulated Hill-Sachs defects. Am J Sports Med 2010;38(3):594–9.
49. Burkhart SS, De Beer JF. Traumatic glenohumeral bone defects and their relationship to failure of arthroscopic Bankart repairs: significance of the inverted-pear glenoid and the humeral engaging Hill-Sachs lesion. Arthroscopy 2000; 16(7):677–94.
50. Provencher MT, LeClere LE, King S, et al. Posterior instability of the shoulder: diagnosis and management. Am J Sports Med 2011;39(4):874–86.
51. Bradley JP, Baker CL 3rd, Kline AJ, et al. Arthroscopic capsulolabral reconstruction for posterior instability of the shoulder: a prospective study of 100 shoulders. Am J Sports Med 2006;34(7):1061–71.
52. Fronek J, Warren RF, Bowen M. Posterior subluxation of the glenohumeral joint. J Bone Joint Surg Am 1989;71(2):205–16.
53. Robinson CM, Aderinto J. Recurrent posterior shoulder instability. J Bone Joint Surg Am 2005;87(4):883–92.
54. Bigliani LU, Pollock RG, McIlveen SJ, et al. Shift of the posteroinferior aspect of the capsule for recurrent posterior glenohumeral instability. J Bone Joint Surg Am 1995;77(7):1011–20.
55. Papendick LW, Savoie FH 3rd. Anatomy-specific repair techniques for posterior shoulder instability. J South Orthop Assoc 1995;4(3):169–76.
56. Hawkins RJ, Janda DH. Posterior instability of the glenohumeral joint. A technique of repair. Am J Sports Med 1996;24(3):275–8.
57. Kim SH, Ha KI, Park JH, et al. Arthroscopic posterior labral repair and capsular shift for traumatic unidirectional recurrent posterior subluxation of the shoulder. J Bone Joint Surg Am 2003;85-A(8):1479–87.
58. Caspari RB, Geissler WB. Arthroscopic manifestations of shoulder subluxation and dislocation. Clin Orthop Relat Res 1993;(291):54–66.
59. Antoniou J, Duckworth DT, Harryman DT 2nd. Capsulolabral augmentation for the management of posteroinferior instability of the shoulder. J Bone Joint Surg Am 2000;82(9):1220–30.
60. Dewing CB, McCormick F, Bell SJ, et al. An analysis of capsular area in patients with anterior, posterior, and multidirectional shoulder instability. Am J Sports Med 2008;36(3):515–22.
61. Kim SH, Ha KI, Yoo JC, et al. Kim's lesion: an incomplete and concealed avulsion of the posteroinferior labrum in posterior or multidirectional posteroinferior instability of the shoulder. Arthroscopy 2004;20(7):712–20.
62. Yu JS, Ashman CJ, Jones G. The POLPSA lesion: MR imaging findings with arthroscopic correlation in patients with posterior instability. Skeletal Radiol 2002;31(7):396–9.
63. Van Tongel A, Karelse A, Berghs B, et al. Posterior shoulder instability: current concepts review. Knee Surg Sports Traumatol Arthrosc 2011;19(9):1547–53.

64. Weinberg J, McFarland EG. Posterior capsular avulsion in a college football player. Am J Sports Med 1999;27(2):235–7.
65. Friedman RJ, Hawthorne KB, Genez BM. The use of computerized tomography in the measurement of glenoid version. J Bone Joint Surg Am 1992;74(7): 1032–7.
66. Randelli M, Gambrioli PL. Glenohumeral osteometry by computed tomography in normal and unstable shoulders. Clin Orthop Relat Res 1986;(208):151–6.
67. Gerber C, Ganz R, Vinh TS. Glenoplasty for recurrent posterior shoulder instability. An anatomic reappraisal. Clin Orthop Relat Res 1987;(216):70–9.
68. Hurley JA, Anderson TE, Dear W, et al. Posterior shoulder instability. Surgical versus conservative results with evaluation of glenoid version. Am J Sports Med 1992;20(4):396–400.
69. Norwood LA, Terry GC. Shoulder posterior subluxation. Am J Sports Med 1984; 12(1):25–30.
70. Schwartz E, Warren RF, O'Brien SJ, et al. Posterior shoulder instability. Orthop Clin North Am 1987;18(3):409–19.
71. Weishaupt D, Zanetti M, Nyffeler RW, et al. Posterior glenoid rim deficiency in recurrent (atraumatic) posterior shoulder instability. Skeletal Radiol 2000;29(4): 204–10.
72. Goudie EB, Murray IR, Robinson CM. Instability of the shoulder following seizures. J Bone Joint Surg Br 2012;94(6):721–8.
73. O'Driscoll SW, Evans DC. Contralateral shoulder instability following anterior repair. An epidemiological investigation. J Bone Joint Surg Br 1991;73(6):941–6.
74. Rodeo SA, Suzuki K, Yamauchi M, et al. Analysis of collagen and elastic fibers in shoulder capsule in patients with shoulder instability. Am J Sports Med 1998; 26(5):634–43.
75. Doukas WC, Speer KP. Anatomy, pathophysiology, and biomechanics of shoulder instability. Orthop Clin North Am 2001;32(3):381–91, vii.

Biomechanics of Complex Shoulder Instability

Ryan M. Degen, MD[a], Joshua W. Giles, BESc[b],
Stephen R. Thompson, MD, MEd, FRCSC[a],
Robert B. Litchfield, MD, FRCSC[a], George S. Athwal, MD, FRCSC[a,b,*]

KEYWORDS

- Shoulder instability • Glenoid defect • Humeral head defect • Hill-Sachs
- Remplissage • Latarjet

KEY POINTS

- Recurrent shoulder instability is frequently associated with osseous defects in conjunction with capsulolabral deficiencies.
- Failure to identify these defects has been associated with higher failure rates with isolated soft tissue stabilization procedures.
- Glenoid defects may be addressed with bone grafting or transfer of the coracoid process.
- Humeral head defects may be addressed with bone grafting, soft tissue imbrication, coracoid process transfer, rotational humeral head osteotomy, or resurfacing/arthroplasty.
- Proper identification and treatment of osseous defects resulting in complex shoulder instability is critical in minimizing recurrence.
- Further biomechanical research is required to delineate critical defect values.

INTRODUCTION

The glenohumeral joint relies on a complex interaction between soft tissues and a constraining bony articulation to allow maximal range of motion (ROM) and minimize instability. An applied, external force often sways this balance between mobility and stability, resulting in a traumatic dislocation. Most frequently, this produces an anteroinferior

Disclosures: Nil (R.M. Degen, J.W. Giles, and S.R. Thompson); Smith & Nephew - Institutional education and research support, Zimmer - Educational consultant, Arthrosurface - Royalties, Linvatec - Educational consultant (R.B. Litchfield); Smith & Nephew - Institutional education and research support, Arthrex - Research support, Tornier - Research support, Depuy - Research support, DePuy/Mitek - Educational Consultant, Smith & Nephew - Consultant (G.S. Athwal).
Conflict of Interest: Nil.
[a] Division of Orthopedic Surgery, Western University, 1151 Richmond Street, London, ON N6A 3K7, Canada; [b] Bioengineering Research Laboratory, Hand and Upper Limb Centre, St. Joseph's Health Centre, 268 Grosvenor Road, London, ON N6A 4V2, Canada
* Corresponding author. Department of Orthopedics, St. Joseph's Health Centre, 268 Grosvenor Road, London, Ontario N6A 4V2, Canada.
E-mail address: gsathwal@hotmail.com

Clin Sports Med 32 (2013) 625–636
http://dx.doi.org/10.1016/j.csm.2013.07.002
0278-5919/13/$ – see front matter © 2013 Elsevier Inc. All rights reserved.

capsulolabral avulsion, classically referred to as a soft tissue Bankart lesion, which serves as a contributing factor to recurrent shoulder instability, often necessitating surgical stabilization.[1–5] Complex shoulder instability differs in that in addition to the soft tissue Bankart lesion, recurrent instability is attributable to associated osseous lesions of the glenoid, humeral head, or both.[1,6–9] This article reviews the effect of these lesions and their associated treatment options.

GLENOID DEFECTS

Glenoid bone loss typically occurs at the anterior glenoid rim after a traumatic anterior dislocation. It can occur as an acute fracture, known as a bony Bankart lesion; or, it can be caused by a compression fracture or attritional wear of the glenoid rim with recurrent dislocations (**Fig. 1**).[5,6] These lesions may be present in up to 75% of patients with recurrent shoulder instability.[4–6,10] Biomechanically, loss of a portion of the anterior glenoid rim, making the glenoid concavity less deep, reduces the stabilizing concavity-compression effect and, therefore, reduces the shoulder's ability to resist the translational forces that lead to dislocation.[5,10,11] Additionally, the articular length of the glenoid that is able to contain the humeral head is also reduced, placing more stress on the already deficient capsulolabral structures, predisposing the individual to recurrent instability.[12] An inverse relationship exists between the size of the defect and the associated shoulder stability, with defects of 21% cadaverically shown to contribute to recurrent instability, despite soft tissue stabilization.[6,10]

HUMERAL HEAD DEFECTS

Posterosuperior impaction fractures of the humeral head were first described in 1940 by Hill and Sachs.[13–15] Referred to as Hill-Sachs (HS) lesions, they result from impaction of the posterior, superior aspect of the humeral head against the dense, cortical rim of the anterior, inferior glenoid rim after an anterior dislocation (**Fig. 2**). They are

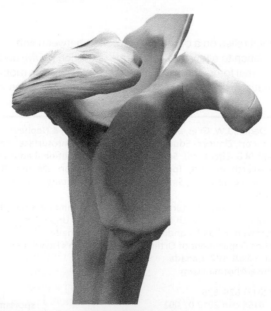

Fig. 1. Computerized rendering of 30% glenoid defect.

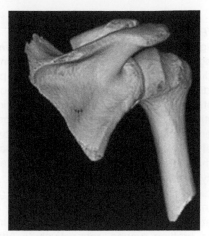

Fig. 2. Humeral head defect (Hill-Sachs defect).

reported to be present following approximately 80% of initial dislocations, and in up to 100% of cases of recurrent instability.[4,6,13,14,16–18] With the humerus in abduction and external rotation, the so-called "position of apprehension," the orientation of these defects may become parallel to the anterior glenoid rim.[7,14] Further external rotation of the humerus in this position may allow the defect to engage the anteroinferior glenoid rim facilitating subsequent glenohumeral dislocation.

PROGNOSIS

Failing to identify and address these osseous defects as part of the treatment protocol for anterior shoulder instability has been demonstrated to lead to rates of recurrent instability as high as 67%.[2,6,7] It is imperative to identify and appropriately address these lesions to improve outcomes after shoulder stabilization. Several treatment options have been described for each of these lesions and they are briefly reviewed here.

GLENOID DEFECTS

Itoi and colleagues[10] studied the effect that the size of the glenoid defect had on shoulder stability. They created a cadaveric model of anterior shoulder instability with progressively larger lesions, initially starting with an intact joint, then an isolated capsulolabral tear; and subsequent glenoid defects of 9%, 21%, 34%, and 46%. In each state they performed a capsular repair, followed by a translation test in the abducted, externally rotated position. They found in most cases that defects of less than 21% were adequately stabilized with an isolated soft tissue Bankart repair.[10] Beyond that size, an isolated Bankart repair was inadequate in restoring joint stability, resulting in treatment failure and recurrent instability. This was corroborated in the findings of Burkhart and colleagues,[7] where a review of their patients after arthroscopic Bankart repair found that those with significant glenoid defects had recurrence rates as high as 67%. Therefore, when a defect of the glenoid exceeds 20% to 25% of its width, it is recommended to proceed with surgical management of these defects beyond the traditional soft tissue Bankart stabilization.[5]

Anatomic Procedures

Glenoid bone grafting (Eden-Hybinette procedure)

Contoured bone grafting of the anteroinferior glenoid rim was originally described by Eden in 1918, and again by Hybinette in 1932.[6] Occasionally referred to as the Eden-Hybinette procedure, several permutations of the procedure have been described with the only difference being the material used as bone graft for the glenoid reconstruction. Graft options include iliac crest autograft or allograft.[1] The procedure itself involves reconstituting the glenoid rim with bone graft, positioned along the deficient segment of the glenoid, with the capsule interposed between this graft and the glenoid rim.[1,4,6,19] This effectively makes the graft extra-articular, where it is then contoured appropriately to match the glenoid articular surface.[6] Alternatively, the graft may be placed intra-articularly with the capsule closed around this.[12] Biomechanical testing of this construct in the setting of a capsular injury and 25% glenoid defect demonstrated a reduction in anterior translation from approximately 346% at 30 degree of abduction and 345% at 60 degree of abduction in the injury state to 179% and 159% in the post–bone grafting groups, respectively.[12] Although this procedure reduced glenohumeral translation compared with the injury state, it did not adequately stabilize all specimens, and paled in comparison with the Latarjet coracoid transfer performed in the same testing protocol. The efficacy of the contoured-bone graft seemed to decrease in external rotation, because three of eight specimens subluxated in the anteroinferior direction with the limb in 60 degree of abduction and external rotation.[12]

Nonanatomic Procedures

Bristow coracoid transfer

Described in 1958 by Helfet, and named after his mentor Rowley Bristow, the Bristow procedure involves transfer of the tip of the coracoid with its associated conjoined tendon through a subscapularis split. The initial description, however, used suture fixation. May in 1970 modified the Bristow to include screw fixation passed along the axis of the coracoid 1 cm medial to the anteroinferior glenoid rim (**Fig. 3**).[8,20] Although it

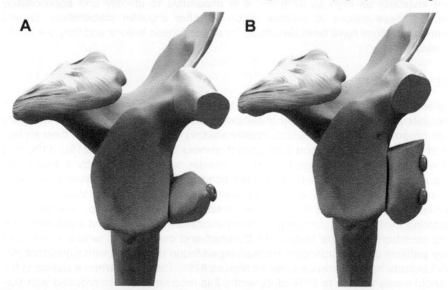

A   B

Fig. 3. Computer rendering of Bristow (A) and Latarjet (B) coracoid transfers for glenoid defect (conjoined tendon omitted).

seemingly represents a bone block transfer, based on the original description, and its location of fixation medial to the joint surface, it was intended to only create a sling effect.[8] Over the years, its description has been slightly modified such that the fragment is now fixed flush with the glenoid surface to serve as a bone block, additionally providing a resistive force to anterior shear forces that typically lead to dislocation.[6] A cadaveric study performed by Thomas and colleagues[21] compared the stabilizing effect of a contemporarily described Bristow versus isolated transfer of the conjoined tendon, or effectively, the classically described Bristow. Both were found to sufficiently improve shoulder stability after creation of a soft tissue Bankart lesion by decreasing anterior translation from 12 ± 4.2 and 12.2 ± 5.9 mm in the injury state to 5.2 ± 2.3 and 4.9 ± 1.4 mm in the posttreatment groups, respectively.[21] This returned stability to near baseline levels, suggesting that perhaps the stabilizing effect of the Bristow procedure is attributable mostly to the sling effect of the conjoined tendon and lower subscapularis fibers, both of which are tensioned in the position of abduction and external rotation. The caveat here was that the glenoid rim remained intact in this study with the exception of the soft tissue Bankart injury; the bone block may prove to have a more significant role in glenoid bone-defect scenarios.

Latarjet coracoid transfer
First described in 1954, the Latarjet coracoid transfer differs from the Bristow in that a larger segment of the coracoid process is transferred to the anteroinferior glenoid rim.[22] The Latarjet involves exposing and osteotomizing the coracoid so that the entire horizontal component of the coracoid is harvested and then passed through a horizontal split in the subscapularis with the associated conjoined tendon left attached. The inferior surface of the coracoid is then fixed flush with the glenoid neck to reconstitute the glenoid arc, and it is secured with a screw. Subsequent descriptions have demonstrated larger coracoid grafts with two screw fixation (see **Fig. 3**). Patte described the principles of the stabilizing effect of the Latarjet being threefold: (1) it provides a static bony resistance to anterior translation, (2) the dynamic sling effect of the conjoint tendon provides restraint to translation in the position of abduction and external rotation, and (3) it allows for repair of the capsulolabral structures with incorporation of the stump of the coracoacromial ligament (CAL) to augment this repair.[12,23,24] Biomechanical testing revealed that, in the setting of a 25% glenoid defect, the Latarjet was able to restore stiffness (resistance to translation) back to baseline parameters after the initial capsulotomy, outperforming the contoured bone-grafting, or Eden-Hybinette procedure.[12] The effect was maximally noted in abduction and 60 degrees of external rotation with tensioning of the conjoint tendon and lower subscapularis fibers increasing the sling effect in this position.[12] This "belt-suspension" stabilization was found to be most significant in this position, whereas the bone block itself had minimal effect.[25] Interestingly, in abduction and neutral rotation, the capsular repair with CAL incorporation was found to have the most significant stabilizing effect.[25] In comparative testing, the Latarjet outperformed contoured bone grafting in the treatment of anteroinferior glenoid defects, suggesting the conjoined tendon plays a significant role in stabilizing the shoulder.[12]

Capsular repair with inclusion of the resected CAL may have a more substantial effect than initially expected, because a significant decrease in stiffness was found between the traditional Latarjet and its arthroscopic modification, which omits this capsular repair.[26] Duplication of the capsule, with incorporation of the CAL, allowed increased tension in the anterior soft tissues with the arm abducted and externally rotated, providing a greater resistive force to anterior translation.[12,25,26] This relates to the concept initially addressed by Hovelius and colleagues[27] where they noted improved stability after Bristow coracoid transfer if an anterior capsular plication was added, increasing the tension in the anterior soft tissue restraints and reducing recurrence rates from 18% in those without to 4% in those with an added plication.

HUMERAL DEFECTS

In contrast to glenoid defects, there is little biomechanical evidence defining critical sizes of humeral head defects associated with recurrent instability.[13,28] It is anecdotally accepted that humeral head defects of less than 20% of the total width have been shown to be adequately stabilized with repair of the associated soft tissue Bankart lesion alone.[13,14,29] Lesions between 20% and 40% of the overall width confer varying degrees of instability, and are not well understood because additional factors may increase the significance of these defects, such as concurrent bony Bankart lesions or the orientation and location of the HS defect on the humeral head.[14,18,28,30] In a study by Sekiya and colleagues,[28] four different sized HS defects (12.5%, 25%, 37.5%, and 50% of humeral head width) were created to biomechanically delineate what size of lesion may benefit from surgical management. From their results, it was noted that defects as small as 12.5% may have significant biomechanical consequences on joint stability, although they may not require surgical attention. However, lesions of 37.5% and 50% had profound destabilizing effects, and should warrant surgical intervention.[28] Additional studies echo their findings that lesions greater than 40% contribute to recurrent shoulder instability, and should be managed surgically, with one of the options discussed next.[13,14,31]

Anatomic Procedures

Humeral head bone augmentation

The goal of this particular procedure is to restore native anatomy, reconstituting the humeral head articular arc, preventing the defect from engaging the anteroinferior glenoid rim while in the position of apprehension, and thus avoiding a dislocation event.[14] This can be done using a variety of materials including autograft from the iliac crest; fresh frozen allograft (ie, humeral head or femoral head); or even metallic partial resurfacing implants (ie, arthrosurface hemi-cap).[14,18,28,32,33]

In a biomechanical analysis by Giles and colleagues,[18] comparative testing was performed looking at the effect of humeral head allograft reconstruction versus partial resurfacing in the treatment of moderate and large HS defects of 30% and 45% of the humeral head width. Coupled with a soft tissue Bankart repair, the allograft reconstruction group was found to prevent defect engagement and dislocation in all specimens regardless of defect size, while not significantly altering ROM or joint stiffness (**Fig. 4**). In contrast, the metallic partial resurfacing group experienced residual defect engagement in 50% of specimens for the 30% defect and 75% of specimens for the 45% defect, because the metallic circular implant did not completely fill the wedge-shaped HS defect, allowing the remaining superior defect to continue to engage the glenoid rim.[18] The metallic resurfacing group slightly increased joint stiffness, but not to statistical significance, whereas ROM was restored to baseline levels of the intact specimen. Both procedures restored joint ROM, but it seems that matched-defect sized allograft reconstruction provided superior outcomes in terms of preventing further instability.[18]

Nonanatomic Procedures

Soft tissue transfer

Mostly historical, the Magnusson-Stack and Putti-Platt procedures were soft tissue procedures that were frequently used in recurrent anterior instability with humeral

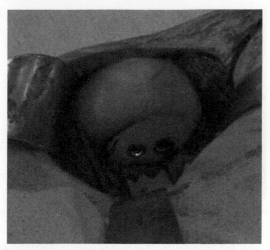

Fig. 4. Allograft bone graft for Hill-Sachs defect.

head defects to limit external rotation and thus prevent HS defect engagement.[8,16] The Magnusson-Stack procedure consists of transferring the subscapularis tendon insertion from the lesser tuberosity to the greater tuberosity, whereas the Putti-Platt procedure involves a medial capsular advancement of the lateral joint capsule along with a subscapularis tenodesis.[8,16] Although initially effective at preventing anterior dislocations, these procedures have fallen out of favor because they have been associated with restricted ROM, altered joint kinematics, and accelerated joint wear with the development of early osteoarthritis.[8,16,34]

Remplissage
Remplissage is the French word meaning "to fill." This term was coined by Purchase and colleagues in 2008.[35] The procedure, however, was originally described by Connolly in 1972, which involved open tenodesis of the posterior joint capsule and infraspinatus tendons into the abraded humeral defect.[36] This converts the lesion to an extra-articular defect, and prevents it from engaging the anterior glenoid rim; in addition, the tenodesis acts as a "check-rein" to limit anterior translation and subsequent dislocation.[17,29,36] In 2008, Purchase and colleagues[35] described an arthroscopic modification of the same procedure with a concomitant Bankart repair, where suture anchors are placed into the "valley" of the HS defect to then imbricate the posterior soft tissues (**Figs. 5** and **6**). Biomechanical analysis of the effect of a combined Bankart repair and remplissage procedure was conducted in 15% and 30% HS defects.[29] This study revealed that the Bankart repair alone was enough to stabilize shoulders with a small (15%) defect and that addition of the remplissage in this group only served to significantly limit internal-external rotational ROM. This restriction in motion predominantly occurred in the adducted position, whereas the effect in abduction was not significant. In the 30% HS defect group, all specimens dislocated in abduction after isolated Bankart repair; addition of the remplissage prevented all defects from engaging the glenoid rim and no dislocations occurred. Internal-external rotational ROM, however, was significantly reduced in adduction, and not in abduction. Despite remplissage being thought of as a procedure designed for treating instability with associated small HS defects, this biomechanical research highlights that it may actually be used best in the setting of a moderately sized defect.[29]

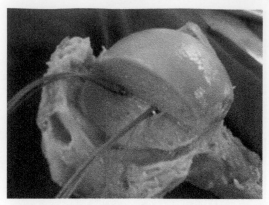

Fig. 5. Suture anchor placement in valley of Hill-Sachs defect for remplissage.

Additional study into the technique of remplissage anchor placement and suture passage has demonstrated that the position of the anchor itself is of less importance, with no difference in stability identified between anchors placed in the rim of the defect or at the base, in the so-called "valley."[37] However, the position of the sutures through the soft tissue can significantly limit ROM.[37] Elkinson and colleagues[37] demonstrated that passing sutures 1 cm more medial than the desired position through the infraspinatus and posterior capsule resulted in a significant decrease in the internal-external rotation ROM, therefore stressing the importance of precise suture passage to reduce potential complications.

Coracoid transfer (Bristow/Latarjet)

As described in previous sections, the coracoid transfer offers several benefits. In the setting of an engaging HS defect, the primary purpose of the Bristow/Latarjet procedure is to provide the resistive forces of the conjoined tendon and inferior subscapularis fibers, or the so-called "sling-effect," while additionally increasing the articular arc length of the glenoid to prevent engagement of the humeral head defect (**Fig. 7**).[8,14] Currently, no biomechanical studies testing their efficacy in the setting of an engaging HS defect are available.

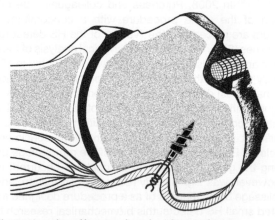

Fig. 6. Diagram illustrating the effect produced with remplissage.

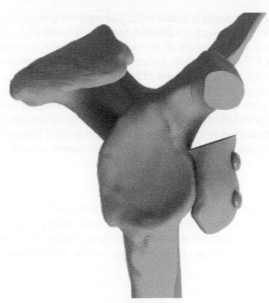

Fig. 7. Latarjet coracoid transfer with an intact glenoid, increasing glenoid arc length in the setting of an engaging Hill-Sachs defect.

Rotational humeral osteotomy

Weber and colleagues[38] described a rotational humeral osteotomy to treat large posterolateral humeral head defects associated with recurrent anterior instability. A surgical neck humeral osteotomy is performed and the shaft is then externally rotated, creating relative internal rotation of the humeral head, and secured with a plate to the humeral head.[38] The principal behind this procedure is to increase the retroversion of the humeral head, so that the HS defect is moved farther posteriorly; this effectively moves the intact anterior portion of the humeral head into the articulating zone and prevents engagement of the posterior defect.[6,8,38] The original description involved shortening the subscapularis tendon and anterior capsule, serving to further reduce the amount of external rotation to again help avoid defect engagement.[8,38] Although few long-term follow-up studies exist, 5-year preliminary results indicated no functional limitations on ROM, although internal rotation was significantly decreased postoperatively (79 ± 21.8 degrees preoperative; 71 ± 17 degrees postoperative).[39] Because of concerns regarding nonunion or delayed union, this procedure is not commonly performed.[14]

Shoulder arthroplasty (hemi/total)

For HS defects greater than 40% of the humeral head width, consideration should be given to resurfacing or joint replacement. Generally, joint-preserving techniques should be favored in younger patients, because implant survivability becomes a long-term issue with hemiarthroplasty and total shoulder arthroplasty.[14] Partial resurfacing HemiCap (Arthrosurface, Franklin, MA) incompletely fills the HS defect, likely attributable to the geometric differences between the circular implant and wedge-shaped defect. Although significantly increasing joint stiffness relative to the unstable state, residual defect engagement occurred in four of eight specimens in the 30% HS defect group and six of eight in the 45% HS defect state.[18] Choosing a larger implant, with the disadvantage of greater host humeral head bone removal, may prevent the observed phenomenon of partial engagement.

The indications for arthroplasty in the setting of traumatic instability with a large HS defect are not clear. Typically, it is reserved for elderly patients, usually greater than 50 years old; those with chronic dislocations; and those with arthritic changes in the glenohumeral joint.[6,8,14] Small case series have shown reasonable success rates with improved stability, ROM, and levels of function after arthroplasty.[40] In this setting, stability was improved by intentionally retroverting the humeral component, bone grafting of anterior glenoid bone defects, and protected postoperative rehabilitation.[40] However, it should be noted that the aforementioned arthroplasty procedures serve as a last resort in the treatment of instability-related arthropathy, because implant surviv-ability is an issue as are permanent restrictions from heavy activity.

SUMMARY

Identification and treatment of the osseous lesions associated with complex shoulder instability remains challenging. Further biomechanical testing is required to delineate critical defect values and determine which treatments provide improved glenohumeral joint stability for the various defect sizes, while minimizing the associated complications.

REFERENCES

1. Provencher MT, Bhatia S, Ghodadra NS, et al. Recurrent shoulder instability: cur-rent concepts for evaluation and management of glenoid bone loss. J Bone Joint Surg Am 2010;92(Suppl 2):133–51. http://dx.doi.org/10.2106/JBJS.J.00906.
2. Boileau P, Villalba M, Héry JY, et al. Risk factors for recurrence of shoulder insta-bility after arthroscopic Bankart repair. J Bone Joint Surg Am 2006;88(8): 1755–63. http://dx.doi.org/10.2106/JBJS.E.00817.
3. Black KP, Schneider DJ, Yu JR, et al. Biomechanics of the Bankart repair: the relationship between glenohumeral translation and labral fixation site. Am J Sports Med 1999;27(3):339–44. Available at: http://www.ncbi.nlm.nih.gov/pubmed/10352770. Accessed December 2, 2012.
4. Anakwenze OA, Hsu JE, Abboud JA, et al. Recurrent anterior shoulder instability associated with bony defects. Orthopedics 2011;34(7):538–44. http://dx.doi.org/10.3928/01477447-20110526-21 [quiz: 545–6].
5. Piasecki DP, Verma NN, Romeo AA, et al. Glenoid bone deficiency in recurrent anterior shoulder instability: diagnosis and management. J Am Acad Orthop Surg 2009;17(8):482–93. Available at: http://www.ncbi.nlm.nih.gov/pubmed/19652030. Accessed November 26, 2012.
6. Lynch JR, Clinton JM, Dewing CB, et al. Treatment of osseous defects associated with anterior shoulder instability. J Shoulder Elbow Surg 2009;18(2):317–28. http://dx.doi.org/10.1016/j.jse.2008.10.013.
7. Burkhart SS, De Beer JF. Traumatic glenohumeral bone defects and their relation-ship to failure of arthroscopic Bankart repairs: significance of the inverted-pear glenoid and the humeral engaging Hill-Sachs lesion. Arthroscopy 2000;16(7): 677–94. Available at: http://www.ncbi.nlm.nih.gov/pubmed/11027751. Accessed November 3, 2012.
8. Chen AL, Hunt SA, Hawkins RJ, et al. Management of bone loss associated with recurrent anterior glenohumeral instability. Am J Sports Med 2005;33(6):912–25. http://dx.doi.org/10.1177/0363546505277074.
9. Bushnell BD, Creighton RA, Herring MM. Bony instability of the shoulder. Arthros-copy 2008;24(9):1061–73. http://dx.doi.org/10.1016/j.arthro.2008.05.015.

10. Itoi E, Lee SB, Berglund LJ, et al. The effect of a glenoid defect on anteroinferior stability of the shoulder after Bankart repair: a cadaveric study. J Bone Joint Surg Am 2000;82(1):35–46. Available at: http://www.ncbi.nlm.nih.gov/pubmed/10653082. Accessed December 2, 2012.

11. Lazarus MD, Sidles JA, Harryman DT, et al. Effect of a chondral-labral defect on glenoid concavity and glenohumeral stability. A cadaveric model. J Bone Joint Surg Am 1996;78(1):94–102. Available at: http://www.ncbi.nlm.nih.gov/pubmed/8550685. Accessed December 7, 2012.

12. Wellmann M, Petersen W, Zantop T, et al. Open shoulder repair of osseous glenoid defects: biomechanical effectiveness of the Latarjet procedure versus a contoured structural bone graft. Am J Sports Med 2009;37(1):87–94. http://dx.doi.org/10.1177/0363546508326714.

13. Kaar SG, Fening SD, Jones MH, et al. Effect of humeral head defect size on glenohumeral stability: a cadaveric study of simulated Hill-Sachs defects. Am J Sports Med 2010;38(3):594–9. http://dx.doi.org/10.1177/0363546509350295.

14. Provencher MT, Frank RM, Leclere LE, et al. The Hill-Sachs lesion: diagnosis, classification, and management. J Am Acad Orthop Surg 2012;20(4):242–52. http://dx.doi.org/10.5435/JAAOS-20-04-242.

15. Hill HA, Sachs MD. The grooved defect of the humeral head: a frequently unrecognized complication of dislocations of the shoulder joint. Radiology 1940;35(6):690–700. http://dx.doi.org/10.1148/35.6.690.

16. Skendzel JG, Sekiya JK. Diagnosis and management of humeral head bone loss in shoulder instability. Am J Sports Med 2012;40(11):2633–44. http://dx.doi.org/10.1177/0363546512437314.

17. Boileau P, O'Shea K, Vargas P, et al. Anatomical and functional results after arthroscopic Hill-Sachs remplissage. J Bone Joint Surg Am 2012;94(7):618–26. http://dx.doi.org/10.2106/JBJS.K.00101.

18. Giles JW, Elkinson I, Ferreira LM, et al. Moderate to large engaging Hill-Sachs defects: an in vitro biomechanical comparison of the remplissage procedure, allograft humeral head reconstruction, and partial resurfacing arthroplasty. J Shoulder Elbow Surg 2012;21(9):1142–51. http://dx.doi.org/10.1016/j.jse.2011.07.017.

19. Provencher MT, Ghodadra N, LeClere L, et al. Anatomic osteochondral glenoid reconstruction for recurrent glenohumeral instability with glenoid deficiency using a distal tibia allograft. Arthroscopy 2009;25(4):446–52. http://dx.doi.org/10.1016/j.arthro.2008.10.017.

20. May VR. A modified Bristow operation for anterior recurrent dislocation of the shoulder. J Bone Joint Surg Am 1970;52:1010–6.

21. Thomas PR, Parks BG, Douoguih WA. Anterior shoulder instability with Bristow procedure versus conjoined tendon transfer alone in a simple soft-tissue model. Arthroscopy 2010;26(9):1189–94. http://dx.doi.org/10.1016/j.arthro.2010.01.033.

22. Latarjet M. Treatment of recurrent dislocation of the shoulder. Lyon Chir 1954;49(8):994–7. Available at: http://www.ncbi.nlm.nih.gov/pubmed/13234709. Accessed November 11, 2012.

23. Burkhart SS, De Beer JF, Barth JR, et al. Results of modified Latarjet reconstruction in patients with anteroinferior instability and significant bone loss. Arthroscopy 2007;23(10):1033–41. http://dx.doi.org/10.1016/j.arthro.2007.08.009.

24. Patte D. Instabilité antérieure de l'épaule. Cahier des enseignements de la Sofcot 1981;(55):55–66.

25. Wellmann M, De Ferrari H, Smith T, et al. Biomechanical investigation of the stabilization principle of the Latarjet procedure. Arch Orthop Trauma Surg 2012;132(3):377–86. http://dx.doi.org/10.1007/s00402-011-1425-z.

26. Schulze-Borges J, Agneskirchner JD, Bobrowitsch E, et al. Biomechanical comparison of open and arthroscopic Latarjet procedures. Arthroscopy 2013;29(4): 630–7. http://dx.doi.org/10.1016/j.arthro.2012.12.003.

27. Hovelius L, Sandström B, Olofsson A, et al. The effect of capsular repair, bone block healing, and position on the results of the Bristow-Latarjet procedure (study III): long-term follow-up in 319 shoulders. J Shoulder Elbow Surg 2012;21(5): 647–60. http://dx.doi.org/10.1016/j.jse.2011.03.020.

28. Sekiya JK, Wickwire AC, Stehle JH, et al. Hill-Sachs defects and repair using osteoarticular allograft transplantation: biomechanical analysis using a joint compression model. Am J Sports Med 2009;37(12):2459–66. http://dx.doi.org/10.1177/0363546509341576.

29. Elkinson I, Giles JW, Faber KJ, et al. The effect of the remplissage procedure on shoulder stability and range of motion: an in vitro biomechanical assessment. J Bone Joint Surg Am 2012;94(11):1003–12. http://dx.doi.org/10.2106/JBJS.J.01956.

30. Yamamoto N, Itoi E, Abe H, et al. Contact between the glenoid and the humeral head in abduction, external rotation, and horizontal extension: a new concept of glenoid track. J Shoulder Elbow Surg 2007;16(5):649–56. http://dx.doi.org/10.1016/j.jse.2006.12.012.

31. Armitage MS, Faber KJ, Drosdowech DS, et al. Humeral head bone defects: remplissage, allograft, and arthroplasty. Orthop Clin North Am 2010;41(3):417–25. http://dx.doi.org/10.1016/j.ocl.2010.03.004.

32. Miniaci A, Gish M. Management of anterior glenohumeral instability associated with large Hill Sachs defects. Techniques in Shoulder & Elbow Surgery 2004; 5(3):170–5.

33. Gerber C, Lambert SM. Allograft reconstruction of segmental defects of the humeral head for the treatment of chronic locked posterior dislocation of the shoulder. J Bone Joint Surg Am 1996;78(3):376–82. Available at: http://www.ncbi.nlm.nih.gov/pubmed/8613444. Accessed March 3, 2013.

34. Hawkins RJ, Angelo RL. Glenohumeral osteoarthrosis. A late complication of the Putti-Platt repair. J Bone Joint Surg Am 1990;72(8):1193–7. Available at: http://www.ncbi.nlm.nih.gov/pubmed/2204630. Accessed March 3, 2013.

35. Purchase RJ, Wolf EM, Hobgood ER, et al. Hill-Sachs "remplissage": an arthroscopic solution for the engaging hill-sachs lesion. Arthroscopy 2008;24(6): 723–6. http://dx.doi.org/10.1016/j.arthro.2008.03.015.

36. Connolly J. Humeral head defects associated with shoulder dislocations: their diagnostic and surgical significance. Instr Course Lect 1972;21:42–54.

37. Elkinson I, Giles JW, Boons HW, et al. The shoulder remplissage procedure for Hill-Sachs defects: does technique matter? J Shoulder Elbow Surg 2012;22(6): 835–41. http://dx.doi.org/10.1016/j.jse.2012.08.015.

38. Weber BG, Simpson LA, Hardegger F. Rotational humeral osteotomy for recurrent anterior dislocation of the shoulder associated with a large Hill-Sachs lesion. J Bone Joint Surg Am 1984;66(9):1443–50. Available at: http://www.ncbi.nlm.nih.gov/pubmed/6501339. Accessed December 17, 2012.

39. Kronberg M, Broström LA. Rotation osteotomy of the proximal humerus to stabilise the shoulder. Five years' experience. J Bone Joint Surg Br 1995;77(6):924–7. Available at: http://www.ncbi.nlm.nih.gov/pubmed/7593108. Accessed February 24, 2013.

40. Flatow EL, Miller SR, Neer CS. Chronic anterior dislocation of the shoulder. J Shoulder Elbow Surg 1993;2(1):2–10. http://dx.doi.org/10.1016/S1058-2746(09)80131-6.

Mechanics and Pathomechanics in the Overhead Athlete

W. Ben Kibler, MD, Trevor Wilkes, MD, Aaron Sciascia, MS, ATC, PES*

KEYWORDS

- Shoulder injury • Mechanics of throwing • Pathomechanics of throwing
- Kinetic chain

KEY POINTS

- Overhead throwing motions are accomplished through activation of the kinetic chain, which produces the normal mechanics.
- It is imperative to be able to identify normal mechanics in order to recognize abnormal mechanics which are known to contribute to injury.
- Since the body works and fails a unit, it should be comprehensively evaluated in order to detect deficits and/or impairments either proximally or distally to the site of symptoms, which then can be restored to allow normal kinetic chain function.

INTRODUCTION

The overhead throwing or serving motion is a complex dynamic activity involving the entire body. It results in the performance of a task that requires repetitive high velocity, high load, and a large range of motion activities with a high degree of precision. It is necessary to have knowledge about the normal mechanics of this motion to understand optimum function of this motion in creating performance, and it is necessary to have knowledge of the altered mechanics or pathomechanics, that exist and contribute to the dysfunction of this motion, creating poor performance and injury.

This article illustrates current knowledge regarding the mechanics of the overhead motion in normal function and discusses the known pathomechanics and how they seem to relate to altered performance, injury, and injury risk. This knowledge has implications for clinical evaluation, treatment guidelines, and rehabilitation protocols.

MECHANICS OF THE OVERHEAD MOTION: WHAT MAKES THE BALL GO

The overhead throwing motion is developed and regulated through a sequentially co-ordinated and task-specific kinetic chain of force development and a sequentially activated kinematic chain of body positions and motions.[1] The kinematics of both the

Shoulder Center of Kentucky, Lexington Clinic, 1221 South Broadway, Lexington, KY 40504, USA
* Corresponding author.
E-mail address: ascia@lexclin.com

Clin Sports Med 32 (2013) 637–651
http://dx.doi.org/10.1016/j.csm.2013.07.003
0278-5919/13/$ – see front matter © 2013 Elsevier Inc. All rights reserved.

baseball throw and tennis serve have been well described and may be broken down into phases.[2–4] These descriptions show how muscles can move the individual segments and show the temporal sequence of the motions. The kinetics are not as well described but are important due to the forces and motions that are developed. These forces and motions are applied to all the body segments to allow their summation, regulation, and transfer throughout the segments, resulting in performance of the task of throwing or hitting the ball. The term, *kinetic chain*, is used to collectively describe both of these mechanical linkages. Using these definitions and terminology allows a unifying concept to understand the overall mechanics.

An effective athletic kinetic chain is characterized by 3 components[4]: (1) optimized anatomy in all segments; (2) optimized physiology (muscle flexibility and strength and well-developed, efficient, task-specific motor patterns for muscle activation); and (3) optimized mechanics (sequential generation of forces appropriately distributed across motions that result in the desired athletic function).

The kinetic chain has several functions: (1) using integrated programs of muscle activation to temporarily link multiple body segments into one functional segment (eg, the back leg in cocking stance and push-off and the arm in long axis rotation prior to ball release or ball impact) to decrease the degrees of freedom (DOFs) in the entire motion[2,5,6]; (2) providing a stable proximal base for distal arm mobility; (3) maximizing force development in the large muscles of the core and transferring it to the hand[2,7,8]; (4) producing interactive moments at distal joints that develop more force and energy than the joint itself could develop and decrease the magnitude of the applied loads at the distal joint[9–14]; and (5) producing torques that decrease deceleration forces.[12–16]

Several studies have clearly established the basic roles of the kinetic chain, both in baseball and tennis.[7,9–11,14,17–21] Each body part has specific roles in the entire motion.[2] The feet are contact points with the ground and allow maximum ground reaction force for proximal stability and force generation. The legs and core are the mass for the stable base and the engine for the largest amount of force generation. The shoulder is the funnel for force regulation and transmission and the fulcrum for stability during the rapid motion of the arm. The arm and hand is the rapidly moving delivery mechanism of the force to the ball or racquet.

To achieve its role in kinetic chain function, the shoulder must develop precise ball-and-socket kinematics to create maximum concavity-compression[22] that optimizes functional stability throughout the entire range of rapid motion. Requirements for functional stability include optimum alignment of the humerus and glenoid within ±30° angulation,[16] co-contraction and compression force couples of the rotator cuff and shoulder muscles,[23,24] a stable scapular base,[25] adequate balanced rotational range of motion,[26–28] and labral integrity to act as a washer, allowing best fit of the humerus into the glenoid.[29]

Tasks performed in baseball and tennis occur as a result of the summation of speed principle, which states that in order to maximize the speed at the distal end of a linked system, the movement should start with the proximal segments (the hips and core) and progress to the distal segments (shoulder, elbow, and wrist).[12] Each segment in this linked system can influence motions of its adjacent segments. For example, during a baseball pitch, stability of the back and stride legs allow rotation of the trunk, which, in turn, allows for maximal throwing arm external rotation. The stable lower extremity serves as a platform for trunk and upper extremity motion, where the amount of trunk rotation is proportionate to the amount of arm motion, which can occur. Variations in motor control and physical fitness components, such as strength, flexibility, and muscle endurance, can affect the efficiency and effectiveness of all segments of the linked system.[5,6,30]

Efficient mechanics can be improved by decreasing the possible DOFs throughout the entire motion.[5,6,31,32] There are 244 possible DOFs in the body from the foot to the hand.[5] Most models of maximum efficiency in body motions find that limiting DOFs to approximately 6 to 8 maximizes the total force output and minimizes effort and load.[32] DOFs can be limited by coordinated muscle activation coupling, called *integrative complexes*, that constrain and couple positions and motions so that several segments move as one.[31] Examples include the back leg stance position in baseball cocking, where the body is stabilized over the planted leg,[2] and the long axis rotation motion in baseball or tennis, where shoulder internal rotation, a minimally moving elbow, and forearm pronation allow the hand to rotate around the long axis from shoulder to wrist.[20]

The few independent DOFs are called nodes and represent key positions and motions in the overhead tasks.[2] These key positions are correlated with optimum force development and minimal applied loads and are considered the most efficient methods of coordinating kinetic chain activation. There may be multiple individual variations in other parts of the kinetic chain, but these are the most basic and the ones required to be present in all motions. The baseball pitching motion can be evaluated by analyzing a set of 8 progressive positions and motions (**Fig. 1**, **Table 1**).[18] These include trunk control over the back leg, hand in pronation "on top of the ball" in cocking, front leg directly toward home plate, control of lumbar lordosis in acceleration, hips facing home plate, arm cocking–scapular retraction/arm horizontal abduction/shoulder external rotation to maintain cocked arm in the scapular plane, "high" elbow above shoulder, and long axis rotation—coupled shoulder internal rotation/forearm pronation—at ball release.[2,9–11,14,17,33] The tennis serve motion can be evaluated by analyzing a set of 8 nodes or positions and motions that are correlated with optimum biomechanics (**Fig. 2**, **Table 2**).[2] These include optimum foot placement, adequate knee flexion in cocking progressing to knee extension at ball impact, hip/trunk counter-rotation away from the court in cocking, back hip tilt downwards in cocking, hip/trunk rotation with a separation at approximately 30°, coupled scapular retraction/arm rotation to achieve cocking in the scapular plane, back leg to front leg motion to create a shoulder-over-shoulder motion at ball impact, and long axis rotation into ball impact and follow-through.[2–4] These nodes can be evaluated by visual observation or by video recording and analysis. An example of tennis-specific pathomechanics is illustrated in **Fig. 3**, with detailed descriptions of the deleterious motions listed in **Table 2**.

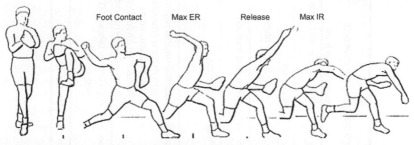

Fig. 1. The phases of throwing. The proper nodes are illustrated throughout the sequence. They include back hip and leg loading, hand on top of the ball, controlled lumbar lordosis, lead foot toward home plate, both hips facing home plate, and long axis rotation. *Abbreviations:* Max ER, maximal external rotation; Max IR, maximal internal rotation. (*From* Fleisig GS, Escamilla RF, Andrews JR, et al. Kinematic and kinetic comparison between pitching and football passing. Journal of Applied Biomechanics 1996;12:207–24; with permission.)

Table 1
Baseball nodes and possible consequences

	Node	Normal Mechanics	Pathomechanics	Result	To be Evaluated
1	Foot position	Directly toward home plate	Open or closed	Increased load on trunk or shoulder	Hip and/or trunk flexibility and strength
2	Knee motion	Stand tall	Increased knee flexion	Decreased force to arm	Hip and knee strength
3	Hip motion	Facing home plate	Rotation away from home plate	Increased load on shoulder and elbow	Hip and trunk strength
4	Trunk motion	Controlled lordosis	Hyperlordosis and back extension	Increased load on abdominals and "slow arm"	Hip and trunk strength
5	Scapular position	Retraction	Scapular dyskinesis	Increased internal and external impingement with increased load on rotator cuff muscles	Scapular strength and mobility
6	Shoulder/scapular motion	Scapulohumeral rhythm with arm motion (scapular retraction/humeral horizontal abduction/ humeral external rotation)	Hyper angulation of humerus in relation to glenoid	Increase load on anterior shoulder with potential internal impingement	Scapular and shoulder flexibility and strength
7	Elbow position	High elbow (above 90° abduction)	Dropped elbow (below 90° abduction)	Increased valgus load on elbow	Scapular position and strength, trunk and hip flexibility and strength
8	Hand position	On top of ball	Under or on side of ball	Increased valgus load on elbow	Shoulder and elbow position

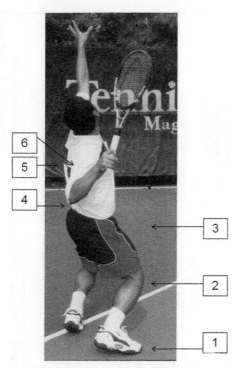

Fig. 2. Proper tennis serve nodes for optimal performance. The number sequence correlates with the normal description in **Table 2**. There is proper foot position and loading, adequate knee bend, back hip counter-rotation and tilt away from the court, X-angle of approximately 30°, trunk rotation, and arm cocking in line with the scapula. (*Adapted from* Lintner D, Noonan TJ, Kibler WB. Injury patterns and biomechanics of the athlete's shoulder. Clin Sports Med 2008;27(4):527–52.)

Adequate performance of the kinetic chain requires optimum anatomy and physiology. Optimum anatomy must be present in all of the joints in the kinetic chain. Joint injury (such as sprained ankles, unresolved knee injury or stiffness, hip tightness, and back injury) can have deleterious effects for core stability, force production, interactive moment production, and arm position.[4,30] Optimum physiology requires adequate muscle strength, flexibility, and endurance throughout the kinetic chain. It also requires proper muscle activation patterns for core stability, force development, integrative complexes, joint stabilization, and segment deceleration.[4] The optimized anatomy can then be acted on by the optimized physiology to create task-specific mechanics to achieve the kinematics and kinetics that produce the desired result of optimal performance in throwing or hitting the ball, creating the lowest possible risk of injury.

PATHOMECHANICS IN THE OVERHEAD MOTION: WHAT HAPPENS WHEN THE BALL DOES NOT GO

Overhead athletes with a painful shoulder have been shown to have a multitude of possible causative factors contributing to the presenting complaints of pain and decreased function, either by causing the anatomic injury or increasing the dysfunction from the injury. They may be alterations in anatomy, physiology, and/or

Table 2
Tennis nodes and possible consequences

	Node	Normal Mechanics	Pathomechanics	Result	To be Evaluated
1	Foot position	In line, foot back	Foot forward	Increased load on trunk or shoulder	Hip and/or trunk flexibility and strength
2	Knee motion	Knee flexion greater than 15°	Decreased knee flexion less than 15°	Increased load on anterior shoulder and medial elbow	Hip and knee strength
3	Hip motion	Counter-rotation with posterior hip tilt	No hip rotation or tilt	Increased load on shoulder and trunk; inability to push through increasing load on abdominals	Hip and trunk flexion flexibility and strength
4	Trunk motion	Controlled lordosis; X-angle ~30°	Hyperlordosis and back extension; X-angle <30° (hypo), X-angle >30° (hyper)	Increased load on abdominals and "slow arm"; Increase load on anterior shoulder	Hip, trunk, and shoulder flexibility
5	Scapular position	Retraction	Scapular dyskinesis	Increased internal and external impingement with increased load on rotator cuff muscles	Scapular strength and mobility
6	Shoulder/scapular motion	Scapulohumeral rhythm with arm motion (scapular retraction/humeral horizontal abduction/humeral external rotation)	Hyperangulation of humerus in relation to glenoid	Increase load on anterior shoulder with potential internal impingement	Scapular and shoulder strength and flexibility
7	Shoulder over shoulder	Back shoulder moving up and through the ball at impact, then down into follow-through	Back shoulder staying level	Increased load on abdominals	Front hip strength and flexibility, back hip weakness
8	Long axis rotation	Shoulder internal rotation/forearm pronation	Decreased shoulder internal rotation	Increased load on medial elbow	Glenohumeral rotation

X-angle, measurement of hip/trunk separation angle, the angle between a horizontal line between anterior aspect of both acromions and horizontal line between both anterior superior iliac spines when viewed from above, first described by McLean and Andrisani.[62]
Note: Numbers 1–6 occur prior to the acceleration phase of the service motion whereas numbers 7 and 8 occur after ball impact.

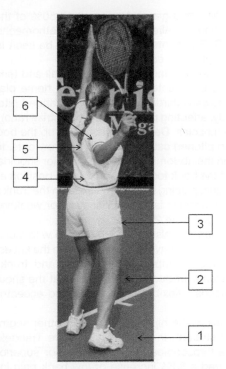

Fig. 3. Improper tennis serve nodes suggested to negatively affect function. The number sequence correlates with the pathomechanics description in **Table 2**. There is minimal foot loading, minimal knee flexion, ho hip rotation or tilting, no trunk rotation, and X-angle of 0°. (*Adapted from* Lintner D, Noonan TJ, Kibler WB. Injury patterns and biomechanics of the athlete's shoulder. Clin Sports Med 2008;27(4):527–52.)

biomechanics. They can combine to produce an alteration in the normal mechanics, resulting in pathomechanics that may create decreased efficiency in the kinetic chains, impaired performance, increased injury risk, or actual injury.[12,21,34] These pathomechanics contribute to the disabled throwing shoulder (DTS),[35] a general term that describes the limitations of function that exist in symptomatic overhead athletes—from baseball players to tennis players—in that they cannot optimally perform the task of throwing or hitting the ball. In a large percentage of cases, DTS is the result of a cascade to injury,[35] a process in which the body's response to the inherent demands of throwing or hitting results in a series of alterations throughout the kinetic chain that can affect the optimal function of all segments in the chain. The most common sites of pathomechanics include the legs and core, scapula, and shoulder. In a closed system, such as the kinetic chain, alteration in one area creates changes throughout the entire system.[29] This is known as the catch-up phenomenon, where the changes in the interactive moments alter the forces in the distal segments.[12,36] The increased forces place extra stress on the distal segments, which often result in the sensation of pain or actual anatomic injury.

Legs/Core

The legs and core connect the body to the ground, producing the ground reaction force that is important for force development, create the proximal base of stability required for distal mobility, and generate more than 50% of the kinetic energy and force delivered to the hand.[7,36] Alterations creating pathomechanics in this area are seen in up to 50% of DTS patients.[1] Alterations can be seen in foot position, knee motion, hip motion/strength, and core stability.

Altered foot position can be a factor in both baseball and tennis. Lead foot placement in baseball should be directed straight toward home plate.[18] Deviations that close the body (stride toward third base for a right-handed pitcher) cause a pitcher to throw across the body, affecting performance (ball/strike ratio) and increasing loads on the hip and oblique muscles. Deviations that open up the body (stride toward first base for a right-handed pitcher) cause a pitcher to throw outside the target area and place increased load on the abdominal muscles, anterior shoulder, and medial elbow. In tennis, positioning of the back foot in a foot forward position alters the ability of the body to rotate into cocking, placing increased stress on the trunk and shoulder (**Fig. 4**). A commonly altered foot position is a compensation for weakness in hip and in trunk flexibility and strength (see **Table 2**).

Alteration of knee flexion has also been associated with increased stresses in the arm. Tennis players who did not have adequate bend in the knees, breaking the kinetic chain and decreasing the contribution by the hip and trunk, had 23% to 27% increased loads in horizontal adduction and rotation at the shoulder and valgus load at the elbow.[21] Quadriceps inflexibility and decreased eccentric strength may alter knee motion.

Weakness or tightness at the hip can also affect other segments. Decreased hip flexibility in rotation or strength in abduction (positive Trendelenburg) was seen in 49% of athletes with arthroscopically proved posterior superior–labral tears.[37] Vad and colleagues[38] reported a 33% increase of low back pain in professional golfers with tight hip muscles. Altered hip and trunk motion was found to increase shoulder loads.[39] The musculoskeletal alterations could potentially be due to tissue maladaptations from repetitively imposed loads.[40] Strength imbalances around the hip and lumbar spine have been demonstrated by many studies, suggesting that these deficits may play a role in the dysfunction of the kinetic chain.[41,42]

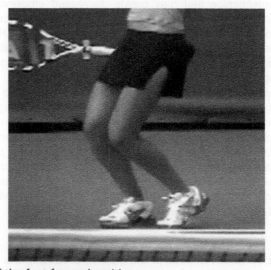

Fig. 4. Example of the foot forward position.

Scapula

Scapular dyskinesis is also seen in virtually every athlete with DTS. Dyskinesis represents an alteration of static scapular position or dynamic scapular motion in coordination with arm motion. The altered position and motions create a loss of control of retraction and posterior tilt, resulting in protraction, anterior tilt, and excessive internal rotation. Functional problems include external impingement due to anterior tilt,[43–45] internal impingement due to internal rotation and glenoid antetilting,[46] decreased rotator cuff strength,[47,48] and increased anterior capsular strain.[49] Dyskinesis is associated with 67% to 100% of shoulder injuries.[50]

Shoulder

Alterations in glenohumeral rotation are consistently found in overhead athletes with DTS and are the factors most highly associated with shoulder pain and injury.[1,34,51] They create multiple problems in and around the throwing shoulder, including scapular dyskinesis due to a wind-up of the tight posterior structures,[25] external impingement due to anterior superior humeral head translation in follow-through,[26,52] and posterior superior humeral head translation in cocking and anterior superior translation in flexion, which increase labral shear.[27,35] Increased evidence suggests that both glenohumeral internal rotation deficit (GIRD) and total range-of-motion deficit (TROMD) create the pathomechanics.[34,51]

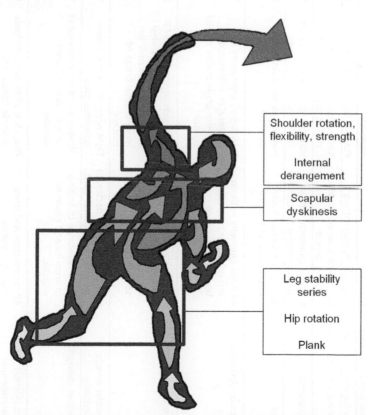

Fig. 5. Illustration of the kinetic chain and the areas of clinical evaluation, as described in Table 3.

Table 3
Proximal to distal kinetic chain evaluation

Examination Emphasis	Normal	Abnormal	Result	Evaluation
One leg stability: stance	Negative Trendelenburg	Positive Trendelenburg	Decrease force to shoulder	Gluteus medius strength
One leg stability: squat	Control of knee varus/valgus during decent	Knee valgus or corkscrewing during decent	Alters arm position during task	Dynamic postural control
Hip rotation	Bilateral symmetry within known normal limits	Side-to-side asymmetry and/or not within normal limits	Decrease trunk flexibility and rotation	Internal and external rotation of hip
Plank	Ability to maintain body position for at least 30 s	Inability to maintain body position	Decreased core stability and strength	Dynamic postural control in suspended horizontal position
Scapular dyskinesis	Bilateral symmetry with no inferior angle or medial border prominence	Side-to-side asymmetry or bilateral prominence of inferior angle and/or medial border	Decreased rotator cuff function and increased risk of internal and/or external impingement	Scapular muscle control of scapular position ("yes/no" clinical evaluation,[63,64] manual corrective maneuvers[25,47])
Shoulder rotation	Side-to-side symmetry or internal and external rotation values less than 15° or less than 5°	Side-to-side asymmetry of 15° or more in internal and/or external rotation or 5° or more of total range of motion	Altered kinematics and increased load on the glenoid labrum	Internal and external rotation of glenohumeral joint
Shoulder muscle flexibility	Normal mobility of pectoralis minor and latissimus dorsi	Tight pectoralis minor and/or latissimus dorsi	Scapular protraction	Palpation of pectoralis minor and latissimus dorsi
Shoulder strength	Normal resistance to testing in anterior and posterior muscles	Weakness and/or imbalance of anterior and posterior muscles	Scapular protraction, decreased arm elevation, strength, and concavity-compression	Muscle strength from a stabilized scapula
Joint internal derangement	All provocative and stress testing negative	Pop, click, slide, pain, stiffness, possible "dead arm"	Loss of concavity-compression and functional stability	Labral injury, rotator cuff injury or weakness, glenohumeral instability, biceps tendinopathy

Also, multiple muscles around the shoulder have been found to develop tightness as a result of throwing. The most commonly affected muscles are the pectoralis minor, subscapularis, and latissimus dorsi. The pathophysiology is believed to result from chronic tensile overload and resulting scar or from a muscle adaptive response.[53] The tight pectoralis minor creates a tendency for scapular anterior tilt and acromial downward tilt, decreasing the arm's ability to cock or reach maximal abduction.[43,54,55] The tight subscapularis decreases arm external rotation, limiting arm cocking. The tight latissimus dorsi limits overhead positioning and cocking.

The ultimate pathomechanical factor in the DTS is loss of optimal concavity-compression and functional glenohumeral stability. This can result from a combination of malalignment of the humerus on the glenoid,[56] alteration of muscle force couples, scapular dyskinesis,[49,57] GIRD/TROMD,[26,27] rotator cuff disease,[1] and/or labral injury.[1,58] This results in the performance symptoms of loss of velocity and accuracy and the "dead arm"[37] and in the clinical symptoms of pain, clicking, sliding, weakness, and injury.

CLINICAL IMPLICATIONS

The body works as a unit to achieve optimum overhead throwing function and can fail as a unit in altered performance or the DTS. Therefore, the evaluation of overhead athletes with DTS needs to be comprehensive and can involve evaluation of the pertinent normal mechanics, evaluation of possible pathomechanics, identification of physiologic and biomechanical factors contributing to the pathomechanics, and the kinetic chain examination as well as identification of all pathoanatomic factors that may exist in the shoulder. Similarly, treatment should include optimization of the pathoanatomy as well as restoration of the pathophysiology and pathomechanics.[1]

Evaluation of mechanics and pathomechanics can be clinically accomplished by direct observation and/or video analysis of the motion. Specific methods for evaluation and criteria for determining presence (yes) or absence (no) of the nodes have been developed for baseball[18] and tennis[2,3] and are summarized in **Tables 1** and **2**. This examination can identify anatomic areas and mechanical motions that may be contributing to the symptoms and suggest areas for more detailed evaluation.

The kinetic chain examination should include a screening evaluation of leg and core stability, observational evaluation for scapular dyskinesis, and evaluation of various elements in the shoulder. It should be supplemented by a detailed examination of the areas highlighted by the symptoms or evaluation[30] (**Fig. 5, Table 3**).

The shoulder examination should be comprehensive, emphasizing evaluation of the anatomy (labrum, biceps, and/or rotator cuff internal derangement), physiology (muscle weakness/imbalance and flexibility), and mechanics (scapular dyskinesis, GIRD, and TROMD).

Treatment should also involve a comprehensive approach, including restoration of all kinetic chain deficits, altered mechanics, and functional joint stability. Rehabilitation should address all the physiologic and mechanical factors.[1,59–61] These include restoration of hip range of motion and leg strength, core stability and strength, scapular control, shoulder muscle flexibility and strength, and glenohumeral rotation. Surgery should address repairing joint structures to optimize the capability for functional stability.[1]

SUMMARY

Optimal performance of the overhead throwing task requires precise mechanics that involve coordinated kinetic and kinematic chains to develop, transfer, and regulate the forces the body needs to withstand the inherent demands of the task and to allow optimal performance. These chains have been evaluated and the basic components, called nodes, have been identified.

Impaired performance and/or injury, the DTS, is associated with alterations in the mechanics that are called pathomechanics. They can occur at multiple locations throughout the kinetic chain. They must be evaluated and treated as part of the overall problem.

Observational analysis of the mechanics and pathomechanics using the node analysis method can be useful in highlighting areas of alteration that can be evaluated for anatomic injury or altered physiology. The comprehensive kinetic chain examination can evaluate sites of kinetic chain breakage, and a detailed shoulder examination can assess joint internal derangement of altered physiology that may contribute to the pathomechanics.

Treatment of the DTS should be comprehensive, directed toward restoring physiology and mechanics and optimizing anatomy. This maximizes the body's ability to develop normal mechanics to accomplish the overhead throwing task.

REFERENCES

1. Kibler WB, Kuhn JE, Wilk KE, et al. The disabled throwing shoulder - Spectrum of pathology: 10 year update. Arthroscopy 2013;29(1):141–61.
2. Lintner D, Noonan TJ, Kibler WB. Injury patterns and biomechanics of the athlete's shoulder. Clin Sports Med 2008;27(4):527–52.
3. Kovacs M, Ellenbecker T. An 8-stage model for evaluating the tennis serve: implications for performance enhancement and injury prevention. Sports Health 2011;3:504–13.
4. Sciascia AD, Thigpen CA, Namdari S, et al. Kinetic chain abnormalities in the athletic shoulder. Sports Med Arthrosc 2012;20(1):16–21.
5. Davids K, Glazier PS, Araujo D, et al. Movement systems as dynamical systems: the functional role of variability and its implications for sports medicine. Sports Med 2003;33(4):245–60.
6. Sporns O, Edelman GM. Solving Bernstein's problem: a proposal for the development of coordinated movement by selection. Child Dev 1993;64:960–81.
7. Elliott BC, Marshall R, Noffal G. Contributions of upper limb segment rotations during the power serve in tennis. J Appl Biomech 1995;11:443–7.
8. Toyoshima S, Miyashita M. Force-velocity relation in throwing. Res Q 1973;44(1): 86–95.
9. Hirashima M, Kadota H, Sakurai S, et al. Sequential muscle activity and its functional role in the upper extremity and trunk during overarm throwing. J Sports Sci 2002;20:301–10.
10. Hirashima M, Kudo K, Watarai K, et al. Control of 3D limb dynamics in unconstrained overarm throws of different speeds performed by skilled baseball players. J Neurophysiol 2007;97(1):680–91.
11. Hirashima M, Yamane K, Nakamura Y, et al. Kinetic chain of overarm throwing in terms of joint rotations revealed by induced acceleration analysis. J Biomech 2008;41:2874–83.
12. Putnam CA. Sequential motions of body segments in striking and throwing skills: description and explanations. J Biomech 1993;26:125–35.
13. Fleisig GS, Andrews JR, Dillman CJ, et al. Kinetics of baseball pitching with implications about injury mechanisms. Am J Sports Med 1995;23(2):233–9.
14. Fleisig GS, Barrentine SW, Escamilla RF, et al. Biomechanics of overhand throwing with implications for injuries. Sports Med 1996;21:421–37.

15. Young JL, Herring SA, Press JM, et al. The influence of the spine on the shoulder in the throwing athlete. J Back Musculoskelet Rehabil 1996;7:5–17.

16. Nieminen H, Niemi J, Takala EP, et al. Load-sharing patterns in the shoulder during isometric flexion tasks. J Biomech 1995;28(5):555–66.

17. Fleisig GS, Barrentine SW, Zheng N, et al. Kinematic and kinetic comparison of baseball pitching among various levels of development. J Biomech 1999; 32(12):1371–5.

18. Davis JT, Limpisvasti O, Fluhme D, et al. The effect of pitching biomechanics on the upper extremity in youth and adolescent baseball pitchers. Am J Sports Med 2009;37(8):1484–91.

19. Toyoshima S, Hoshikawa T, Miyashita M. Contributions of body parts to throwing performance. In: Nelson RC, Morehouse CA, editors. Biomechanics IV. Baltimore (MD): University Park Press; 1974. p. 169–74.

20. Marshall R, Elliott BC. Long axis rotation: the missing link in proximal to distal segment sequencing. J Sports Sci 2000;18(4):247–54.

21. Elliott B, Fleisig G, Nicholls R, et al. Technique effects on upper limb loading in the tennis serve. J Sci Med Sport 2003;6(1):76–87.

22. Lippitt S, Vanderhooft JE, Harris SL, et al. Glenohumeral stability from concavity-compression: a quantitative analysis. J Shoulder Elbow Surg 1993;2(1):27–35.

23. DiGiovine NM, Jobe FW, Pink M, et al. An electromyographic analysis of the upper extremity in pitching. J Shoulder Elbow Surg 1992;1(1):15–25.

24. Speer KP, Garrett WE. Muscular control of motion and stability about the pectoral girdle. In: Matsen Iii FA, Fu F, Hawkins RJ, editors. The shoulder: a balance of mobility and stability. Rosemont (IL): American Academy of Orthopaedic Surgeons; 1994. p. 159–73.

25. Kibler WB. The role of the scapula in athletic function. Am J Sports Med 1998; 26:325–37.

26. Harryman DT II, Sidles JA, Clark JM, et al. Translation of the humeral head on the glenoid with passive glenohumeral motion. J Bone Joint Surg Am 1990;72(9): 1334–43.

27. Grossman MG, Tibone JE, McGarry MH, et al. A cadaveric model of the throwing shoulder: a possible etiology of superior labrum anterior-to-posterior lesions. J Bone Joint Surg Am 2005;87(4):824–31.

28. Wilk KE, Meister K, Andrews JR. Current concepts in the rehabilitation of the overhead throwing athlete. Am J Sports Med 2002;30(1):136–51.

29. Veeger HE, van der Helm FC. Shoulder function: the perfect compromise between mobility and stability. J Biomech 2007;40:2119–29.

30. Kibler WB, Press J, Sciascia AD. The role of core stability in athletic function. Sports Med 2006;36(3):189–98.

31. Glazier PS, Davids K. Constraints on the complete optimization of human motion. Sports Med 2009;39(1):16–28.

32. Bernstein N. The coordination and regulation of movement. London: Pergamon; 1967.

33. Dillman CJ, Fleisig GS, Andrews JR. Biomechanics of pitching with emphasis upon shoulder kinematics. J Orthop Sports Phys Ther 1993;18:402–8.

34. Wilk KE, Macrina LC, Fleisig GS, et al. Loss of internal rotation and the correlation to shoulder injuries in professional baseball pitchers. Am J Sports Med 2011;39(2):329–35.

35. Burkhart SS, Morgan CD, Kibler WB. The disabled throwing shoulder: spectrum of pathology Part I: pathoanatomy and biomechanics. Arthroscopy 2003;19(4): 404–20.

36. Kibler WB. Biomechanical analysis of the shoulder during tennis activities. Clin Sports Med 1995;14:79–85.
37. Burkhart SS, Morgan CD, Kibler WB. Shoulder injuries in overhead athletes, the "dead arm" revisited. Clin Sports Med 2000;19(1):125–58.
38. Vad VB, Bhat AL, Basrai D, et al. Low back pain in professional golfers: the role of associated hip and low back range-of-motion deficits. Am J Sports Med 2004; 32(2):494–7.
39. Robb AJ, Fleisig GS, Wilk KE, et al. Passive ranges of motion of the hips and their relationship with pitching biomechanics and ball velocity in professional baseball pitchers. Am J Sports Med 2010;38(12):2487–93.
40. Kibler WB, McMullen J. Scapular dyskinesis and its relation to shoulder pain. J Am Acad Orthop Surg 2003;11:142–51.
41. Nadler SF, Malanga GA, Feinberg JH, et al. Relationship between hip muscle imbalance and occurrence of low back pain in collegiate athletes: a prospective study. Am J Phys Med Rehabil 2001;80(8):572–7.
42. Nadler SF, Malanga GA, Bartoli LA, et al. Hip muscle imbalance and low back pain in athletes: influence of core strengthening. Med Sci Sports Exerc 2002; 34(1):9–16.
43. Lukasiewicz AC, McClure P, Michener L, et al. Comparison of 3-dimensional scapular position and orientation between subjects with and without shoulder impingement. J Orthop Sports Phys Ther 1999;29(10):574–86.
44. Ludewig PM, Cook TM. Alterations in shoulder kinematics and associated muscle activity in people with symptoms of shoulder impingement. Phys Ther 2000; 80(3):276–91.
45. Michener LA, McClure PW, Karduna AR. Anatomical and biomechanical mechanisms of subacromial impingement syndrome. Clin Biomech 2003;18:369–79.
46. Kibler WB, Dome DC. Internal impingement: concurrent superior labral and rotator cuff injuries. Sports Med Arthrosc 2012;20(1):30–3.
47. Kibler WB, Sciascia AD, Dome DC. Evaluation of apparent and absolute supraspinatus strength in patients with shoulder injury using the scapular retraction test. Am J Sports Med 2006;34(10):1643–7.
48. Tate AR, McClure P, Kareha S, et al. Effect of the scapula reposition test on shoulder impingement symptoms and elevation strength in overhead athletes. J Orthop Sports Phys Ther 2008;38(1):4–11.
49. Weiser WM, Lee TQ, McQuade KJ. Effects of simulated scapular protraction on anterior glenohumeral stability. Am J Sports Med 1999;27:801–5.
50. Warner JJ, Micheli LJ, Arslanian LE, et al. Scapulothoracic motion in normal shoulders and shoulders with glenohumeral instability and impingement syndrome. Clin Orthop Relat Res 1992;285(191):199.
51. Kibler WB, Sciascia AD, Thomas SJ. Glenohumeral internal rotation deficit: pathogenesis and response to acute throwing. Sports Med Arthrosc 2012;20(1):34–8.
52. Silliman JF, Hawkins RJ. Classification and physical diagnosis of instability of the shoulder. Clin Orthop Relat Res 1993;291:7–19.
53. Butterfield TA. Eccentric exercise in vivo: strain-induced muscle damage and adaptation in a stable system. Exerc Sport Sci Rev 2010;38(2):51–60.
54. Borstad JD, Ludewig PM. The effect of long versus short pectoralis minor resting length on scapular kinematics in healthy individuals. J Orthop Sports Phys Ther 2005;35(4):227–38.
55. Kebaetse M, McClure PW, Pratt N. Thoracic position effect on shoulder range of motion, strength, and three-dimensional scapular kinematics. Arch Phys Med Rehabil 1999;80:945–50.

56. Mihata T, McGarry MH, Kinoshita M, et al. Excessive glenohumeral horizontal abduction as occurs during the late cocking phase of the throwing motion can be criticial for internal impingement. Am J Sports Med 2010;38(2):369–82.

57. Mihata T, Jun BJ, Bui CN, et al. Effect of scapular orientation on shoulder internal impingement in a cadaveric model of the cocking phase of throwing. J Bone Joint Surg Am 2012;94(17):1576–83.

58. Pagnani MJ, Warren RF. Instability of the shoulder. In: Nicholas JA, Hershman EB, editors. The upper extremity in Sports Medicine, vol. 2. St Louis (MO): Mosby; 1995. p. 173–208.

59. McMullen J, Uhl TL. A kinetic chain approach for shoulder rehabilitation. J Athl Train 2000;35(3):329–37.

60. Wilk KE, Macrina LC, Arrigo C. Passive range of motion characteristics in the overhead baseball pitcher and their implications for rehabilitation. Clin Orthop Relat Res 2012;470:1586–94.

61. Ellenbecker TS, Cools A. Rehabilitation of shoulder impingement syndrome and rotator cuff injuries: an evidence-based review. Br J Sports Med 2010;44: 319–27.

62. McLean J, Andrisani J. The X-factor swing. New York: Harper Collins; 1997.

63. McClure PW, Tate AR, Kareha S, et al. A clinical method for identifying scapular dyskinesis: part 1: reliability. J Athl Train 2009;44(2):160–4.

64. Uhl TL, Kibler WB, Gecewich B, et al. Evaluation of clinical assessment methods for scapular dyskinesis. Arthroscopy 2009;25(11):1240–8.

Imaging Instability in the Athlete
The Right Modality for the Right Diagnosis

Aaron J. Bois, MD, MSc, FRCSC[a],*, Richard E.A. Walker, MD, FRCPC[b],
Pradeep Kodali, MD[c], Anthony Miniaci, MD, FRCSC[d,e]

KEYWORDS

- Shoulder • Instability • Imaging • Bone loss • Radiography • CT • MR imaging

KEY POINTS

- Intra-articular contrast and direct magnetic resonance (MR) arthrography, even on high-field strength 3-T systems, provides added benefit over conventional MR imaging when evaluating an athlete with shoulder instability.
- Computed tomographic (CT) arthrography is a reliable diagnostic alternative in those patients with a contraindication to MR imaging.
- Accurate imaging assessment with CT or MR imaging of humeral head defects can help in preoperative planning for treatment of these complex bone defects.
- Sagittal and axial plane measurements are more accurate than coronal plane measurements of Hill-Sachs lesions.
- Three-dimensional CT is more reliable and accurate at quantifying glenoid bone loss than two-dimensional CT.
- Surface area measurements seem most valid at quantifying glenoid bone loss.

Funding Sources: There were no funding sources for this study.
Conflicts of Interest: All authors, their immediate families, and any research foundations with which they are affiliated have not received any financial payments or other benefits from any commercial entity related to the subject of this article.
[a] Section of Orthopaedic Surgery, Department of Surgery, University of Calgary, 3330 Hospital Drive NW, Calgary, Alberta T2N 4N1, Canada; [b] Department of Radiology, Faculty of Medicine, University of Calgary, Rm 812, North Tower, Foothills Medical Centre, 1403 29th Street NW, Calgary, AB T2N 2T9, Canada; [c] Department of Orthopaedic Surgery, Ironman Sports Medicine Institute, University of Texas Health Sciences Center at Houston, 6400 Fannin Street, Suite 1700, Houston, TX 77030, USA; [d] Department of Orthopaedic Surgery, Orthopaedic and Rheumatologic Institute, Cleveland Clinic, 9500 Euclid Avenue, Cleveland, OH 44125, USA; [e] Department of Biomedical Engineering, Lerner Research Institute, Cleveland Clinic, 9500 Euclid Avenue, Cleveland, OH 44125, USA
* Corresponding author.
E-mail address: ajmbois@gmail.com

INTRODUCTION

The glenohumeral joint is one of the most frequently dislocated joints in the human body.[1] Shoulder instability is best understood as a spectrum of disease: traumatic unidirectional instability exists at one end of the spectrum, whereas atraumatic and multidirectional instability (MDI) lies at the other extreme.[2]

This article reviews the commonly used imaging modalities for evaluating the athlete with symptoms of shoulder instability, including radiography, computed tomography (CT), and CT arthrography, with an initial focus on magnetic resonance (MR) imaging and MR arthrography. Examples of common soft tissue and osseous lesions associated with instability are provided, concentrating on those lesions seen in unidirectional posttraumatic anterior and posterior instability.

SOFT TISSUE DEFECTS/DISEASE

Technological advancements in cross-sectional imaging, including MR pulse-sequence design, high field strength 3-T platforms, advancements in multidetector CT technology, and the ability to manipulate and reconstruct large imaging data sets has revolutionized imaging of the shoulder girdle. Although radiographic evaluation remains an important and often overlooked and underused diagnostic tool in the evaluation of shoulder instability,[3] MR arthrography is considered the gold standard for soft tissue evaluation before arthroscopy.[4]

MR Imaging and MR Arthrography

MRI affords excellent evaluation of the osseous structures and soft tissue constraints of the glenohumeral joint in the setting of instability. The combination of high spatial resolution, high contrast resolution, and multiplanar two-dimensional (2D) and three-dimensional (3D) imaging techniques has made conventional MR imaging and MR arthrography the tests of choice for the preoperative evaluation of the injured athlete.[4–6] Visualization of the labroligamentous structures, articular cartilage, and the articular surface of the rotator cuff are enhanced by the presence of intra-articular fluid. In the setting of acute trauma, a hemarthrosis provides this distention.[5,6] In the subacute or chronic setting, joint distention can be achieved by performing conventional arthrography (using 10–15 mL of a 2 to 2.5 mM concentration of gadolinium-DTPA contrast at 1.5T) before MR imaging.[5]

Although imaging parameters vary amongst institutions, MR arthrography studies typically include a combination of multiplanar T1-weighted images with frequency-selective fat suppression and fluid-sensitive sequences.[5] The T1 shortening effect of gadolinium-based contrast agents results in high signal joint fluid, which on a background of low signal osseous and soft tissue structures afforded by fat suppression results in a wide range of dynamic image contrast, which improves visualization of subtle intra-articular abnormalities. Most advocate performing a conventional T1-weighted sequence without fat suppression to assess the rotator cuff muscles for atrophy and fatty infiltration and to further evaluate bone marrow.[5,7] We prescribe this technique in the oblique sagittal plane and find it particularly helpful for identifying small osseous Bankart lesions.

An additional advantage of MR arthrography over conventional MR imaging may be the ability to image in a position of abduction external rotation (ABER), in which the anterior-inferior glenohumeral ligament (aIGHL) is taut, resulting in tension on the anterior labrum. In this position, the oblique axial T1-weighted images obtained may improve detection of subtle anteroinferior labral tears as well as partial-thickness articular-sided tears of the supraspinatus and infraspinatus tendons.[5,8,9]

Conventional MR imaging of the labroligamentous complex has reported sensitivities and specificities ranging from 44% to 100% and 66% and 95%, respectively.[9] MR arthrography is reported to be more accurate than conventional MR imaging in detection of labral tears.[10] Waldt and colleagues,[11] in a study by comparing MR arthrography at 1.0 T with arthroscopic correlation, correctly diagnosed an anteroinferior labroligamentous injury in 91 of 104 cases, with a sensitivity of 88%, specificity of 91%, accuracy of 89%, and negative and positive predictive values of 88% and 91%, respectively. In that study, a Perthes lesion was correctly categorized in only 50% of cases, but the investigators suggest that imaging in an ABER position perhaps could improve those results. In a study by Magee and colleagues,[12] MR arthrography at 1.5 T detected 14 additional abnormalities not seen on conventional MR imaging in 20 consecutive baseball players imaged for shoulder pain. With the installation of high field strength clinical 3-T whole-body MR imaging systems, which provide improved signal-to-noise ratio and higher spatial resolution, the need to perform direct MR arthrography is again being debated. In a retrospective study of 150 consecutive patients who underwent conventional MR imaging and MR arthrography at 3 T with arthroscopic correlation,[10] the sensitivity of MR arthrography at 3 T for anterior labral tears was 98%, posterior labral tears 95%, SLAP (superior labral anterior posterior) tears 98%, and partial-thickness articular surface supraspinatus tendon tears 97%. Major and colleagues[13] reported similar results, indicating that tears of the superior and anterior labrum were more often identified on 3-T MR arthrography when compared with conventional 3-T MR imaging. The current literature therefore suggests that even on high field strength 3-T systems, intra-articular contrast with direct MR arthrography provides added benefit over conventional MR imaging when evaluating an athlete with shoulder instability.

Although seemingly limited by a lack of joint distention, indirect MR arthrography, a technique in which MR imaging is performed after an intravenous injection of gadolinium-based contrast, represents an alternate, less invasive method of MR arthrography. In a study by Jung and colleagues[14] comparing indirect MR arthrography and direct MR arthrography of the shoulder at 3 T, no significant difference was detected between the techniques for tears of the rotator cuff, labrum, and long head of biceps tendon, although the study population was small (19 patients).

CT and CT Arthrography

The potential benefits of CT of the shoulder include rapid acquisition of isotropic images with high spatial resolution that can be easily manipulated to provide multiplanar 2D and 3D volume-rendered reconstructions, decreased metal artifact when compared with MR imaging, and acceptability by the claustrophobic patient. Limitations include the use of ionizing radiation for image acquisition and limited soft tissue contrast resolution when compared with MR imaging. The addition of intra-articular contrast with CT arthrography improves soft tissue contrast required for assessment of the glenoid labrum and articular cartilage, and studies comparing CT arthrography and MR arthrography have shown similar performance in evaluating patients with shoulder instability (**Fig. 1**).[9] Shoulder CT is ideal for visualizing small fracture fragments of the glenoid rim and for assessing glenoid bone loss related to recurrent anterior instability.[9,15] CT arthrography is a reliable diagnostic alternative in those patients with a contraindication to MR imaging and for the assessment of recurrent shoulder instability after a surgical stabilization procedure incorporating ferromagnetic fixation devices.[5]

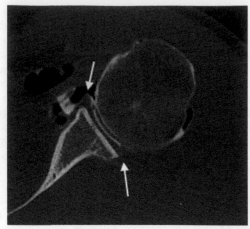

Fig. 1. Axial CT arthrogram of the left shoulder. The air-contrast arthrogram effect shows the normal anterior labrum (*yellow arrow*). High-density contrast fills a tear toward the base of the posterior labrum (*white arrow*).

ANTERIOR INSTABILITY

In most athletes, traumatic subluxation or dislocation of the glenohumeral joint occurs in an anterior or anteroinferior direction, with the arm abducted, externally rotated, and extended. Once the threshold of resistance provided by both static and dynamic stabilizers has been exceeded, shoulder dislocation occurs.[16] Because the union between the collagen fibers of the IGHL and the glenoid labrum is stronger than the union between the labrum and the glenoid rim, failure typically manifests as a labral avulsion from the glenoid and a Bankart or Bankart variant lesion.[17,18] Differentiation of Bankart and Bankart variants with MR arthrography is summarized in **Table 1**. In a few such injuries, failure occurs at the humeral attachment of the capsule, resulting in a humeral avulsion of the glenohumeral ligament (HAGL) lesion. In both instances, the result can be recurrent posttraumatic shoulder instability.

Table 1
Differentiation of Bankart and Bankart variants with MR arthrography

Lesion	Labrum	Displaced	Periosteum	Chondral Lesion	Instability	Provocative MR Arthrography Position
Fibrous Bankart	Detached	Yes	Disrupted	±	Yes	None
Osseous Bankart	Detached with bone fragment	Yes	Disrupted	±	Yes	None
Perthes	Detached	No	Intact ± stripped medially	−	Yes	ABER
ALPSA	Detached	Yes (Medially)	Intact and stripped medially	±	Yes	Adduction-internal-rotation
GLAD	Torn	No	Intact	+	No	ABER

Bankart and Bankart Variants

Fibrous Bankart lesion

The fibrous Bankart lesion represents a tear of the anteroinferior labrum, in which the labroligamentous complex is completely detached from the glenoid rim with disruption of the scapular periosteum.[18] On axial MR images, high signal fluid or contrast extends beneath the detached anteroinferior labrum, which remains in continuity with the aIGHL. Normal labral morphology may or may not be preserved (**Fig. 2**). Because of displacement from the glenoid rim, the fibrous Bankart lesion shows little tendency to heal.[9]

Osseous Bankart lesion

The osseous or bony Bankart lesion represents a fracture of the anteroinferior glenoid rim in which the labroligamentous complex remains attached to the fracture fragment.[19] When small or minimally displaced, the fracture fragment can be difficult to visualize both at routine MR imaging and MR arthrography, particularly if frequency-selective fat suppression is used on all sequences. When interpreting shoulder MR imaging in the setting of anterior instability, it is imperative to carefully evaluate the anterior glenoid margin for cortical irregularity or disruption in each imaging plane, with the size and extent of the Bankart fracture best determined on the oblique sagittal images.[8] CT or CT arthrography is superior to MR imaging/MR arthrography for the detection of small osseous fragments.[8]

Perthes lesion

The Perthes lesion represents a nondisplaced tear of the anterior-inferior labrum characterized by disruption of the osteochondral attachment of the labrum, but an intact scapular periosteal sleeve.[20] Although the periosteal sleeve is typically stripped anteromedially, its integrity helps to maintain an anatomic position of the torn labrum (**Fig. 3**). With time, a chronic Perthes lesion may partially heal, making it difficult to identify on both conventional MR imaging and MR arthrography examinations and at arthroscopy.[8] In a study by Wischer and colleagues,[21] the labral tear was not visualized on the axial MR arthrography images in 50% of arthroscopically proven Perthes

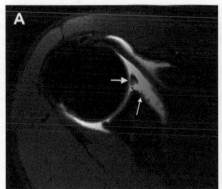
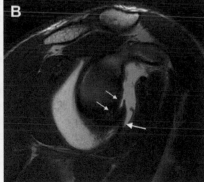

Fig. 2. Fibrous Bankart lesion. (A) Axial fat-suppressed T1-weighted image from an MR arthrogram of the right shoulder. There is complete detachment of the anterior labrum (*yellow arrow*) from the glenoid rim, with disruption of the anterior scapular periosteum (*white arrow* in A). (B) Oblique sagittal T1-weighted image (B) shows the extent of the anteroinferior capsulolabral injury (*yellow arrows*). The aIGHL remains attached to the displaced labrum (*white arrow* in B).

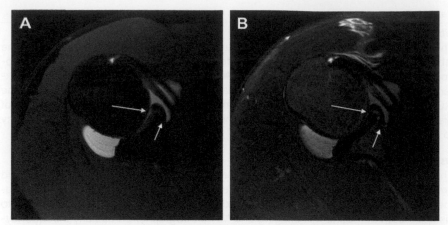

Fig. 3. Perthes lesion. (*A*) Axial fat-suppressed T1-weighted image and (*B*) Axial fat-suppressed T2-weighted image from an MR arthrogram of the right shoulder shows a subtle, nondisplaced tear of the anterior-inferior labrum (*yellow arrow* in [*A*] and [*B*]). Little contrast enters the tear, which is better seen on the fat-suppressed T2-weighted image (*B*). The anterior scapular periosteum is thickened but remains intact (*white arrow* in [*A*] and [*B*]). Imaging in ABER position was not performed.

lesions, although detection was improved by imaging the shoulder in ABER. In this position, traction placed on the aIGHL can elevate the labrum from the glenoid rim, allowing high signal contrast to insinuate into the tear and be visible on the oblique axial T1-weighted image.

Anterior labral periosteal sleeve avulsion
First described by Neviaser in 1993,[22] the anterior labral periosteal sleeve avulsion (ALPSA) lesion is characterized by stripping, medial displacement, and inferior rotation of the anteroinferior labrum along with the aIGHL, with medial stripping but without complete disruption of the scapular periosteum.[22–24] Although easily detected in the acute setting, with time the medialized labral fragment may heal and resynovialize on the glenoid neck. At MR imaging, the ALPSA lesion is often best visualized in the axial and coronal oblique imaging planes, with the low signal, displaced, and deformed labroligamentous complex tightly opposed to the glenoid neck with intact scapular periosteum. A fluid-filled or contrast-filled cleft may be visible between the medially displaced labrum and the glenoid rim, with the glenoid rim notably devoid of labral tissue (**Fig. 4**). Song and colleagues[24] reported that imaging the shoulder in a position of adduction-internal-rotation in addition to neutral-position MR arthrography improved visualization of complex ALPSA lesions. In this position, the intra-articular contrast is displaced preferentially into the anterior joint space, providing separation between the adherent labroligamentous complex and the anterior capsule.

Glenolabral articular disruption
A glenolabral articular disruption (GLAD) lesion consists of a superficial tear of the anteroinferior labrum in combination with an articular cartilage injury of the adjacent glenoid. Because the aIGHL remains intact and there is no associated capsular-periosteal stripping, the anterior labrum remains firmly attached to the glenoid rim, and unlike other Bankart variants, the GLAD lesion is not typically associated with anterior instability.[7,25] The mechanism of injury is a fall on an outstretched, externally

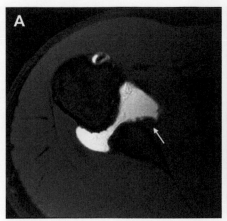
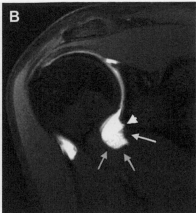

Fig. 4. ALPSA lesion. (*A*) Axial and (*B*) oblique coronal fat-suppressed T1-weighted image from an MR arthrogram of the right shoulder. The anterior-inferior labrum is detached from the glenoid rim and inferomedially displaced (*yellow arrow* in *A* and *B*). The anterior scapular periosteum remains attached to the glenoid neck, but is medially stripped along with the aIGHL (*orange arrows* in *B*). Note the contrast-filled cleft between the displaced labrum and the glenoid rim (*white arrowhead* in *B*).

rotated, and abducted arm, resulting in an osteochondral impaction injury of the glenoid articular surface by the humeral head.[25] Two distinct patterns of cartilage injury were described by Sanders and colleagues,[25] including a flap tear and a focal round or oval chondral defect with subjacent cortical depression, both visualized to best vantage on axial images. In both instances, the high signal fluid or contrast either fills the cleft undermining the chondral flap or the focal defect. Larger lesions may also be visible on the oblique coronal images (**Fig. 5**).[25] Like the Perthes lesion, MR arthrography in the ABER position may improve identification of the labral tear (**Fig. 6**).[25]

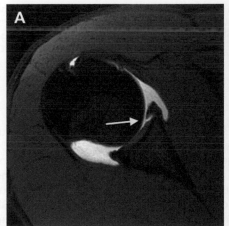
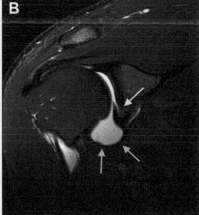

Fig. 5. GLAD lesion. (*A*) Axial fat-suppressed T1-weighted image and (*B*) oblique coronal fat-suppressed T2-weighted image from an MR arthrogram of the right shoulder. High signal fluid is seen filling a chondral flap tear at the base of the anteroinferior labrum (*yellow arrow* in *A* and *B*). The aIGHL (*orange arrows* in *B*) is intact.

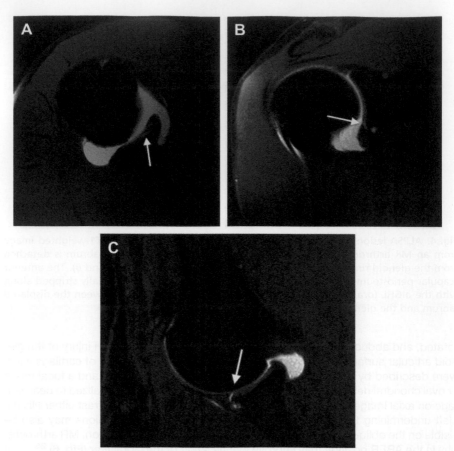

Fig. 6. GLAD lesion with ABER. (*A*) Axial and (*B*) oblique coronal fat-suppressed T1-weighted image from an MR arthrogram of the right shoulder. The chondral flap tear at the base of the anteroinferior labrum (*yellow arrow* in *A* and *B*) is poorly visualized when imaged in the neutral position. Traction placed on the aIGHL distracts the apposed margins of the chondral flap tear and improves visualization on the oblique axial fat-suppressed T1-weighted image performed in ABER position (*yellow arrow* in *C*). (*Courtesy of* Shamir Patel, MD, FRCPC, Calgary, AB, Canada).

HAGL/bony HAGL

Either soft tissue HAGL or bony HAGL (BHAGL) is reported to be an infrequent but important injury after anterior glenohumeral dislocation, reported in less than 10% of patients undergoing arthroscopic surgery for anterior instability.[26,27] Despite clinical findings of anterior instability, HAGL injuries can be difficult to visualize at the time of arthroscopic and open shoulder surgery, highlighting the importance of accurate preoperative imaging identification of this lesion.[9,17] Identification of a HAGL lesion on MR imaging requires joint distention, either by effusion in the acute setting or the use of MR arthrography. The humeral avulsion of the aIGHL is best appreciated on the oblique coronal images, where fluid or arthrographic contrast breaches the humeral attachment site, with displacement of the torn end of the ligament medially. The result is an abnormal, J-shaped rather than the normal U-shaped configuration of the axillary recess (**Fig. 7**).[17,27,28] An osseous avulsion (BHAGL) is identified in a few cases.

POSTERIOR INSTABILITY

Traumatic posterior glenohumeral subluxation or dislocation is less common and typically requires a posteriorly directed force with the arm flexed, adducted, and internally rotated.[8,9] Unlike anterior glenohumeral instability, posterior instability is not predictable simply based on the presence of a posterior labral tear, but typically

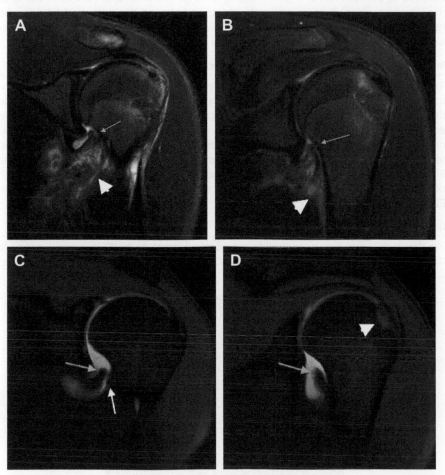

Fig. 7. HAGL lesions. (*A, B*) Oblique coronal fat-suppressed T2-weighted MR images of the left shoulder. In the acute setting, the posttraumatic joint effusion enhances visualization of the humeral avulsion of the IGHL (*orange arrow* in A and B), with high signal soft tissue edema extending along the medial margin of the humerus, inferior to the torn capsule, and into the quadrilateral space (*white arrowheads* in A and B). (*C, D*) Oblique coronal fat-suppressed T1-weighted images from an MR arthrogram of the left shoulder in another patient with a HAGL lesion. In the chronic setting, the high signal arthrographic contrast outlines the torn end of the aIGHL (*orange arrow* in C and D), with contrast undermining the humeral attachment (*white arrow* in C). A Hill-Sachs deformity (*white arrowhead*) is noted in (*D*).

requires the addition of stretching or stripping of the joint capsule and posterior scapular periosteum from the glenoid neck.[9,29] The longer the detached labroligamentous complex segment, the closer the association of the lesion with symptomatic posterior instability.[9]

Reverse Bankart Lesion

Unlike its anterior counterpart, a complete avulsion of the posterior labrum from the glenoid rim with disruption of the posterior scapular periosteum (the reverse Bankart lesion) is rare, because the periosteum, albeit medially stripped, frequently remains attached to the torn labrum.[9] MR imaging findings are best appreciated in the axial plane as high signal fluid or contrast extending between the detached labrum and the posterior glenoid margin. A reverse Hill-Sachs lesion or associated posterior glenoid rim fracture (reverse bony Bankart) may also be visualized (**Fig. 8**).

Posterior Labrocapsular Periosteal Sleeve Avulsion

The posterior labrocapsular periosteal sleeve avulsion (POLPSA) is similar to a non-displaced ALPSA lesion, characterized by an avulsion of the posterior labrum by the attached posterior capsule with medial stripping of the posterior scapular periosteum.[9,30] Unlike the reverse Bankart lesion, the posterior scapular periosteum remains intact, producing a patulous recess beneath the detached labrum and periosteal sleeve.[30] At MR imaging, high signal joint fluid or contrast may be visible dissecting between the posterior labrum and its posterior glenoid attachment, with focal thickening of the low signal, medially stripped posterior scapular periosteum (**Fig. 9**).[9,30]

Kim Lesion

The Kim lesion was first described in the surgical literature in 2004, when Seung-Ho Kim and colleagues[29] described a potentially arthroscopically occult lesion of the

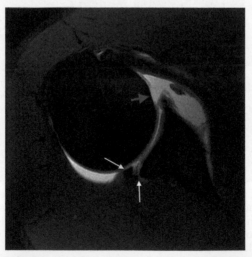

Fig. 8. Reverse Bankart lesion. Axial fat-suppressed T1-weighted image from an MR arthrogram of the right shoulder. There is complete detachment of the posterior labrum from the glenoid rim (*yellow arrow*) with disruption of the posterior scapular periosteum (*white arrow*). Note the subtle flattening of the anteromedial aspect of the humeral head and associated chondral defect (*red arrow*), consistent with a reverse Hill-Sachs deformity.

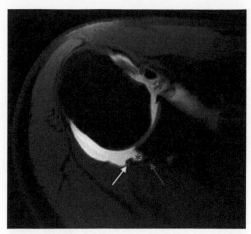

Fig. 9. POLPSA lesion. Axial fat-suppressed T1-weighted image from an MR arthrogram of the right shoulder. The posterior labrum is detached from the glenoid rim (*yellow arrow*) with medial stripping of the posterior scapular periosteum without complete disruption (*red arrow*). Note the patulous, contrast-filled recess (*asterisk*) created deep to the detached labrum and medially stripped periosteal sleeve.

posterior labrum characterized by a superficial, concealed, or incomplete tear at the base of the posteroinferior labrum, resulting in abnormal flattening of the posterior labrum with retroversion of the chondrolabral junction. In that series, all 15 patients had a posterior labral tear visible at MR arthrography, with the lesion characterized by a combination of the following: (1) incomplete avulsion or abnormal contour of the posterior labrum, (2) loss of labral height, and (3) intact junction between the glenoid articular cartilage and posterior labrum (**Fig. 10**).[29]

Posterior HAGL and Reverse HAGL

Posterior dislocation of the shoulder may result in failure of the posterior capsule at its humeral insertion, either as a humeral avulsion of the posterior band of the inferior glenohumeral ligament (IGHL) (PHAGL) or a humeral avulsion of the posterior capsule above the level of the posterior band, with or without extension inferiorly to involve the posterior band of the IGHL (RHAGL) (**Fig. 11**).[31] These acronyms are frequently used interchangeably in the radiologic and surgical literature. A muscle strain injury or partial-thickness tear of the tendon of the teres minor muscle has been described in association with these posterior capsular injuries, and the presence of such an injury should prompt a search for either a PHAGL or RHAGL lesion.[31]

BONE DEFICIENCY/LOSS

Glenohumeral bone loss plays a critical role in recurrent instability by altering joint contact area, congruency, and function of the static restraints.[16,32,33] Both biomechanical[34–38] and clinical[19,39–48] studies have shown that when bone loss approaches a critical threshold, Bankart repairs have a high failure rate when performed alone. Valid preoperative assessment of bone loss in shoulder instability is therefore crucial for surgical decision making, because unrecognized critical bone loss predisposes the patient to recurrent shoulder instability.

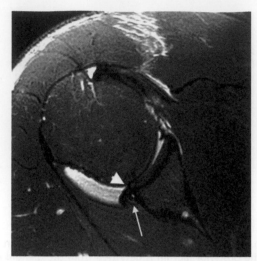

Fig. 10. Kim lesion. Axial fat-suppressed T2-weighted image from an MR arthrogram of the right shoulder. There is a superficial incomplete tear of the posterior labrum (*yellow arrow*) resulting in an abnormal flattened appearance to the posterior labrum (*white arrowhead*). Because the tear does not extend to the articular surface, it is potentially concealed at arthroscopy. (*Courtesy of* Shamir Patel, MD, FRCPC, Calgary, AB, Canada).

In addition to the routine radiographic views of the shoulder, specialized views and advanced imaging techniques have been developed to detect and quantify bone defects of the humeral head and glenoid rim. Although multiple radiographic methods have been described for detecting glenohumeral bone loss (ie, screening radiographs), there is no universally accepted method to quantify such defects.

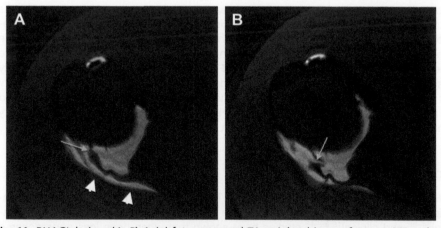

Fig. 11. RHAGL lesion. (*A, B*) Axial fat-suppressed T1-weighted image from an MR arthrogram of the right shoulder. There is a humeral avulsion of the posterior capsule (*orange arrows* in *A* and *B*). Contrast leaks through the capsular defect and can be seen extending superficial to the posterior capsule (*white arrowheads* in *A*). (*Courtesy of* Ian K.Y. Lo, MD, FRCSC, Calgary, AB, Canada).

HUMERAL BONE LOSS
Prevalence/Morphology/Classification

In 1861, Flower[49] was one of the first to describe humeral lesions commonly found with recurrent anterior shoulder instability. In 1940, Hill and Sachs[50] performed a radiologic analysis of humeral head compression fractures, which is known as a Hill-Sachs lesion. This lesion was found in 74% of patients in their series with recurrent anterior shoulder instability.[50] Since then, similar rates of radiologically evident humeral head defects have been found, ranging from 67% to 81% of patients after an initial dislocation[51–53] and from 70% to 87% of patients after recurrent instability.[52–54]

Richards and colleagues[55] used transaxial MR imaging with a 360° frame of reference to document the location and depth of arthroscopically confirmed Hill-Sachs lesions. Using this imaging technique, a Hill-Sachs defect was clearly visible within the boundaries of 170° to 260°, with an average midpoint of 209° (**Fig. 12**A). Hill-Sachs defects were found within the top 5-mm of the humeral head and extended an average of 12-mm distally. Depth varied in relation to overall lesion size, ranging from 2 to 6-mm (average 4-mm). In a more recent study, Saito and colleagues[56] used axial CT imaging to map the location and size of Hill-Sachs lesions in reference to the location of the bare area of the proximal humerus. Using the top of the humeral head as a reference point, Hill-Sachs lesions were observed between 0 and 24-mm, whereas the bare area started to appear at 19 to 21 mm and extended to the 37-mm to 39-mm slice level (see **Fig. 12**B).

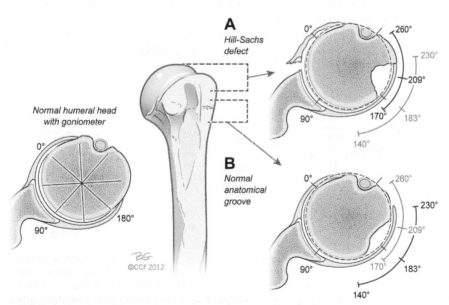

Fig. 12. (A) Typical location of Hill-Sachs lesion and (B) anatomic groove. (*Adapted from* Richards RD, Sartoris DJ, Pathria MN, et al. Hill-Sachs lesion and normal humeral groove: MR imaging features allowing their differentiation. Radiology 1994;190(3):665–8; and Bois AJ, Miniaci A. Surgical management of instability with bone loss. In: Iannotti J, Miniaci A, Williams G, et al. editors. Disorders of the shoulder: diagnosis and management, vol. 2: sports injuries. 3rd edition. Philadelphia: Lippincott Williams & Wilkins; 2013; p. 228–54. *Courtesy of* Cleveland Clinic Center for Medical Art & Photography; with permission.)

Rowe and colleagues[39] classified humeral head lesions into 3 categories according to defect size (length and depth): mild lesions represented defects that were 2 × 0.3 cm; moderate, 4 × 0.5 cm; severe, 4 × 1 cm or larger. Bigliani and colleagues[57] classified Hill-Sachs defects according to the percentage of head involvement using 1 axial image slice using CT or MR imaging: less than 20% (mild defect); between 20% and 45% (moderate defect); and greater than 45% (severe defect). Burkhart and De Beer[41] found a high failure rate of soft tissue stabilization procedures when performed in isolation in patients with engaging Hill-Sachs lesions (**Fig. 13**). Since this landmark study, most investigators have classified Hill-Sachs defects using this system; such defects can be classified using either dynamic arthroscopy (gold standard)[58] or preoperative CT imaging.[48]

Noninvasive Evaluation of Humeral Bone Loss

Recently, there has been increased awareness of the significance of humeral head defects on shoulder instability, with the acceptance that bone loss is a bipolar problem.[37,38,56] Humeral head bone loss has been ignored, in part, because there is no universally accepted imaging technique or criteria to define what is significant. Multiple studies have tried to clearly visualize and detect Hill-Sachs lesions, although no consistent way of measurement has been adopted.[59,60] In addition, not only is the size of the lesion important but also the amount of articular surface involvement, location of the defect relative to the glenoid track, and presence of associated glenoid bone loss (**Fig. 14**).[61] A large, deep defect that does not involve the articulating component of the humeral head may not be as significant as a smaller defect with a significant articular cartilage involvement that creates an engaging lesion with the glenoid rim. This mode of failure, defined as a humeral articular arc length deficit, was assessed using dynamic arthroscopy only[58]; however, other investigators have attempted to make such measurements radiographically.[44] A similar concept was described in 1948 by Palmer and Widen.[62]

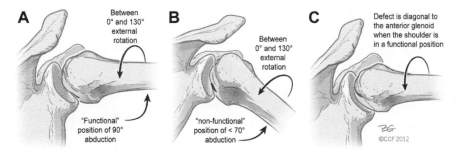

Fig. 13. Engaging and nonengaging Hill-Sachs lesions. (*A*) An engaging lesion is parallel to the anterior glenoid rim when the shoulder is in a functional position. (*B*) The engagement point of a nonengaging lesion occurs with the arm in a nonfunctional position. (*C*) In a functional position, a nonengaging lesion is diagonal and nonparallel to the anterior glenoid rim. (*Adapted from* Burkhart SS, De Beer JF. Traumatic glenohumeral bone defects and their relationship to failure of arthroscopic Bankart repairs: significance of the inverted-pear glenoid and the humeral engaging Hill-Sachs lesion. Arthroscopy 2000;16(7):677–94; and Bois AJ, Miniaci A. Surgical management of instability with bone loss. In: Iannotti J, Miniaci A, Williams G, et al. editors. Disorders of the shoulder: diagnosis and management, vol. 2: sports injuries. 3rd edition. Philadelphia: Lippincott Williams & Wilkins; 2013; p. 228–54. *Courtesy of* Cleveland Clinic Center for Medical Art & Photography; with permission.)

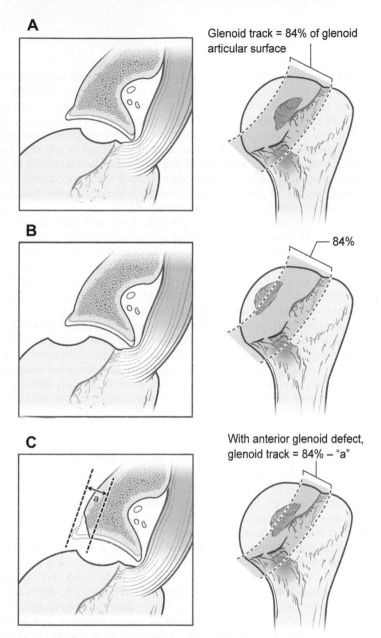

Fig. 14. Glenoid track concept and the interaction of combined glenohumeral bone loss. (*A*) If a Hill-Sachs lesion remains within the glenoid track, there is no chance that the lesion will engage on the anterior glenoid rim. (*B*) If the medial margin of the Hill-Sachs lesion is outside the glenoid track, there is a risk that the humeral head defect will engage the glenoid rim. (*C*) The risk of lesion engagement is dramatically increased when there is an associated defect of the anterior glenoid rim. (*Adapted from* Yamamoto N, Itoi E, Hidekazu A, et al. Contact between the glenoid and the humeral head in abduction, external rotation, and horizontal extension: a new concept of glenoid track. J Shoulder Elbow Surg 2007;16(5):649–56, with permission; and Bois AJ, Miniaci A. Surgical management of instability with bone loss. In: Iannotti J, Miniaci A, Williams G, et al. editors. Disorders of the shoulder: diagnosis and management, vol. 2: sports injuries. 3rd edition. Philadelphia: Lippincott Williams & Wilkins; 2013; p. 228–54. *Courtesy of* Cleveland Clinic Center for Medical Art & Photography; with permission.)

Radiography

The ideal imaging technique is easy to reproduce, with excellent reliability amongst physicians, and would predict clinically significant bone defects. Multiple studies have attempted to address this issue. Hill and Sachs[50] were the first to point out the importance of shoulder rotation for detecting humeral head impression fractures, suggesting that only in marked internal rotation does the posterolateral aspect of the head become viewed in profile for proper evaluation of defect length and depth. In 1959, Hall and colleagues[63] reported one of the best views for identifying Hill-Sachs lesions, known today as the Stryker notch view. Both the anteroposterior (AP) view in internal rotation and the Stryker notch view have been found to be the most sensitive for detecting humeral head lesions on plain radiographs.[64]

With respect to determining the size of the defect, Ito and colleagues[65] tried to quantify the size in 30 shoulders with anterior shoulder instability using a view that they described in a previous study.[60] The arm was placed in 135° of flexion and 15° of internal rotation, with the cassette placed underneath the shoulder and the beam aimed vertically through the humeral head. These investigators believed that this projection provided a clear view without distortion of the Hill-Sachs lesion. They found the shallower lesions correlated with a greater degree of joint laxity.

Kralinger and colleagues[66] measured the length, width, and depth using a 60° internal rotation view and a view described by Bernageau and colleagues[67] and calculated a Hill-Sachs quotient as a product of these 3 measurements. Although they found a correlation with grade III (Hill-Sachs quotient >2.5 cm^2) and recurrent instability, this method has not been universally accepted. This situation is likely because of the learning curve required to obtain these radiographic projections in addition to the inconsistency often seen in special radiographic views.

Advanced imaging

Although plain radiographs offer a relatively inexpensive screening tool to identify these defects, 2D and 3D imaging using CT or MR imaging theoretically provides a more accurate depiction of these lesions by visualizing them in 3 different planes. CT at many institutions can offer the added value of providing better bony detail, with 1-mm slices and 3D reconstructions improving the accuracy of determining the true location and size of the defect.

We performed a study that evaluated the reliability and accuracy of making width and depth measurements of different-sized Hill-Sachs lesions using axial, sagittal, and coronal 2D CT images.[68] Using a technique similar to Saito and colleagues,[56] lesion width was calculated as an edge-to-edge measurement and depth calculated using a best-fit circle method. Measurements were made by 5 physicians to assess reliability and compared with a 3D laser scanner to assess accuracy. We found these measurements to be reproducible, with the sagittal and axial planes being the most accurate.

More recently, Cho and colleagues[48] correlated the size and location of lesions on CT to predict engaging Hill-Sachs lesions. These investigators found that lesion width of 52% and depth of 14% of the diameter of the humeral head on the axial plane and width of 42% and depth of 13% on the coronal plane correlated with engagement of the lesion. Measurement of Hill-Sachs angle on 3D CT also correlated with engaging lesions. This study is valuable and attempts should be made preoperatively to predict lesions that will engage to assist in surgical decision making.

Given the literature, our preferred technique is to use a method similar to Cho and colleagues[48] using sagittal (**Fig. 15**) and axial (**Fig. 16**) planes on CT or MR imaging to quantify defect size. Coronal plane analysis has not shown to be as accurate as the

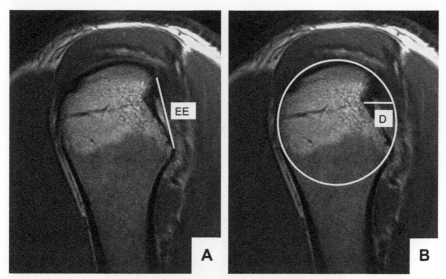

Fig. 15. MR imaging measurements. (*A*) Sagittal length (EE). (*B*) Sagittal depth (D).

other planes and is likely caused by the typical orientation of a Hill-Sachs lesion being parallel to the coronal plane. This situation increases the risk of potentially missing small lesions; however, this plane may be useful for more superior lesions. A best-fit circle method is used to calculate depth, and a direct edge-to-edge width measurement is made on the slice that shows the largest defect. If 3D CT reconstructions are available, they can be valuable to quantify defect parameters for preoperative planning (**Fig. 17**). Patients with lesions measuring wider than 16-mm in the axial or sagittal plane, deeper than 4-mm in the sagittal plane, and deeper than 5-mm in the axial plane may require bone augmentation procedures, because these patients have a higher likelihood of failed soft tissue stabilization (Gerson et al, 2011, unpublished data).[60]

Humeral head defects are an often ignored lesion in shoulder instability. Careful analysis of the lesion can help surgeons predict those that engage or that may fail a

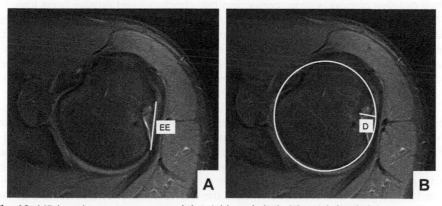

Fig. 16. MR imaging measurements. (*A*) Axial length (EE). (*B*) Axial depth (D).

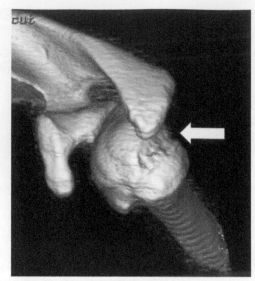

Fig. 17. 3D CT reconstruction with Hill-Sachs lesion (*arrow*).

soft tissue stabilization procedure. Defect size and location seem to be the most prognostically important variables related to failed soft tissue surgery. Once identified, several methods have been described to quantify humeral head lesions and are summarized in (**Fig. 18**).

GLENOID BONE LOSS
Prevalence/Morphology/Classification

Containment of the humeral head by the glenoid is a result of both the deepening effect of its concave surface and the articular arc length or safe zone of the articular surface.[16,41] One of the earliest reports of glenoid bone loss was in 1961, when Rowe and Sakellarides[19] discussed glenoid bone deficiency in the form of a rim fracture after anterior instability and proposed that such a lesion could be a possible cause of recurrent instability.

In a radiographic study of glenohumeral bone loss, Edwards and colleagues[54] identified osseous glenoid lesions, comprising both fractures and erosive bone loss, in 87% of patients with recurrent dislocations. Using more advanced imaging techniques such as 2D CT, Griffith and colleagues[70] found that the predominant form of glenoid bone loss was a compressive or attritional injury (91%), whereas only 22% of patients had evidence of a glenoid rim fracture. Conversely, using 3D CT to assess glenoid bone loss in 100 patients with recurrent instability, Sugaya and colleagues[71] found that only 40% of patients had erosive or attritional bone loss.

Contrary to previous descriptions, when viewing the glenoid fossa en face, the clinical appearance of glenoid bone loss occurs in a line nearly parallel to the long axis of the glenoid.[72] Using a clock face for orientation, Saito and colleagues[72] found that glenoid defects were located between 12:08 and 6:32, with the average orientation of the defect pointing toward 3:01 (**Fig. 19**). However, clinical bone loss can still occur in more anteroinferior locations.

In 1998, Bigliani and colleagues[40] were the first to classify lesions of the anterior glenoid rim: type I, a displaced avulsion fracture with attached capsule; type II, a

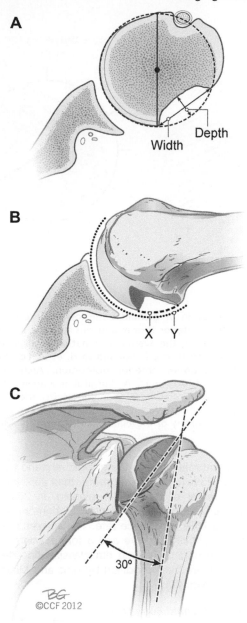

Fig. 18. Methods used to quantify Hill-Sachs lesions. (*A*) Such defects may be quantified using depth or width measurements, (*B*) percentage of humeral head involvement [(X/Y) × 100], where x = defect length, and y = total articular arc length or (*C*) by measuring the Hill-Sachs angle. (*Adapted from* Cho SH, Cho NS, Rhee YG. Preoperative analysis of the Hill-Sachs lesion in anterior shoulder instability: how to predict engagement of the lesion. Am J Sports Med 2011;39(11):2389–95; Chen AL, Hunt SA, Hawkins RJ, et al. Management of bone loss associated with recurrent anterior glenohumeral instability. Am J Sports Med 2005;33(6):912–25; and Bois AJ, Miniaci A. Surgical management of instability with bone loss. In: Iannotti J, Miniaci A, Williams G, et al. editors. Disorders of the shoulder: diagnosis and management, vol. 2: sports injuries. 3rd edition. Philadelphia: Lippincott Williams & Wilkins; 2013; p. 228–54. *Courtesy of* Cleveland Clinic Center for Medical Art & Photography; with permission.)

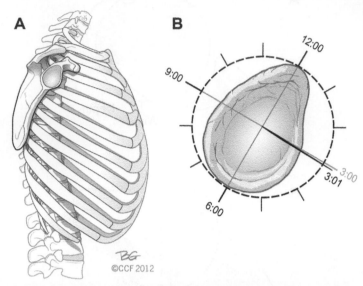

Fig. 19. Location and orientation of glenoid bone loss in anterior shoulder instability. (*A*) The scapula rests on the posterior thorax and tilts forward in the sagittal plane. (*B*) Using a clock face for orientation, the average orientation of a glenoid defect points toward 3:01. (*Adapted from* Saito H, Itoi E, Minagawa H, et al. Location of the Hill-Sachs lesion in shoulders with recurrent anterior dislocation. Arch Orthop Trauma Surg 2009;129(10):1327–34; and Bois AJ, iniaci A. Surgical management of instability with bone loss. In: Iannotti J, Miniaci A, Wlliams G, et al. editors. Disorders of the shoulder: diagnosis and management, vol. 2: sports injuries. 3rd edition. Philadelphia: Lippincott Williams & Wilkins; 2013; p. 228–54. *Courtesy of* Cleveland Clinic Center for Medical Art & Photography; with permission.)

medially displaced fragment malunited to the glenoid rim; and type III, erosion of the glenoid rim with less than 25% (type IIIA) or greater than 25% (type IIIB) bone loss in reference to the AP diameter of the inferior glenoid. In 2006, Boileau and colleagues[45] found that the association of a glenoid compression fracture and a stretched IGHL leads to a 75% recurrence rate. The authors believe that this combined pathology is prognostically additive and a formal contraindication to arthroscopic Bankart repair. The original glenoid rim classification described by Bigliani and associates[40] has therefore been modified by Bois and Miniaci[73] to account for this pathologic distinction (**Fig. 20**).

Noninvasive Evaluation of Glenoid Bone Loss

Multiple methods have been described to both detect and quantify glenoid bone loss using noninvasive imaging. Similar to humeral bone loss imaging techniques, a universally accepted preoperative method to quantify glenoid bone loss does not exist, and surgical decision making regarding glenoid deficiency is commonly based on subjective assessments; such methods have been shown to be inaccurate and should be avoided.[74]

Radiography

Specialized radiographic views have been developed to detect glenoid rim lesions, and most involve variations of the traditional axillary lateral view, including the West Point axillary,[75] Bernageau,[67] apical oblique (Garth),[76] and Didiee views.[64]

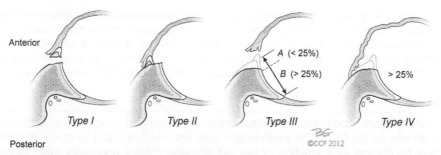

Fig. 20. Glenoid rim lesion types associated with anterior glenohumeral instability. Type I, a displaced avulsion fracture with attached capsule. Type II, a medially displaced fragment malunited to the glenoid rim. Type III, erosion of the glenoid rim with less than 25% (type IIIA) or greater than 25% (type IIIB) deficiency. Type IV, erosion of the glenoid rim with greater than 25% deficiency combined with a stretched IGHL. (*Adapted from* Bigliani LU, Newton PM, Steinmann SP, et al. Glenoid rim lesions associated with recurrent anterior dislocation of the shoulder. Am J Sports Med 1998;26(1):41–5; and Bois AJ, Miniaci A. Surgical management of instability with bone loss. In: Iannotti J, Miniaci A, Williams G, et al. editors. Disorders of the shoulder: diagnosis and management, vol. 2: sports injuries. 3rd edition. Philadelphia: Lippincott Williams & Wilkins; 2013. p. 228–54. *Courtesy of* Cleveland Clinic Center for Medical Art & Photography; with permission.)

Using the Bernageau glenoid profile view,[67] Edwards and colleagues[54] described the cliff sign and blunted angle sign to represent anteroinferior glenoid deficiency after resorption of an avulsion fragment and microimpaction fractures, respectively. Murachovsky and colleagues[77] recently assessed the accuracy and reproducibility of the Bernageau view using a cohort of 10 patients with unilateral traumatic anterior instability. Each subject underwent a 3D CT of both shoulders, which served as the gold standard. The investigators reported that the percentage differences (ie, accuracy) of bone loss between radiography and 3D CT were, on average 2.28% (range 0%–6.05%). In addition, the average interobserver statistics (ie, reproducibility) was 0.81 (very good) for the right side and 0.76 (good) for the left side.

The West Point axillary view has also had high accuracy for detecting glenoid bone loss when compared with CT.[64,78] More recently, the anterior sclerotic glenoid line sign as assessed on a true AP (Grashey) radiograph has been described and has moderate sensitivity (60%) and high specificity (100%) for the detection of anterior glenoid bone loss when compared with CT; however, this technique was not able to detect posterior glenoid rim lesions.[79]

Despite the multitude of specialized views, conventional radiographs often fail to detect or accurately quantify bone deficiency; this is likely a reflection of the combined inexperience shared by radiology technicians in obtaining these specialized views and by clinicians attempting to interpret and quantify bone loss on 2D projections. When a high level of clinical suspicion remains, advanced imaging techniques are recommended.

Advanced imaging

The standard imaging modality for quantifying glenoid bone loss is CT. Bone loss parameters obtained can be classified into 2 categories: indicators of bone loss (ie, methods that detect that there is a problem) and quantifiers of bone loss (ie, methods that quantify how much bone is missing and its location). The latter can be further subdivided into linear and surface area methods of measurement and are summarized in **Table 2**. The role of CT arthrography and MR arthrography has been well described and although they can be used for assessment of osseous defects, such techniques are more sensitive for detecting soft tissue lesions associated with glenohumeral instability.[80,81] The role of MR imaging for quantifying glenoid bone loss is inconclusive.

2D CT

Linear indicators of bone loss have been previously described using an en face view of the glenoid on 2D CT.[70] The width/length ratio (normal 0.7)[70] and length of glenoid defect expressed as a function of glenoid diameter[35] have previously been found most predictive of glenoid bone loss and recurrent instability after soft tissue repairs, respectively. Gerber and Nyffeler[35] assessed glenohumeral dislocation resistance using a biomechanical model of anteroinferior glenoid bone loss, and found that when the glenoid defect length was larger than half of the widest AP diameter of the glenoid (ie, larger than the radius), the dislocation resistance decreased to approximately 70% of an intact joint (**Fig. 21**). In such cases, soft tissue repairs alone were more likely to fail, leading to recurrent instability.

In 2012, Sommaire and colleagues[82] determined that the risk of failing an arthroscopic Bankart repair was significantly increased when the ratio of defect length/maximum glenoid width reached or exceeded 40%.

In our recent anatomic study,[15] the reliability and accuracy of standard 2D and 3D CT measurements of glenoid bone loss was evaluated. We found variable agreement and accuracy for all 6 observers using 2D CT to measure defect length and calculate the width/length ratio (ie, indicators of bone loss). We believe that this variability may be because of the difficulty of choosing the correct image slice and selecting appropriate 3D anatomic landmarks on a 2D plane. Overall, none of the methods assessed in this study using 2D CT was found to be valid. We therefore recommend using 3D CT to make linear measurements on the glenoid surface.

3D CT

CT with multiplanar reconstructions and digital subtraction of the humeral head allows an en face view of the glenoid.[83] Such imaging provides a complete 3D representation

Table 2
Summary of imaging techniques for assessment of glenoid bone loss

	Technique Description	Imaging Modality
Linear Method		
Gerber & Nyffeler,[35] 2002	Dislocation resistance (x/w)	CT arthrography
Griffith et al,[70] 2003	Indicators of bone loss	2D CT of en face glenoid
Barchilon et al,[84] 2008	Ratio method (d/D)	2D and 3D CT of en face glenoid
Chuang et al,[85] 2008	Glenoid index	3D CT of en face glenoid
Surface Area Method		
Sugaya et al,[71] 2003	Glenoid fragment surface area	3D CT of en face glenoid
Baudi et al,[86] 2005	Pico method	2D CT of en face glenoid
Nofsinger et al,[87] 2011	Anatomic glenoid index	3D CT of en face glenoid
Dumont et al,[88] 2012	Glenoid arc angle	3D CT of en face glenoid
Bois et al,[95] 2013	Regression modeling method	3D CT of en face glenoid

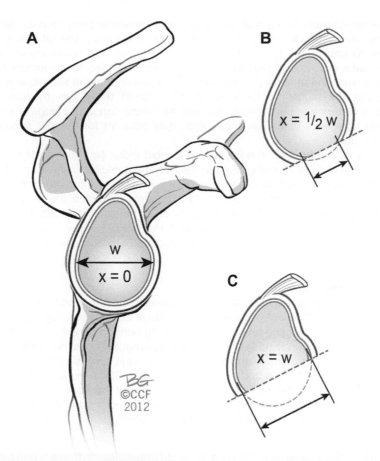

Fig. 21. Biomechanical relationship between anteroinferior glenoid bone loss and dislocation resistance. (*A*) Normal glenoid width (w) without bone loss (x). (*B*) Glenoid bone loss equal to the radius or half the AP diameter of the glenoid. (*C*) Glenoid bone loss involving more than half of the AP diameter of the glenoid results in a 30% loss of dislocation resistance. (*Adapted from* Gerber C, Nyffeler RW. Classification of glenohumeral joint instability. Clin Orthop Relat Res 2002;400:65–76; and Bois AJ, Miniaci A. Surgical management of instability with bone loss. In: Iannotti J, Miniaci A, Williams G, et al. editors. Disorders of the shoulder: diagnosis and management, vol. 2: sports injuries. 3rd edition. Philadelphia: Lippincott Williams & Wilkins; 2013; p. 228–54. *Courtesy of* Cleveland Clinic Center for Medical Art & Photography; with permission.)

of the glenoid fossa morphology without requiring a standardized CT scanner gantry position for image analysis. Using this technique, multiple methods have been developed to quantify glenoid deficiency, and are based on either linear[35,70,84,85] or surface area[71,86–88] measurements that become expressed as a percentage of the normal inferior glenoid circle. 3D CT is the most reliable and accurate imaging modality for assessment of glenoid bone loss.[15,89,90]

Linear techniques

In 2008, Barchilon and colleagues[84] described the ratio method (ie, using distance from the center of the inferior glenoid circle to the bone defect edge and the radius of the circle) for quantification of the percentage of glenoid bone loss. In the same study, the investigators compared the results obtained using the ratio method on unilateral 2D and 3D CT with those obtained using the Pico technique on 3D CT. Similar results were found between all 3 methods. We also found almost perfect agreement using the ratio method on 3D CT,[15] indicating that the technique is reproducible, but the highest percent errors were found using this method. Small changes in distance measurements (as little as 1-mm) can cause large changes in calculated bone loss measurements, which may account for the low accuracy of this technique.

Chuang and colleagues[85] developed the glenoid index (ie, ratio of the maximum inferior diameter of the injured glenoid to the maximum inferior diameter of the uninjured contralateral glenoid) to quantify bone loss in patients with anterior glenohumeral instability and found that this method accurately predicted the necessity of a bone grafting procedure in 96% of cases (24 of 25 patients) (**Fig. 22**). In our study assessing technique validity,[15] we found that the glenoid index is useful only for the more clinically relevant anterior defects that are parallel to the long axis of the glenoid.

Surface area techniques

In 2003, Sugaya and colleagues[71] were the first investigators to report the use of a surface area technique to quantify bone loss. The size of the osseous fragment (ie, bony Bankart) was calculated as a ratio of the area of the bone fragment to the area of the intact inferior glenoid circle. In 2005, Baudi and colleagues[86] described the Pico surface area technique to quantify attritional or erosive bone loss using a similar method to that described by Sugaya and colleagues (**Fig. 23**). Since the advent of the Pico technique, several investigators, including the authors of this review article, have reported that this technique provides a reproducible, precise, and accurate method for measuring glenoid bone loss.[15,91–94] However, there are potential problems that

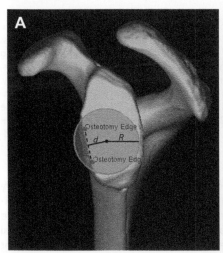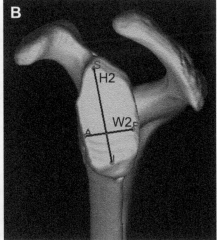

Fig. 22. Linear quantification techniques using custom 3D CT image analysis and visualization software (ImageIQ, Cleveland, Ohio). (*A*) Ratio method. The ratio between the depth to the defect margin (d) and radius (R) of the inferior glenoid circle is used to calculate the percentage of glenoid bone loss. (*B*) Glenoid index. Height (H2) and adjusted width (W2) measurements are used to determine the glenoid index.

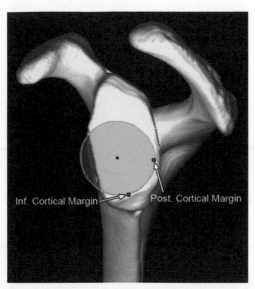

Fig. 23. Pico surface area quantification technique using custom 3D CT image analysis and visualization software (ImageIQ, Cleveland, Ohio). The circumference of the normal inferior glenoid circle is manually positioned on the pathologic glenoid using the remaining intact glenoid rim as a reference. Surface area measurements for regions of bone loss (*red*) and intact bone (*green*) are used to calculate bone loss.

arise from using surface area measurements (ie, area measurements) to quantify bone loss, because most biomechanical and clinical data defining critical thresholds of bone loss are based on linear measurements of defect width or length at the level of the inferior glenoid circle. Thus, caution should be exercised when attempting to make comparisons between linear and surface area techniques because such measurements cannot be interchanged (**Fig. 24**). Little is known of the importance of the depth of glenoid bone loss and how volumetric measurements may contribute to surgical decision making.

More recently, 3 additional surface area methods have been described using unilateral 3D CT of the injured (ie, ipsilateral) en face glenoid, including the anatomic glenoid index[87] (AGI) and glenoid arc angle.[88] Using the AGI, Nofsinger and colleagues[87] reported better interrater reliability for measurements performed on patients with minimal bone loss undergoing Bankart repair (0.73) compared with those patients with critical bone loss undergoing a Laterjet procedure (0.63). In 2013, Bois and colleagues[95] developed a quantification method that uses simple linear measurements on the injured glenoid to predict the amount of bone loss by means of regression modeling. Overall, more work is required to evaluate the reliability and accuracy of these recent techniques (see **Table 2**).

Despite the known advantages of 3D CT imaging techniques, the disadvantages include the financial burden to the institution and possibly the patient, the need for specialized computer software to quantify bone loss, and the lack of awareness in the orthopedic and radiology communities of the multiple measurement methods available and their general validity. This situation has led to an overall lack of agreement and consistency among the orthopedic community regarding glenoid bone loss quantification.

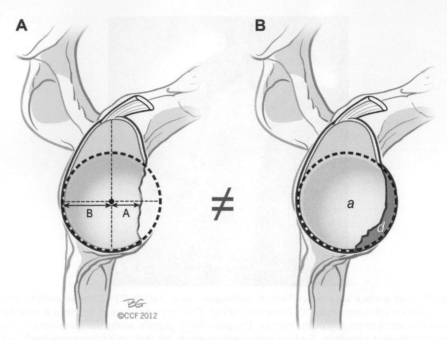

Fig. 24. Methods used to quantify glenoid bone loss. Computer software-assisted calculations of glenoid bone loss using (*A*) linear method (A = distance from center of glenoid to defect edge, B = distance from center of glenoid to posterior rim) and (*B*) surface area method. (a = surface area of normal inferior glenoid, d = surface area of defect or missing region of glenoid). Although calculated bone loss between the 2 methods is similar (ie, absolute value of ~20%–25%), the measurements represent different dimensions and locations of bone loss. (*Adapted from* Burkhart SS, De Beer JF, Tehrany AM, et al. Quantifying glenoid bone loss arthroscopically in shoulder instability. Arthroscopy 2002;18(5):488–91; Baudi P, Righi P, Bolognesi D, et al. How to identify and calculate glenoid bone deficit. Chir Organi Mov 2005;90(2):145–52; and Bois AJ, Miniaci A. Surgical management of instability with bone loss. In: Iannotti J, Miniaci A, Williams G, et al. editors. Disorders of the shoulder: diagnosis and management, vol. 2: sports injuries. 3rd edition. Philadelphia: Lippincott Williams & Wilkins; 2013; p. 228–54. *Courtesy of* Cleveland Clinic Center for Medical Art & Photography; with permission.)

SUMMARY

The imaging evaluation of an athlete with glenohumeral instability encompasses multiple modalities, including radiography, CT, and MRI. There remains an overall lack of agreement and consistency among the orthopedic community regarding techniques used to quantify glenohumeral bone loss. When a high level of clinical suspicion remains, advanced imaging techniques are strongly recommended to ensure reliable and accurate assessment of defect size and location.

REFERENCES

1. Zacchilli MA, Owens BD. Epidemiology of shoulder dislocations presenting to emergency departments in the United States. J Bone Joint Surg Am 2010; 92(3):542–9.

2. Lo IK, Bishop JY, Miniaci A, et al. Multidirectional instability: surgical decision making. Instr Course Lect 2004;53:565–72.
3. Sanders TG, Jersey SL. Conventional radiography of the shoulder. Semin Roentgenol 2005;40(3):207–22.
4. Bak K, Wiesler ER, Poehling GG, ISAKOS Upper Extremity Committee. Consensus statement on shoulder instability. Arthroscopy 2010;26(2): 249–55.
5. Omoumi P, Teixeira P, Lecouvet F, et al. Glenohumeral joint instability. J Magn Reson Imaging 2011;33(1):2–16.
6. Dumont GD, Russell RD, Robertson WJ. Anterior shoulder instability: a review of pathoanatomy, diagnosis and treatment. Curr Rev Musculoskelet Med 2011; 4(4):200–7.
7. Bergin D. Imaging shoulder instability in the athlete. Magn Reson Imaging Clin N Am 2009;17(4):595–615.
8. Sanders TG, Zlatkin M, Montgomery J. Imaging of glenohumeral instability. Semin Roentgenol 2010;45(3):160–79.
9. Macmahon PJ, Palmer WE. Magnetic resonance imaging of glenohumeral instability. Magn Reson Imaging Clin N Am 2012;20(1):295–312.
10. Magee T. 3-T MRI of the shoulder: is MR arthrography necessary? AJR Am J Roentgenol 2009;192(1):86–92.
11. Waldt S, Burkart A, Imhof AB, et al. Anterior shoulder instability: accuracy of MR arthrography in the classification of anteroinferior labroligamentous injuries. Radiology 2005;237(2):578–83.
12. Magee T, Williams D, Mani N. Shoulder MR arthrography: which patient group benefits most? AJR Am J Roentgenol 2004;183(4):669–74.
13. Major NM, Browne J, Domzalski T, et al. Evaluation of the glenoid labrum with 3-T MRI: is intraarticular contrast necessary. Am J Roentgenol 2011;196(5): 1139–44.
14. Jung JY, Yoon YC, Yi SK, et al. Comparison study of indirect MR arthrography and direct MR arthrography of the shoulder. Skeletal Radiol 2009;38(7): 659–67.
15. Bois AJ, Fening SD, Polster J, et al. Quantifying glenoid bone loss in anterior shoulder instability: reliability and accuracy of 2-dimensional and 3-dimensional computed tomography measurement techniques. Am J Sports Med 2012; 40(11):2569–77.
16. Matsen FA 3rd, Chebli C, Lippitt S. Principles for the evaluation and management of shoulder instability. J Bone Joint Surg Am 2006;88(3):648–59.
17. Bencardino JT, Beltran J. MR imaging of the glenohumeral ligaments. Radiol Clin North Am 2006;44(4):489–502.
18. Bankart AS. The pathology and treatment of recurrent instability of the shoulder-joint. Br J Surg 1938;26:23–9.
19. Rowe CR, Sakellarides HT. Factors related to recurrence of anterior dislocations of the shoulder. Clin Orthop Relat Res 1961;20:40–8.
20. Perthes G. Über Operationen bei habitueller Schulterluxation. Deutsche Zeitschrift für Chirurgie 1906;85:199–227 [in German].
21. Wischer TK, Bredella MA, Genant HK, et al. Perthes lesion (a variant of the Bankart lesion): MR imaging and MR arthrographic findings with surgical correlation. Am J Roentgenol 2002;178(1):233–7.
22. Neviaser TJ. The anterior labroligamentous periosteal sleeve avulsion lesion: a cause of anterior instability of the shoulder. Arthroscopy 1993; 9(1):17–21.

23. Atay OA, Aydingoz U, Doral MN, et al. Anterior labroligamentous periosteal sleeve avulsion lesion at the superior glenoid labrum. Knee Surg Sports Traumatol Arthrosc 2002;10(2):122–5.

24. Song HT, Huh YM, Kim S, et al. Anterior-inferior labral lesions of recurrent shoulder dislocation evaluated by MR arthrography in an adduction internal rotation (ADIR) position. J Magn Reson Imaging 2006;23(1):29–35.

25. Sanders TG, Tirman PF, Linares R, et al. The glenolabral articular disruption: MR arthrography with arthroscopic correlation. Am J Roentgenol 1999;172(1):1171–5.

26. Wolf EM, Cheng JC, Dickson K. Humeral avulsion of glenohumeral ligaments as a cause of anterior shoulder instability. Arthroscopy 1995;11(5):600–7.

27. Liavaag S, Stiris MG, Svenningsen S, et al. Capsular lesions with glenohumeral ligament injuries in patients with primary shoulder dislocation: magnetic resonance imaging and magnetic resonance arthrography evaluation. Scand J Med Sci Sports 2001;21(6):e291–7.

28. George MS, Khazzam M, Kuhn JE. Humeral avulsion of glenohumeral ligaments. J Am Acad Orthop Surg 2011;19(3):127–33.

29. Kim SH, Ha KI, Yoo JC, et al. Kim's lesion: an incomplete and concealed avulsion of the posteroinferior labrum in posterior or multidirectional posteroinferior instability of the shoulder. Arthroscopy 2004;20(7):712–20.

30. Yu JS, Ashman CJ, Jones G. The POLPSA lesion: MR imaging findings with arthroscopic correlation in patients with posterior instability. Skeletal Radiol 2002;31(7):396–9.

31. Bokor DJ, Fritsch BA. Posterior shoulder instability secondary to a reverse humeral avulsion of the glenohumeral ligament. J Shoulder Elbow Surg 2010;19(6):853–8.

32. Greis PE, Scuderi MG, Mohr RA, et al. Glenohumeral articular contact areas and pressures following labral and osseous injury to the anteroinferior quadrant of the glenoid. J Shoulder Elbow Surg 2002;11(5):442–51.

33. Ghodadra N, Gupta A, Romeo AA, et al. Normalization of glenohumeral articular contact pressures after Latarjet or iliac crest bone-grafting. J Bone Joint Surg Am 2010;92(6):1478–89.

34. Itoi E, Lee SB, Berglund LJ, et al. The effect of a glenoid defect on anteroinferior stability of the shoulder after Bankart repair: a cadaveric study. J Bone Joint Surg Am 2000;82(1):35–46.

35. Gerber C, Nyffeler RW. Classification of glenohumeral joint instability. Clin Orthop Relat Res 2002;400:65–76.

36. Yamamoto N, Itoi E, Abe H, et al. Effect of an anterior glenoid defect on anterior shoulder stability: a cadaveric study. Am J Sports Med 2009;37(5):949–54.

37. Sekiya JK, Wickwire AC, Stehle JH, et al. Hill-Sachs defects and repair using osteoarticular allograft transplantation: biomechanical analysis using a joint compression model. Am J Sports Med 2009;37(12):2459–66.

38. Kaar SG, Fening SD, Jones MH, et al. Effect of humeral head defect size on glenohumeral instability: a cadaveric study of simulated Hill-Sachs defects. Am J Sports Med 2010;38(3):594–9.

39. Rowe CR, Zarins B, Ciullo JV. Recurrent anterior dislocation of the shoulder after surgical repair. Apparent causes of failure and treatment. J Bone Joint Surg Am 1984;66(2):159–68.

40. Bigliani LU, Newton PM, Steinmann SP, et al. Glenoid rim lesions associated with recurrent anterior dislocation of the shoulder. Am J Sports Med 1998;26(1):41–5.

41. Burkhart SS, De Beer JF. Traumatic glenohumeral bone defects and their relationship to failure of arthroscopic Bankart repairs: significance of the inverted-pear glenoid and the humeral engaging Hill-Sachs lesion. Arthroscopy 2000; 16(7):677–94.

42. Lo IKY, Parten PM, Burkhart SS. The inverted pear glenoid: an indicator of significant glenoid bone loss. Arthroscopy 2004;20(2):169–74.

43. Miniaci A, Gish M. Management of anterior glenohumeral instability associated with large Hill-Sachs defects. Tech Shoulder Elbow Surg 2004;5:170–5.

44. Chen AL, Hunt SA, Hawkins RJ, et al. Management of bone loss associated with recurrent anterior glenohumeral instability. Am J Sports Med 2005;33(6):912–25.

45. Boileau P, Villalba M, Hery JY, et al. Risk factors for recurrence of shoulder instability after arthroscopic Bankart repair. J Bone Joint Surg Am 2006;88(8):1755–63.

46. Cetik O, Uslu M, Ozsar BK. The relationship between Hill-Sachs lesion and recurrent anterior shoulder dislocation. Acta Orthop Belg 2007;73(2):175–8.

47. Mologne TS, Provencher MT, Menzel KA, et al. Arthroscopic stabilization in patients with an inverted pear glenoid: results in patients with bone loss of the anterior glenoid. Am J Sports Med 2007;35(8):1276–83.

48. Cho SH, Cho NS, Rhee YG. Preoperative analysis of the Hill-Sachs lesion in anterior shoulder instability: how to predict engagement of the lesion. Am J Sports Med 2011;39(11):2389–95.

49. Flower WH. On the pathological changes produced in the shoulder-joint by traumatic dislocation, as derived from an examination of all the specimens illustrating this injury in the museums of London. Transactions of the Pathological Society of London 1861;12:179–201.

50. Hill HA, Sachs MD. The grooved defect of the humeral head: a frequently unrecognized complication of dislocations of the shoulder joint. Radiology 1940;35: 690–700.

51. Antonio GE, Griffith JF, Yu AB, et al. First-time shoulder dislocation: high prevalence of labral injury and age-related differences revealed by MR arthrography. J Magn Reson Imaging 2007;26(4):983–91.

52. Griffith JF, Antonio GE, Yung PS, et al. Prevalence, pattern, and spectrum of glenoid bone loss in anterior shoulder dislocation: CT analysis of 218 patients. AJR Am J Roentgenol 2008;190(5):1247–54.

53. Widjaja AB, Tran A, Bailey M, et al. Correlation between Bankart and Hill-Sachs lesions in anterior shoulder dislocation. ANZ J Surg 2006;76(6):436–8.

54. Edwards TB, Boulahia A, Walch G. Radiographic analysis of bone defects in chronic anterior shoulder instability. Arthroscopy 2003;19(7):732–9.

55. Richards RD, Sartoris DJ, Pathria MN, et al. Hill-Sachs lesion and normal humeral groove: MR imaging features allowing their differentiation. Radiology 1994; 190(3):665–8.

56. Saito H, Itoi E, Minagawa H, et al. Location of the Hill-Sachs lesion in shoulders with recurrent anterior dislocation. Arch Orthop Trauma Surg 2009;129(10): 1327–34.

57. Bigliani LU, Flatow EL, Pollock RG. Fractures of the proximal humerus. In: Rockwood CA, Green DP, Bucholz RW, et al, editors. Fractures in adults. 4th edition. Philadelphia: Lippincott-Raven; 1996. p. 1055–107.

58. Burkhart SS, De Beer JF, Tehrany AM, et al. Quantifying glenoid bone loss arthroscopically in shoulder instability. Arthroscopy 2002;18(5):488–91.

59. Workman TL, Burkhard TK, Resnick D, et al. Hill-Sachs lesion: comparison of detection with MR imaging, radiography, and arthroscopy. Radiology 1992; 185(3):847–52.

60. Ito H, Shirai Y, Takayama A, et al. A new radiographic projection for the postero-lateral notch in cases of recurrent dislocation of the shoulder. Nihon Ika Daigaku Zasshi 1996;63(6):499–501.
61. Yamamoto N, Itoi E, Hidekazu A, et al. Contact between the glenoid and the humeral head in abduction, external rotation, and horizontal extension: a new concept of glenoid track. J Shoulder Elbow Surg 2007;16(5):649–56.
62. Palmer I, Widen A. The bone block method for recurrent dislocation of the shoulder joint. J Bone Joint Surg Br 1948;30(1):53–8.
63. Hall RH, Isaac F, Booth CR. Dislocation of the shoulder with special reference to accompanying small fractures. J Bone Joint Surg Am 1959;41(3):489–94.
64. Pavlov H, Warren RF, Weiss CB, et al. The roentgenographic evaluation of anterior shoulder instability. Clin Orthop Relat Res 1985;194:153–8.
65. Ito H, Takayama A, Shirai Y. Radiographic evaluation of the Hill-Sachs lesion in patients with recurrent anterior shoulder instability. J Shoulder Elbow Surg 2000; 9(6):495–7.
66. Kralinger FS, Golser K, Wischatta R, et al. Predicting recurrence after primary anterior shoulder dislocation. Am J Sports Med 2002;30(1):116–20.
67. Bernageau J, Patte D, Debeyre J, et al. Value of the glenoid profile in recurrent luxations of the shoulder. Rev Chir Orthop Reparatrice Appar Mot 1976; 62(Suppl 2):142–7.
68. Kodali P, Jones MH, Polster J, et al. Accuracy of measurement of Hill-Sachs lesions with computed tomography. J Shoulder Elbow Surg 2011;20(8): 1328–34.
69. Gerson J, Kodali P, Fening S, et al. The effect of humeral head defect size on instability of the shoulder. Canadian Orthopaedic Association (COA) Annual Meeting, St John's, Newfoundland, Canada; Podium Presentation. June, 2011.
70. Griffith JF, Antonio GE, Tong CW, et al. Anterior shoulder dislocation: quantification of glenoid bone loss with CT. AJR Am J Roentgenol 2003;180(5): 1423–30.
71. Sugaya H, Moriishi J, Dohi M, et al. Glenoid rim morphology in recurrent anterior glenohumeral instability. J Bone Joint Surg Am 2003;85(5):878–84.
72. Saito H, Itoi E, Sugaya H, et al. Location of the glenoid defect in shoulders with recurrent anterior dislocation. Am J Sports Med 2005;33(6):889–93.
73. Bois AJ, Miniaci A. Surgical management of instability with bone loss. In: Iannotti J, Miniaci A, Williams G, et al, editors. Disorders of the shoulder: diagnosis and management, vol. 2. Sports injuries. 3rd edition. Philadelphia: Lippincott Williams & Wilkins; 2013. p. 228–54.
74. Huijsmans PE, de Witte PB, de Villiers RV, et al. Recurrent anterior shoulder instability: accuracy of estimations of glenoid bone loss with computed tomography is insufficient for therapeutic decision-making. Skeletal Radiol 2011; 40(10):1329–34.
75. Rokous JR, Feagin JA, Abbott HG. Modified axillary roentgenogram: a useful adjunct in the diagnosis of recurrent instability of the shoulder. Clin Orthop Relat Res 1972;82:84–6.
76. Garth WP Jr, Slappey CE, Ochs CW. Roentgenographic demonstration of instability of the shoulder: the apical oblique projection. A technical note. J Bone Joint Surg Am 1984;66(9):1450–3.
77. Murachovsky J, Bueno RS, Nascimento LG, et al. Calculating anterior glenoid bone loss using the Bernageau profile view. Skeletal Radiol 2012;41(10): 1231–7.

78. Itoi E, Lee SB, Amrami KK, et al. Quantitative assessment of classic anterioinferior bony Bankart lesions by radiography and computed tomography. Am J Sports Med 2003;31(1):112–8.
79. Jankauskas L, Rudiger HA, Pfirrmann CW, et al. Loss of the sclerotic line of the glenoid on anteroposterior radiographs of the shoulder: a diagnostic sign for an osseous defect of the anterior glenoid rim. J Shoulder Elbow Surg 2010;19(1):151–6.
80. Lecouvet FE, Simoni P, Koutaissoff S, et al. Multidetector spiral CT arthrography of the shoulder. Clinical applications and limits, with MR arthrography and arthroscopic correlations. Eur J Radiol 2008;68(1):120–36.
81. Oh JH, Kim JY, Choi JA, et al. Effectiveness of multidetector computed tomography arthrography for the diagnosis of shoulder pathology: comparison with magnetic resonance imaging with arthroscopic correlation. J Shoulder Elbow Surg 2010;19(1):14–20.
82. Sommaire C, Penz C, Clavert P, et al. Recurrence after arthroscopic Bankart repair: is quantitative radiological analysis of bone loss of any predictive value? Orthop Traumatol Surg Res 2012;98(5):514–9.
83. Stevens KJ, Preston BJ, Wallace WA, et al. CT imaging and three-dimensional reconstructions of shoulders with anterior glenohumeral instability. Clin Anat 1999;12(5):326–36.
84. Barchilon VS, Kotz E, Barchilon Ben-Av M, et al. A simple method for quantitative evaluation of the missing area of the anterior glenoid in anterior instability of the glenohumeral joint. Skeletal Radiol 2008;37(8):731–6.
85. Chuang TY, Adams CR, Burkhart SS. Use of preoperative three-dimensional computed tomography to quantify glenoid bone loss in shoulder instability. Arthroscopy 2008;24(4):376–82.
86. Baudi P, Righi P, Bolognesi D, et al. How to identify and calculate glenoid bone deficit. Chir Organi Mov 2005;90(2):145–52.
87. Nofsinger C, Browning B, Burkhart SS, et al. Objective preoperative measurement of anterior glenoid bone loss: a pilot study of a computer-based method using unilateral 3-dimensional computed tomography. Arthroscopy 2011; 27(3):322–9.
88. Dumont GD, Russell RD, Browne MG, et al. Area-based determination of bone loss using the glenoid arc angle. Arthroscopy 2012;28(7):1030–5.
89. Rerko MA, Pan X, Donaldson C, et al. Comparison of various imaging techniques to quantify glenoid bone loss in shoulder instability. J Shoulder Elbow Surg 2013;22(4):528–34.
90. Bishop JY, Jones GL, Rerko MA, et al. 3-D CT is the most reliable imaging modality when quantifying glenoid bone loss. Clin Orthop Relat Res 2013;471(4): 1251–6.
91. Huijsmans PE, Haen PS, Kidd M, et al. Quantification of a glenoid defect with three-dimensional computed tomography and magnetic resonance imaging: a cadaveric study. J Shoulder Elbow Surg 2007;16(6):803–9.
92. d'Elia G, Di Giacomo A, D'Alessandro P, et al. Traumatic anterior glenohumeral instability: quantification of glenoid bone loss by spiral CT. Radiol Med 2008; 113(4):496–503.
93. Magarelli N, Milano G, Sergio P, et al. Intra-observer and interobserver reliability of the 'Pico' computed tomography method for quantification of glenoid bone defect in anterior shoulder instability. Skeletal Radiol 2009;38(11): 1071–5.

94. Magarelli N, Milano G, Baudi P, et al. Comparison between 2D and 3D computed tomography evaluation of glenoid bone defect in unilateral anterior gleno-humeral instability. Radiol Med 2012;117(1):102–11.
95. Bois AJ, Rothy AC, Ghodadra A, et al. Normal glenoid relationships used for unilateral quantification of glenoid bone loss in glenohumeral instability. Canadian Orthopaedic Association (COA) Annual Meeting, Winnipeg, MB, Canada; Podium Presentation. June, 2013.

Decision Making in the In-Season Athlete with Shoulder Instability

James P. Ward, MD[a], James P. Bradley, MD[b],*

KEYWORDS

- Shoulder • Instability • Arthroscopy • In-season athlete

KEY POINTS

- Shoulder injuries result in a significant amount of lost practice and game time, with at least 10 days being lost in almost half the cases.
- Immobilization in internal versus external rotation has not been shown to have a significant effect on recurrence rates.
- Most athletes are able to complete the season with non-operative treatment, however over 1/3rd suffered recurrent instability events during the year.
- No significant difference between open and arthroscopic treatment of shoulder instability in terms of recurrence rates or scoring systems has been found.
- A return to play goal is set at 6 months post-operatively excluding throwing athletes who may expect to return at 9 months.

INTRODUCTION

The glenohumeral joint is the most mobile joint in the body. Its wide range of motion allows for the ability to perform various athletic endeavors, including the precise overhead throwing motion intrinsic to many sports. This mobility comes at the expense of stability, because it is also the most commonly dislocated joint in the body. Most of the anterior dislocations occurring during sports are caused by either a collision with an anteriorly directed force applied to the posterior aspect of the shoulder or via an indirect mechanism with a fall onto an outstretched arm, with a resultant external rotation moment applied to the abducted limb.[1–3] Owens and colleagues[4] reported an injury rate of 0.12 per 1000 exposures, with the highest risk sports being ice hockey, football, and wrestling. The injuries resulted in a significant amount of time lost, with at least 10 days being missed in 45% of cases. Posterior instability is less commonly associated with a frank dislocation, but more commonly seen as recurrent transient subluxation events, resulting in pain and an inability to perform at the athlete's desired level.[5]

[a] University of Pittsburgh Medical Center, 3200 South Water Street, Pittsburgh, PA 15203, USA;
[b] Pittsburgh Steelers, Burke and Bradley Orthopaedics, University of Pittsburgh Medical Center, 200 Medical Arts Building, Suite 4010, 200 Delafield Road, Pittsburgh, PA 15215, USA
* Corresponding author.
E-mail address: bradleyjp@upmc.edu

Clin Sports Med 32 (2013) 685–696
http://dx.doi.org/10.1016/j.csm.2013.07.005
0278-5919/13/$ – see front matter © 2013 Elsevier Inc. All rights reserved.
sportsmed.theclinics.com

ANATOMY AND BIOMECHANICS

The glenohumeral joint is a diarthroidal joint, allowing range of motion in all 6 degrees of freedom. The relative lack of bony congruency, allowing for its wide range of motion, results in an increased reliance on other static and dynamic stabilizers. The rotator cuff, through its concavity-compression model, provides most of the dynamic stability. The labrum serves to deepen the glenoid, acting as an important static stabilizer.[6] The glenohumeral ligaments (superior, middle, and inferior) provide static stability at varying abduction angles. Their functions are listed in **Table 1**.[7] The inferior glenohumeral ligament (IGHL) has been found on cadaveric studies to consist of an anterior band, posterior band, and interposed axillary pouch.[8] It is thought to function as a hammock inferior to the humeral head with anchor points on the anterior and posterior glenoid.[9] The essential lesion in anterior shoulder instability is detachment of the anteroinferior labrum and capsule, including the anterior band of the IGHL. Magnetic resonance imaging (MRI) obtained on 27 patients after primary traumatic dislocation show a 92.5% rate of Hill-Sachs lesions and a 96.3% rate of Bankart lesions. MRI was found to be significantly more sensitive and specific in detecting disease after an instability episode. Not all patients had a frank dislocation, leading to development of the concept of a transient luxation, defined as a substantial translation of the humeral head relative to the glenoid with the development of pathologic findings consistent with complete dislocation but with spontaneous reduction of the joint to its anatomic position.[10]

The posterior aspect of the capsule has no ligamentous support and is the thinnest area of the capsule, making it prone to repetitive stress.[11] Recurrent stress has been postulated to plastically deform the capsule, increasing joint volume, and allowing for instability.[12] More traumatic mechanisms may lead to a reverse Bankart lesion, but this is not encountered at the same frequency as with anterior instability.

EPIDEMIOLOGY OF ANTERIOR INSTABILITY

The incidence of traumatic dislocation ranges from 11.2 to 23.9 per 100,000 person-years.[10,13–16] Shoulder dislocations are more common in men, ages 20 to 29 years, with almost half occurring during sports.[10,13,14] In an epidemiologic study by Owens and colleagues,[17] the 1-year incidence was 2.8%, with 84% of these being subluxations. The inclusion of subluxations yields an incidence that is 1 order of magnitude higher than previously found. Most of these events were anterior and usually caused by contact injuries, in accordance with previous reports. The spectrum of shoulder instability produced a 56.4% rate of labral tears on MRI, which may result in recurrent instability, even without a frank dislocation as the index event.[17] The higher incidence

Table 1 Functions of the glenohumeral ligaments	
Superior glenohumeral ligament	Prevents anterior and inferior displacement when the arm is adducted
Middle glenohumeral ligament	Prevents anterior and inferior displacement when the arm is at 45° of abduction
Anterior band of the inferior glenohumeral ligament	Prevents anterior displacement with the arm abducted to 90° and externally rotated
Posterior band of the inferior glenohumeral ligament	Prevents posterior displacement with the arm abducted to 90° and internally rotated

is partly attributable to the younger, athletic population studied and the high rate of follow-up. Recurrence rate is inversely related to the patient's age at the time of the primary instability event.[18-20] Many studies also find a relation to sports participation or overhead activity; however, in a study by Kralinger and colleagues,[21] the rate of recurrence was found to be unrelated to activity, physical therapy, or length and type of immobilization after being adjusted for age at index event after regression analysis.[22] In a prospective cohort study by Robinson and colleagues,[20] more than 55% of the patients who developed recurrent instability did so within the first 2 years after the index event. An additional 11% developed recurrence between years 2 and 5, implying that recurrence is most likely in the early period after the primary event. Ligamentous laxity has also been implicated as a risk factor for instability. A study defining laxity as external rotation of 85° with the shoulder adducted found a 7-fold increased risk of recurrence, possibly because of altered capsular proprioception.[23]

PHYSICAL EXAMINATION AND ON-FIELD MANAGEMENT OF SHOULDER INSTABILITY

The initial evaluation begins with an assessment of airway, breathing, and circulation. In football or ice hockey, the helmet and shoulder pads are left in place until spinal column injury has been ruled out. An initial history gathers information from the athlete as well as the athletic trainer or other on-field personnel. If video replay is available, this gives better information regarding mechanism of injury, because the athlete may not recall the events leading to shoulder instability. Hand dominance, history of previous instability, and history of shoulder surgery should be obtained. An initial physical examination assesses the presence of deformity, open wounds, and limitations in range of motion. A full assessment of nerve function before any reduction attempt is of paramount importance. Injuries to the axillary nerve occur in 5% to 35% of first-time dislocations.[24] These injuries are most commonly neurapraxic and resolve spontaneously, but are disconcerting to the athlete. In the absence of any obvious proximal limb deformity, a reduction maneuver may be attempted on the field, before the onset of muscle spasm.[25] According to a recent review, no specific recommendations can be made regarding the technique of reduction in terms of effectiveness.[26,27] If the reduction is difficult or if the athlete is unable to tolerate it on the field, he or she is taken to the training room, where an intra-articular block with lidocaine is performed and radiographs may be obtained. The use of intra-articular lidocaine has been associated with lower complication rates and less time in the emergency department. No significant differences exist between this technique and the use of conscious sedation.[26,27] After successful reduction, a thorough postreduction neurovascular examination is carried out to assess for changes in nerve function, especially the axillary nerve. Postreduction radiographs are obtained to document concentric joint reduction and to assess for fractures. A true anteroposterior (AP) view of the glenohumeral joint is obtained, with the beam directed 35° to 45° relative to the chest wall. The AP views may be obtained in internal and external rotation. Axillary and outlet or Y views are necessary to obtain imaging in orthogonal planes. An axillary view is necessary to document acceptable reduction.[28]

In the subacute setting, physical examination includes range of motion and rotator cuff strength testing. Tests for generalized ligamentous laxity are also performed, along with side-to-side testing of both shoulders for multidirectional instability (anterior and posterior load and shift and sulcus sign). The patient is then placed supine and the arm abducted and externally rotated. The sensation of instability is a positive apprehension sign, whereas pain alone is less specific for anterior labral disease. Posteriorly directed pressure applied to the anterior aspect of the glenohumeral joint should result in a cessation of symptoms (positive relief sign). The abrupt removal of the examiner's hand may result in reintroduction of symptoms (positive surprise sign). The apprehension test is a predictor of recurrence after primary traumatic dislocation, with an odds ratio of 4.3 in the presence of a positive test. The test also showed a 41.7% sensitivity and 85.7% specificity in predicting recurrence.[29]

The Kim test has been identified as a method of identifying posterior instability. The patient's arm is placed in 90° of abduction and 45° of forward flexion. With an axial load applied to the elbow, a posterior and inferior force is applied to the arm. The test is positive if pain and a sensation of posterior subluxation are elicited.[30] The jerk test is another diagnostic maneuver for posterior instability. The examiner grasps the superior aspect of the shoulder with 1 hand, whereas the other grasps the elbow. The arm is flexed and internally rotated, and a posterior force is applied to the elbow while an anterior force is applied to the shoulder girdle. The arm is then abducted. The sensation of reduction of the humeral head with discomfort on the patient's part is a positive result. If both the Kim and jerk test are positive, there is 97% sensitivity to diagnose posterior instability.[30]

MRI should be considered to evaluate injuries to the labrum, rotator cuff, and articular cartilage. In the acute phase, hemarthrosis acts a contrast agent to allow for improved diagnosis. In the subacute setting, intra-articular gadolinium is used to highlight the labrum and diagnose subtle tears. The normal labrum has a triangular appearance on axial images, but may appear blunted or rounded as a subtle sign of injury. Obtaining a series in the ABER position (maximally abducted and externally rotated) tensions the anterior band of the IGHL and improves detection of nondisplaced tears and articular sided partial thickness rotator cuff tears (PASTA [partial articular sided tendon avulsion] lesions).[28] Athletes younger than 40 years are more likely to have an injury in the anteroinferior labrum, whereas those older than 40 years are more likely to tear their rotator cuff.[25]

Treatment is based on whether the instability is primary or recurrent, findings on imaging studies, timing in relation to the season, level of play, and desire to return. Although there is a risk of recurrence with nonoperative treatment and early return to play, this is the only option for the in-season athlete wishing to return.

NONOPERATIVE MANAGEMENT OF ANTERIOR INSTABILITY

The in-season athlete who wishes to complete their season after an episode of shoulder instability has no choice but to undergo nonoperative treatment. A discussion regarding the risks and benefits of this choice should be carried out in a frank, direct manner with the athlete and his or her family. Relative and absolute contraindications to continuing play should also be considered (**Box 1**). These considerations are based on lower levels of evidence and expert opinion, because no well-designed studies exist. An athlete may be allowed to return during the season, albeit with increased risk of recurrence, if he or she has have minimal pain, near normal motion, strength, functional ability, and sport-specific skills.[26]

Recent literature debated the position and duration of immobilization after an instability event and its effect on recurrence. Itoi and colleagues,[31] in an MRI study, showed improved reduction of the Bankart lesion when the patient was immobilized in external rotation. A prospective randomized clinical trial of internal versus external rotation immobilization for a period of 3 weeks followed. The compliance rate in the external rotation group was found to be superior along with a significant reduction in recurrence. There was a 38.2% relative risk reduction after an intention to treat analysis in favor of external rotation immobilization.[32] Critics of this study cite the relatively

---

Box 1
Contraindications to nonoperative in-season management of anterior glenohumeral instability

Dominant arm in a throwing or overhead athlete

Failure of nonoperative treatment/brace wear

Recurrent dislocator

Large or engaging Hill-Sachs lesion

Glenoid bone loss greater than 20%

Humeral avulsion of glenohumeral ligament lesion

Large capsular rent

Previous failed surgery

---

low follow-up rate of the patients and the high noncompliance rate in both groups. Subsequent studies have not produced a similar result. Finestone and colleagues[33] evaluated the immobilization positions in a prospective randomized study. No statistically significant difference in recurrence rates was found after immobilization for 4 weeks. Liavaag and colleagues[34] also performed a randomized prospective study, with a minimum follow-up of 2 years, with 97% follow-up. Improved compliance was found in the external rotation immobilization group; however, there was no significant difference in the recurrence rates. A systematic review of 9 level I or II studies[35] was unable to find a significant difference between immobilization in internal or external rotation, although a trend existed for a lower recurrence in the external rotation group. Furthermore, this review was not able to show a difference in recurrence rates between immobilization for 1 versus 3 weeks. The current best available literature does not support immobilization in external rotation after an instability event, although further studies are necessary.

Buss and colleagues[36] studied nonoperative management for the in-season athlete. After each episode of instability, the athletes were treated only with physical therapy and were not immobilized. They found that an average of 10.2 days time was missed per instability episode, with an average of 1.4 events per season. Braces were recommended for the remainder of the season. Most athletes (87%) were able to complete the season with brace wear and therapy; however, 37% experienced at least 1 additional instability event. Almost half of the athletes underwent stabilization procedures in the off-season.[36] No study exists showing the efficacy of in-season brace wear to reduce the number of instability episodes; however, we recommend their use for all athletes, excluding the dominant upper extremity of throwing or overhead athletes.

OPERATIVE MANAGEMENT OF ANTERIOR INSTABILITY

Operative stabilization is indicated for the young athlete with instability because of the high recurrence rate with nonoperative management. Optimally, this treatment is performed in the off-season to minimize lost time and to allow for adequate rehabilitation. Debates persist as to whether arthroscopic stabilization provides equivalent outcomes and success rates compared with open surgery.

Sachs and colleagues[22] have reported risk factors for recurrence and the ability to predict the need for surgery. In a prospective analysis, 91% of patients sustaining a recurrence were younger than 40 years, most of whom had participated in contact or collision sports or performed overhead activities in the normal course of their employment. Of the patients older than 40 years, 90% remained stable during the follow-up period. Risk factors predicting recurrence included age at the time of the initial event, participation in contact or collision sports, and engaging in overhead activities.

Specific indications for open management have been identified. These indications include large or engaging Hill-Sachs lesions or glenoid bone defects greater than 30%. Patients with these lesions have higher recurrence rates after isolated capsulo-labral reconstruction.[37] Open procedures are associated with a greater loss of external rotation, which may be a relative contraindication in the elite overhead athlete.[38] Midterm results of open Bankart reconstruction have been evaluated in a retrospective review with 11-year follow-up.[39] In this study, 84% of patients reported good or excellent outcomes, with a recurrence rate ranging between 6.7% and 9.7%. This recurrence rate increased to 22.6% when subluxations and positive apprehension tests were included. Most patients were able to return to their preoperative work status and level of sporting activity. No significant side-to-side differences in external rotation were identified; however, 29% of follow-up radiographs identified mild osteoarthritis. Longer-term follow-up of 29 years reported by Pelet and colleagues[40] showed a 10% recurrence rate, all within 5 years of surgery. The rate of symptomatic osteoarthritis proved significant, with a 16% rate of conversion to total shoulder arthroplasty. A mean rotational arc loss of 43° was identified with a significant decrease in functional scores. Despite this, 80% of those patients who did not require arthroplasty reported good results. Balg and Boileau[41] developed a scoring system to determine which patients would benefit from open versus arthroscopic reconstruction. They identified risk factors for recurrence and assigned relative values to help guide treatment (**Table 2**). Patients with a score less than 3 had a 5% risk of recurrence using arthroscopic stabilization techniques, whereas scores greater than 6 had a 70% recurrence with arthroscopy and were considered to be candidates for primary stabilization with a Latarjet procedure.

The usefulness of arthroscopic stabilization has garnered mainstream acceptance especially since the advent of modern suture anchor techniques. Certain principles must be adhered to when using an arthroscopic approach for stabilization, including the use of 3 or more suture anchors, providing adequate proximal shift of the anterior capsule along with plication to address laxity and treatment of associated intra-articular disease.[38] Revision surgery is not an absolute contraindication to an arthroscopic approach.[38] Initial reports of recurrence rates after arthroscopy were significantly higher than open techniques,[42–45] but several recent systematic reviews have not found a significant difference.[46–48] These more recent reviews also showed that no significant difference exists between the 2 approaches in most major shoulder scoring systems.

Table 2 Shoulder instability scoring system according to Balg and Boileau[41]	
Age >20 y = 0	Age <20 y = 2
Recreation sport participation = 0	Competitive sport participation = 2
Noncontact sports = 0	Contact sports = 1
No shoulder hyperlaxity = 0	Shoulder hyperlaxity (external rotation >85°) = 1
No Hill-Sachs on AP radiograph = 0	Hill-Sachs on AP radiograph = 2
Normal glenoid contour on AP radiograph = 0	Loss of glenoid contour on AP radiograph = 2

Arthroscopic techniques have been evaluated in special groups, such as adolescents and contact or collision athletes. In 3 retrospective analyses of adolescent athletes, recurrence rates, including both dislocations and subluxations, were approximately 20%, with almost half being secondary to traumatic events. The investigators concluded that arthroscopic techniques were appropriate in the younger patient population.[49–51] Mazzocca and colleagues[52] evaluated the use of arthroscopic techniques in contact and collision athletes, who would be assumed to place greater demands on their stabilization. After a 3-year follow-up, the recurrence rate was 11%, with all recurrences in collision athletes. All athletes had a significant improvement in validated scoring systems and no significant loss of range of motion was detected. Other investigators have corroborated this recurrence rate, with a range of postoperative instability from 10% to 17%, usually related to significant sport-related trauma.[53,54]

OUR PREFERRED MANAGEMENT OF ANTERIOR INSTABILITY

Nonoperative management is pursued in the early season to midseason, in the absence of the contraindications listed in **Box 1**. If the primary event occurs later in the season, early operative management may be considered to allow for adequate rehabilitation time for the ensuing season, depending on the athlete's level of play and eligibility. An arthroscopic approach is used for most patients, even in revision situations. The system developed by Balg and Boileau[41] is useful for determining the relative rates of success between open and arthroscopic approaches. Postoperatively, the athlete is immobilized in a sling for 4 weeks, with pendulum exercises beginning immediately. Formal physical therapy is started at postoperative week 4, with gentle active and passive range of motion and complete discontinuation of the sling by week 6. Strengthening begins 3 months postoperatively, with sport-specific drills beginning at 4 months postoperatively. A goal of return to play in contract sports is set at 6 months. Overhead athletes begin a throwing program at postoperative month 6, with a goal of return to play at 9 months.

EPIDEMIOLOGY OF POSTERIOR INSTABILITY

Frank posterior dislocations are less common. Anterior dislocations are 15.5 to 21.7 times more common, with the incidence of posterior instability estimated at 1.1 events per 100,000 person-years, according to an epidemiologic study by Robinson and colleagues[55] Although electric shock and seizures have been classically associated with posterior dislocations, acute trauma remains the most common mechanism of injury.[55] Predictors of recurrent instability include age greater than 40 years, a large reverse Hill-Sachs lesion, and seizure activity as the cause of the index event.[55] The more common pattern in the in-season athlete is one of recurrent posterior instability and subluxation, likely because of repetitive microtrauma.[5] Athletes at significant risk for posterior instability include those engaging in activities in which a posteriorly directed force is applied to the shoulder in a repetitive fashion. These athletes include football linemen (offensive and defensive), swimmers, gymnasts, weight lifters, and overhead throwers. Reverse Bankart tears and reverse Hill-Sachs lesions may be seen with traumatic dislocations; however, in subluxations, stretching and attenuation of the posterior band of the IGHL are more common.

PHYSICAL EXAMINATION AND ON-FIELD MANAGEMENT

Initial management begins with assessment of the athlete's airway, breathing, and circulation, as noted earlier. The same steps regarding history and physical examination as seen with anterior instability are carried out, along with a careful neurovascular examination of the involved upper extremity. If a frank dislocation is encountered on the field, the method of closed reduction uses cross-body traction applied to the limb while it is flexed, adducted, and internally rotated. Gentle continuous pressure is applied to the posterior aspect of the humeral head to guide it from its position behind the glenoid.[56] If resistance is encountered, prereduction radiographs are recommended along with either intra-articular lidocaine or intravenous sedation for repeated reduction attempts. The examination in the subacute setting along with imaging recommendations are described earlier.

TREATMENT OF POSTERIOR INSTABILITY

Nonoperative treatment is the mainstay for the in-season athlete. Most athletes complain of pain more often than a sensation of recurrent instability and are able to tolerate practice and game play. No clear literature exists regarding the use of a brace to prevent recurrences during game play. A period of at least 6 months of nonoperative treatment has been recommended in most instances, although results are better in those athletes with repetitive microtrauma as opposed to a macrotraumatic event.[57] If surgical management is warranted, it can in most cases be delayed until the off-season. Although the initial described technique was open posterior capsular shifting, most cases may now be managed arthroscopically with similar results.[12,58,59] Kim and colleagues[60] retrospectively reviewed 27 patients using suture anchors for lateral and superior shifting of the posterior band of the IGHL. Ninety-six percent of these athletes reported good or excellent results on UCLA (University of California at Los Angeles) scores. Only 1 patient reported a postoperative recurrence and was unable to return to his original level of play. The investigators noted an average loss of 1 vertebral level of internal rotation. Wolf and Eakin[12] also studied an athletic population reporting 86% good or excellent results with a 90% rate of return to play. Bradley and colleagues[61] have published the largest series of arthroscopically treated posterior instability cases in athletes. In a study of 100 consecutive shoulders, 91% of athletes reported good to excellent results, with 90% returning to sport, 67% at their preoperative level of activity. In a follow-up study of 107 shoulders with a mean follow-up of 27 months, 89% of throwing athletes and 93% of nonthrowing athletes reported good or excellent results. However, the throwing athletes were less likely to return to play at the same level, with only 55% returning to their preinjury level compared with 71% of the nonthrowers. No differences were noted in the subgroups' ASES (American Shoulder and Elbow Surgeons) scores, with both cohorts reporting significant improvement compared with their preoperative state.[62] The senior author's relative and absolute contraindications to arthroscopic management are listed in **Box 2**.

OUR PREFERRED MANAGEMENT OF POSTERIOR INSTABILITY

For most athletes, in-season management includes a formal rehabilitation program. Because most athletes suffer from pain or subluxations rather than frank dislocations, operative management may be deferred until the off-season. If the athlete is unable to compete at their desired level, arthroscopic treatment is indicated, except in the presence of the contraindications listed in **Box 2**. Current data suggest that superior results are obtained when the labrum is taken down from the glenoid rim, even in the presence of a nondisplaced lesion, and fixed with suture anchors, as opposed to a purely capsuloligamentous plication without bony fixation.[61] Postoperatively, the patient is placed in a sling with an abduction pillow for the first 6 weeks postoperatively, which is removed for gentle passive range of motion exercises initially. Active range of

Box 2
Contraindications to arthroscopic management of posterior glenohumeral instability
Surgeon unfamiliarity with operative technique
Patient did not undergo nonoperative treatment
Large, engaging reverse Hill-Sachs lesion
Large reverse bony Bankart lesion
Reverse humeral avulsion of glenohumeral ligament lesion
Voluntary dislocator
Previous failed surgery (relative)

motion is not allowed in the first postoperative month. Once adequate active and passive motion has returned, gentle strengthening exercises are used, usually until 8 weeks postoperatively. Progression to increased resistance training is begun in the fourth postoperative month, with throwing programs (as indicated) beginning at month 6 postoperatively. Return to play for nonthrowers is considered after 6 months, with throwing athletes undergoing a sport-specific throwing program and returning to play 8 to 9 months postoperatively.

SUMMARY

Shoulder instability in the in-season athlete can generally be managed nonoperatively during the season, except when specific contraindications are present, such as bone loss or involvement of the dominant limb in an overhead athlete. Brace wear, although advocated by many investigators, has no proven efficacy in reducing the number or frequency of in-season instability events. Arthroscopic approaches are used for both anterior and posterior instability, with rates of success similar to open approaches but with the advantage of improved postoperative range of motion. Return to play may be considered 6 month postoperatively for the nonthrowing athlete and 9 months postoperatively for the overhead-throwing athlete.

REFERENCES

1. Burra G, Andrews JR. Acute shoulder and elbow dislocations in the athlete. Orthop Clin North Am 2002;33(3):479–95.
2. Rowe CR. Prognosis in dislocations of the shoulder. J Bone Joint Surg Am 1956; 38-A(5):957–77.
3. Wang RY, Arciero RA. Treating the athlete with anterior shoulder instability. Clin Sports Med 2008;27(4):631–48.
4. Owens BD, Agel J, Mountcastle SB, et al. Incidence of glenohumeral instability in collegiate athletics. Am J Sports Med 2009;37(9):1750–4.
5. Bradley JP, Forsythe B, Mascarenhas R. Arthroscopic management of posterior shoulder instability: diagnosis, indications, and technique. Clin Sports Med 2008;27(4):649–70.
6. Matsen FA 3rd, Harryman DT 2nd, Sidles JA. Mechanics of glenohumeral instability. Clin Sports Med 1991;10(4):783–8.
7. Jost B, Koch PP, Gerber C. Anatomy and functional aspects of the rotator interval. J Shoulder Elbow Surg 2000;9(4):336–41.

8. O'Brien SJ, Neves MC, Arnoczky SP, et al. The anatomy and histology of the inferior glenohumeral ligament complex of the shoulder. Am J Sports Med 1990;18(5):449–56.

9. Burkart AC, Debski RE. Anatomy and function of the glenohumeral ligaments in anterior shoulder instability. Clin Orthop Relat Res 2002;(400):32–9.

10. Owens BD, Dawson L, Burks R, et al. Incidence of shoulder dislocation in the United States military: demographic considerations from a high-risk population. J Bone Joint Surg Am 2009;91(4):791–6.

11. Pagnani MJ, Warren RF. Stabilizers of the glenohumeral joint. J Shoulder Elbow Surg 1994;3(3):173–90.

12. Wolf EM, Eakin CL. Arthroscopic capsular plication for posterior shoulder instability. Arthroscopy 1998;14(2):153–63.

13. Simonet WT, Melton LJ 3rd, Cofield RH, et al. Incidence of anterior shoulder dislocation in Olmsted County, Minnesota. Clin Orthop Relat Res 1984;(186):186–91.

14. Zacchilli MA, Owens BD. Epidemiology of shoulder dislocations presenting to emergency departments in the United States. J Bone Joint Surg Am 2010; 92(3):542–9.

15. Nordqvist A, Petersson CJ. Incidence and causes of shoulder girdle injuries in an urban population. J Shoulder Elbow Surg 1995;4(2):107–12.

16. Kroner K, Lind T, Jensen J. The epidemiology of shoulder dislocations. Arch Orthop Trauma Surg 1989;108(5):288–90.

17. Owens BD, Duffey ML, Nelson BJ, et al. The incidence and characteristics of shoulder instability at the United States Military Academy. Am J Sports Med 2007;35(7):1168–73.

18. Mc LH, Cavallaro WU. Primary anterior dislocation of the shoulder. Am J Surg 1950;80(6):615–21 passim.

19. Hovelius L, Olofsson A, Sandstrom B, et al. Nonoperative treatment of primary anterior shoulder dislocation in patients forty years of age and younger. A prospective twenty-five-year follow-up. J Bone Joint Surg Am 2008;90(5): 945–52.

20. Robinson CM, Howes J, Murdoch H, et al. Functional outcome and risk of recurrent instability after primary traumatic anterior shoulder dislocation in young patients. J Bone Joint Surg Am 2006;88(11):2326–36.

21. Kralinger FS, Golser K, Wischatta R, et al. Predicting recurrence after primary anterior shoulder dislocation. Am J Sports Med 2002;30(1):116–20.

22. Sachs RA, Lin D, Stone ML, et al. Can the need for future surgery for acute traumatic anterior shoulder dislocation be predicted? J Bone Joint Surg Am 2007; 89(8):1665–74.

23. Chahal J, Leiter J, McKee MD, et al. Generalized ligamentous laxity as a predisposing factor for primary traumatic anterior shoulder dislocation. J Shoulder Elbow Surg 2010;19(8):1238–42.

24. Perlmutter GS, Apruzzese W. Axillary nerve injuries in contact sports: recommendations for treatment and rehabilitation. Sports Med 1998;26(5):351–61.

25. Hodge DK, Safran MR. Sideline management of common dislocations. Curr Sports Med Rep 2002;1(3):149–55.

26. Kuhn JE. Treating the initial anterior shoulder dislocation–an evidence-based medicine approach. Sports Med Arthrosc 2006;14(4):192–8.

27. Cox CL, Kuhn JE. Operative versus nonoperative treatment of acute shoulder dislocation in the athlete. Curr Sports Med Rep 2008;7(5):263–8.

28. Sanders TG, Zlatkin M, Montgomery J. Imaging of glenohumeral instability. Semin Roentgenol 2010;45(3):160–79.

29. Safran O, Milgrom C, Radeva-Petrova DR, et al. Accuracy of the anterior apprehension test as a predictor of risk for redislocation after a first traumatic shoulder dislocation. Am J Sports Med 2010;38(5):972–5.
30. Kim SH, Park JS, Jeong WK, et al. The Kim test: a novel test for posteroinferior labral lesion of the shoulder–a comparison to the jerk test. Am J Sports Med 2005;33(8):1188–92.
31. Itoi E, Sashi R, Minagawa H, et al. Position of immobilization after dislocation of the glenohumeral joint. A study with use of magnetic resonance imaging. J Bone Joint Surg Am 2001;83-A(5):661–7.
32. Itoi E, Hatakeyama Y, Sato T, et al. Immobilization in external rotation after shoulder dislocation reduces the risk of recurrence. A randomized controlled trial. J Bone Joint Surg Am 2007;89(10):2124–31.
33. Finestone A, Milgrom C, Radeva-Petrova DR, et al. Bracing in external rotation for traumatic anterior dislocation of the shoulder. J Bone Joint Surg Br 2009; 91(7):918–21.
34. Liavaag S, Brox JI, Pripp AH, et al. Immobilization in external rotation after primary shoulder dislocation did not reduce the risk of recurrence: a randomized controlled trial. J Bone Joint Surg Am 2011;93(10):897–904.
35. Paterson WH, Throckmorton TW, Koester M, et al. Position and duration of immobilization after primary anterior shoulder dislocation: a systematic review and meta-analysis of the literature. J Bone Joint Surg Am 2010;92(18):2924–33.
36. Buss DD, Lynch GP, Meyer CP, et al. Nonoperative management for in-season athletes with anterior shoulder instability. Am J Sports Med 2004; 32(6):1430–3.
37. Rowe CR, Zarins B, Ciullo JV. Recurrent anterior dislocation of the shoulder after surgical repair. Apparent causes of failure and treatment. J Bone Joint Surg Am 1984;66(2):159–68.
38. Tjoumakaris FP, Bradley JP. The rationale for an arthroscopic approach to shoulder stabilization. Arthroscopy 2011;27(10):1422–33.
39. Berendes TD, Wolterbeek R, Pilot P, et al. The open modified Bankart procedure: outcome at follow-up of 10 to 15 years. J Bone Joint Surg Br 2007; 89(8):1064–8.
40. Pelet S, Jolles BM, Farron A. Bankart repair for recurrent anterior glenohumeral instability: results at twenty-nine years' follow-up. J Shoulder Elbow Surg 2006; 15(2):203–7.
41. Balg F, Boileau P. The instability severity index score. A simple pre-operative score to select patients for arthroscopic or open shoulder stabilisation. J Bone Joint Surg Br 2007;89(11):1470–7.
42. Cole BJ, L'Insalata J, Irrgang J, et al. Comparison of arthroscopic and open anterior shoulder stabilization. A two to six-year follow-up study. J Bone Joint Surg Am 2000;82-A(8):1108–14.
43. Geiger DF, Hurley JA, Tovey JA, et al. Results of arthroscopic versus open Bankart suture repair. Clin Orthop Relat Res 1997;(337):111–7.
44. Guanche CA, Quick DC, Sodergren KM, et al. Arthroscopic versus open reconstruction of the shoulder in patients with isolated Bankart lesions. Am J Sports Med 1996;24(2):144–8.
45. Steinbeck J, Jerosch J. Arthroscopic transglenoid stabilization versus open anchor suturing in traumatic anterior instability of the shoulder. Am J Sports Med 1998;26(3):373–8.
46. Tjoumakaris FP, Abboud JA, Hasan SA, et al. Arthroscopic and open Bankart repairs provide similar outcomes. Clin Orthop Relat Res 2006;446:227–32.

47. Fabbriciani C, Milano G, Demontis A, et al. Arthroscopic versus open treatment of Bankart lesion of the shoulder: a prospective randomized study. Arthroscopy 2004;20(5):456–62.
48. Godin J, Sekiya JK. Systematic review of arthroscopic versus open repair for recurrent anterior shoulder dislocations. Sports Health 2011;3(4):396–404.
49. Cordischi K, Li X, Busconi B. Intermediate outcomes after primary traumatic anterior shoulder dislocation in skeletally immature patients aged 10 to 13 years. Orthopedics 2009;32(9). pii: orthosupersite.com/view.asp?rID=42855.
50. Castagna A, Delle Rose G, Borroni M, et al. Arthroscopic stabilization of the shoulder in adolescent athletes participating in overhead or contact sports. Arthroscopy 2012;28(3):309–15.
51. Owens BD, DeBerardino TM, Nelson BJ, et al. Long-term follow-up of acute arthroscopic Bankart repair for initial anterior shoulder dislocations in young athletes. Am J Sports Med 2009;37(4):669–73.
52. Mazzocca AD, Brown FM Jr, Carreira DS, et al. Arthroscopic anterior shoulder stabilization of collision and contact athletes. Am J Sports Med 2005;33(1): 52–60.
53. Cho NS, Hwang JC, Rhee YG. Arthroscopic stabilization in anterior shoulder instability: collision athletes versus noncollision athletes. Arthroscopy 2006; 22(9):947–53.
54. Larrain MV, Montenegro HJ, Mauas DM, et al. Arthroscopic management of traumatic anterior shoulder instability in collision athletes: analysis of 204 cases with a 4- to 9-year follow-up and results with the suture anchor technique. Arthroscopy 2006;22(12):1283–9.
55. Robinson CM, Seah M, Akhtar MA. The epidemiology, risk of recurrence, and functional outcome after an acute traumatic posterior dislocation of the shoulder. J Bone Joint Surg Am 2011;93(17):1605–13.
56. Duralde XA, Fogle EF. The success of closed reduction in acute locked posterior fracture-dislocations of the shoulder. J Shoulder Elbow Surg 2006;15(6):701–6.
57. Burkhead WZ Jr, Rockwood CA Jr. Treatment of instability of the shoulder with an exercise program. J Bone Joint Surg Am 1992;74(6):890–6.
58. Mair SD, Zarzour RH, Speer KP. Posterior labral injury in contact athletes. Am J Sports Med 1998;26(6):753–8.
59. Bottoni CR, Franks BR, Moore JH, et al. Operative stabilization of posterior shoulder instability. Am J Sports Med 2005;33(7):996–1002.
60. Kim SH, Ha KI, Park JH, et al. Arthroscopic posterior labral repair and capsular shift for traumatic unidirectional recurrent posterior subluxation of the shoulder. J Bone Joint Surg Am 2003;85-A(8):1479–87.
61. Bradley JP, Baker CL 3rd, Kline AJ, et al. Arthroscopic capsulolabral reconstruction for posterior instability of the shoulder: a prospective study of 100 shoulders. Am J Sports Med 2006;34(7):1061–71.
62. Radkowski CA, Chhabra A, Baker CL, et al. Arthroscopic capsulolabral repair for posterior shoulder instability in throwing athletes compared with nonthrowing athletes. Am J Sports Med 2008;36(4):693–9.

Microinstability and Internal Impingement in Overhead Athletes

Lauchlan Chambers, MD, MPH*, David W. Altchek, MD

KEYWORDS

- Microinstability • Internal impingement • Rotator cuff • Labral debridement
- Arthroscopic suture plication

KEY POINTS

- Overhead athletes require increased shoulder mobility to meet their functional demands in addition to enough stability to prevent joint subluxation.
- While there is no universally accepted definition, microinstability involves pathologic laxity that leads to abnormal mechanics without dislocation.
- Microinstability and internal impingement are diagnosed by a combination of history, physical exam, examination under anesthesia (EUA), and arthroscopic findings.
- Three to six months of physical therapy focused on rotator cuff and scapular stabilizer strengthening with posterior capsule stretching should be performed prior to any surgery. If this fails, arthroscopic suture plication with arthroscopic treatment of other pathology has produced the best clinical outcomes.

INTRODUCTION

As Jobe and colleagues[1] originally described, shoulder pain in the overhead athlete can often be traced to the stabilizing mechanisms of the glenohumeral joint. A complex interplay exists between both the static and dynamic stabilizers of the glenohumeral joint, especially in overhead athletes, in whom a balance of stability and mobility requires the coordination of these stabilizers to meet functional demands. Wilk and Arrigo[2] have referred to this contradictory relationship of a shoulder being hypermobile enough to perform overhead activity yet stable enough to prevent joint subluxation as the *throwers paradox*. Shoulder mobility is characterized by the magnitude of the rotational range of motion (ROM), referred to as "physiologic motion," and translational ROM, referred to as "accessory."[3]

Conflict of Interest: No conflict.
Hospital for Special Surgery, 535 East 70th Street, New York, NY 10021, USA
* Corresponding author.
E-mail address: chambersk@hss.edu

Clin Sports Med 32 (2013) 697–707
http://dx.doi.org/10.1016/j.csm.2013.07.006
0278-5919/13/$ – see front matter © 2013 Elsevier Inc. All rights reserved.

sportsmed.theclinics.com

This coupled motion is necessary for overhead athletes to obtain full ROM and meet the demands of their sport.

No universally accepted definition of *microinstability* exists. A basic description defines microinstability as any rotational or directional pathologic laxity that leads to abnormal mechanics without dislocation.[4] The term *internal impingement* describes pathologic contact between the articular side of the rotator cuff and the margin of the glenoid.[5] Walch and colleagues[5,6] originally reported the case of a young thrower with impingement occurring between the supraspinatus tendon and the posterosuperior edge of the glenoid, and then provided the first clinical evidence to support the concept of internal impingement. With regard to the throwing shoulder of baseball pitchers, some authors have classified internal impingement as microinstability; however, most authors, including Walch, have delineated these 2 entities and suggest that anterior hyperlaxity results in the subsequent development of internal impingement in throwers.[5–8] In their original article, Jobe and colleagues[1] described posterosuperior glenoid impingement and associated anterior instability. They noted limited success with subacromial decompression but clinical improvement with anterior capsulolabral reconstruction, giving credence to the idea that capsular attenuation contributes to glenohumeral abnormality and pain.[9]

Kvitne and Jobe[10] then described the process of progressive attenuation of the static restraints of the shoulder, allowing anterior glenohumeral subluxation, with continued throwing when the repetitive stresses exceed that of tissue repair. Dynamic stabilizers consist of rotator cuff, deltoid, biceps, and periscapular musculature.

Initially, these dynamic stabilizers can compensate for mild instability with increased muscle activity; however, with prolonged activity and muscle fatigue, the humeral head may subluxate anteriorly, allowing the rotator cuff to impinge along the posterosuperior border of the glenoid rim.[10]

To obtain the supraphysiologic ROM critical for successful overhead athletes, adaptations of the glenohumeral joint are necessary. These changes are essential, especially in baseball players, who have been shown to possess the fastest motion in all overhead athletes (7000 degrees per second).[11] These adaptations come in the form of both osseous and soft tissue changes. The position of the upper extremity during the late-cocking stage of throwing involves extreme glenohumeral external rotation, abduction, and extension. In this position, the anterior band of the inferior glenohumeral ligament complex, the primary static stabilizer to anterior translation, is under maximal strain.[12] The stretching of these capsuloligamentous restraints is thought to result in subtle anterior humeral head microinstability and posterosuperior labral tearing; this combination produces a gain in external rotation in overhead athletes.[9,13–15]

Over time this process leads to posterior shoulder tightness and anterior capsule laxity. Some controversy exists as to whether the source of this posterior tightness is from capsular contracture or tightness in the posterior rotator cuff and/or deltoid. Furthermore, the concept that anterior laxity leads to functional microinstability or pathologic instability is not universally accepted. Lengthening of the anterior capsule causes a posterior contracture, resulting in superior and posterior translation of the glenohumeral contact and allowing supraphysiologic external rotation.[16] This process increases contact between the greater tuberosity and posterosuperior glenoid, thereby impinging the posterior rotator cuff and labrum. Scapular dysfunction has also been shown to be a contributor to this pathologic internal impingement. Throwing athletes with internal impingement present with significantly increased posterior scapular tilt and sternoclavicular elevation compared with controls.[17]

Increased humeral and glenoid retroversion in throwing shoulders has been demonstrated in several studies using computed tomography (CT) scans and radiographic analysis.[18–20] Recently, ultrasound assessment of humeral retroversion has been shown to be a reliable and accurate alternative to the traditional gold standard of CT.[21] Repetitive stress to the proximal humeral physis from throwing, between the ages of 12 and 16, is thought to induce an adaptive remodeling response that favors humeral retroversion.[19] This retroversion enables the arm to externally rotate to a greater extent before being constrained by the capsulolabral structures, and is possibly a major contributor toward glenohumeral internal rotation deficit (GIRD).[18,20] Humeral retroversion may not only increase external rotation but also play a role in protecting the static stabilizers through sparing the joint from capsular tension. Osbahr and colleagues[19] suggest that the restraining anteroinferior capsule tissues would undergo less strain per degree of external rotation in the late-cocking phase, thereby sparing the joint from repeated microtrauma. Moreover, Pieper[22] concluded from his study of handball players that chronic shoulder pain in some players was a direct result of lack of retroversion causing repetitive stress on the anteroinferior structures.

CLINICAL EVALUATION

A wide spectrum of shoulder injuries can occur in the overhead athlete, including osteochondral lesions of the glenoid and humeral head, labral tears, partial- and full-thickness rotator cuff tears, and anterior and posterior capsular injury.[1,23–25]

Thus, a thorough history and complete physical examination are essential to obtain the correct diagnosis.

Because a subtle distinction exists between functional microinstability and pathologic laxity, distinguishing between these entities can be difficult.

Internal impingement usually affects adults younger than 40 years who participate in activities involving repetitive abduction and external rotation of their shoulder.[26,27] As with all medical histories, the characteristics of the symptoms are important to delineate, including the timing, location, severity, quality, and alleviating and provocative factors (eg, did the pain begin after an acute incident, such as a missed swing, or was it gradual in onset). The location of the pain and the provocative position of the shoulder are also critical to determine. A symptomatic overhead athlete may report a history of posterior shoulder pain in the late-cocking position. Associated symptoms in patients with microinstability can include a subjective sense of instability, a decrease in velocity, and weakness after throwing.

The most common examination findings in overhead athletes are posterior glenohumeral joint line tenderness, increased external rotation, and decreased internal rotation; however, a complete physical examination should be conducted because of the high prevalence of associated shoulder conditions with internal impingement.[28] Standard shoulder testing for range of motion, classic impingement, and instability, along with specific maneuvers such as apprehension-relocation test and the O'Brien test, should be performed. Evaluation of scapulothoracic motion along with areas of atrophy, especially the supraspinatus and infraspinatus fossa, should also be documented.

Studies have shown that even in healthy overhead athletes, the dominant-sided scapula may be more internally rotated and anteriorly tilted than the nondominant scapula.[29] These athletes may also have increased global laxity or increased anterior translation in their dominant shoulder, and demonstrate apprehension in the provocative position. In general, an adaptive increase in external rotation at the expense of internal rotation is seen. Symptomatic throwing athletes have an average decrease of 10° in the total arc of motion of their dominant arms compared with asymptomatic throwing athletes.[30]

To properly examine posterior shoulder tightness, one must minimize scapular movement and isolate humeral motion. Myers and colleagues[31] described a modified supine assessment, wherein the scapula was stabilized, the arm was brought into horizontal adduction, and the angle formed between the humerus and horizontal plane was measured. This technique yielded higher reliability and validity than the more traditional side-lying technique.[31] In 2000, Meister[32] described "the posterior impingement sign," wherein the injured shoulders were placed into 90° to 110° of abduction, slight extension, and maximal external rotation, showing positive examination results when deep posterior pain was elicited. The overall sensitivity to demonstrate articular-sided rotator cuff tears and/or posterior labrum was found to be 75.5% and the specificity was 85%; however, when only athletes with noncontact injuries were considered, the sensitivity improved to 95% and specificity to 100%.[33]

The final component of the clinical evaluation is a complete examination under anesthesia (EUA), assessing ROM and laxity. Glenohumeral translation is determined by the load-and-shift maneuver, which is graded according to the criteria originally described by Altchek and colleagues.[34] Pathologic glenohumeral laxity is confirmed by a grade II or III finding and a positive drive-through sign on arthroscopic examination (**Fig. 1**).

IMAGING

Because of the common occurrence of concomitant pathologies in the setting of microinstability and internal impingement, a standard series of radiographs should be obtained, including anteroposterior, scapular Y, axillary, West Point, and Stryker Notch views. Although for most patients these will be normal, an ossification on the posteroinferior glenoid rim (*Bennett lesion*), sclerotic changes of greater tuberosity, or rounding of the posterior glenoid rim may be seen (**Fig. 2**).[35]

Although magnetic resonance imaging (MRI) remains a critical component for the workup of any thrower with posterior shoulder pain, findings are usually subtle in the setting of microinstability and internal impingement. Common MRI findings include partial-thickness articular-sided rotator cuff tears of the supraspinatus and/or infraspinatus and posterior and/or superior labral tears (**Fig. 3**). In an effort to better identify the features of small articular-sided tears and labral lesions, some authors have

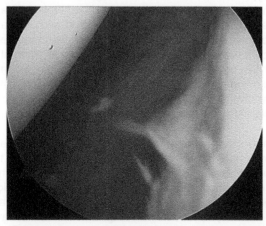

Fig. 1. An arthroscopic image from a posterior viewing portal in a left shoulder showing a positive drive-through sign.

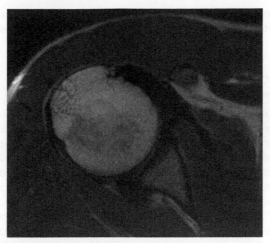

Fig. 2. An axial magnetic resonance imaging slice showing a Bennett lesion, which is an ossi-fication on the posteroinferior glenoid rim.

investigated enhancing imaging with gadolinium. However, Gusmer and colleagues[36] showed that with appropriate pulse sequences, noncontrast MRI was 95% accurate in detecting labral injuries.

Giaroli and colleagues[37] showed a constellation of consistent MRI findings in internal impingement, including undersurface tearing of the supraspinatus or infraspinatus tendon, cystic changes in the posterior humeral head, and posterosuperior labral abnormalities. In abduction and external rotation MRI, physical contact between the undersurface of the rotator cuff and posterosuperior glenoid has been shown to occur in the throwing shoulder and the contralateral nonthrowing shoulder.[24] The authors also noted that MRI showed abnormalities of the rotator cuff and superior labrum in asymptomatic throwing shoulders but not nonthrowing shoulders.[24] Treatment of abnormalities isolated to those seen on MRI in throwing athletes should proceed with prudence.

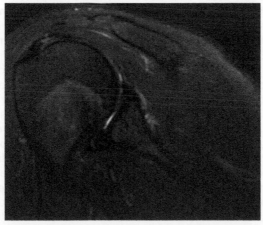

Fig. 3. A coronal MRI slice showing a partial-thickness articular sided rotator cuff tear, a common finding in internal impingement.

Microinstability and internal impingement are diagnosed based on patient history, physical examination, EUA, and pathologic findings during arthroscopy. In the authors' experience, MRI findings are often equivocal.

TREATMENT OPTIONS
Nonoperative Management

As with other shoulder abnormalities, after appropriate imaging and workup to achieve an accurate diagnosis, an adequate trial of conservative management should be attempted. Rest and simple pain relief should be the first-line management. Modalities such as anti-inflammatory drugs, cryotherapy, iontophoresis and phonophoresis, active release techniques, and fascial manipulation may be used to relieve pain. Although a paucity of high-level evidence exists for these techniques, especially for internal impingement, cryotherapy has been supported by level 1 evidence in the postoperative period.[38] Once the shoulder pain has resolved, physical therapy can begin. In general, exercises focused on rotator cuff and scapular stabilizer strengthening combined with posterior capsule stretching should be performed. However, exercises should be dictated by physical examination findings. For example, stretching of the posterior capsule and rotator cuff should be emphasized in patients with GIRD. In high-level tennis players, a prospective study showed that a daily regimen of posterior capsular stretching led in increases in internal and total rotation and a 38% decrease in shoulder problems.[39] In addition to improving posterior flexibility, strengthening of the periscapular musculature and rotator cuff will help achieve the ultimate goal of improving the dynamic stabilization of the glenohumeral joint.[40]

The Authors' Preferred Surgical Technique

For the authors, the indications for surgical intervention is debilitating shoulder pain and instability despite a 3- to 6-month course of the described conservative measures. After appropriate diagnosis based on patient history, physical examination, and imaging, abnormal glenohumeral laxity is confirmed on EUA using the load-and-shift maneuver and based on the presence of a positive drive-through sign on arthroscopic examination.

Regional anesthesia with an interscalene block and sedation are used and the patient is placed in the beach chair position. The EUA is performed to evaluate for ROM and determine the degree and direction of instability. The arm is then placed in a SPIDER Limb Positioner (TENET Medical Engineering, Calgary, Alberta, Canada) or McConnell arm holder (McConnell Orthopedic Manufacturing Company, Greenville, TX, USA) (Fig. 4). Bony landmarks are then drawn, including the spine of the scapula, lateral edge of the acromion, clavicle, acromioclavicular joint, and coracoid process. Supplementary local anesthesia is injected in the area of the posterior portal, which is made 2 cm below and 1 cm medial to the posterolateral corner of the acromion. An anterior portal is established in the rotator interval above the superior border of the subscapularis. A diagnostic arthroscopy is then performed. A third portal is created just inferior to the biceps tendon, in the superolateral aspect of the rotator interval. The portal incisions should be spread by at least 2 to 3 cm to avoid cannula collision. A large bump may be used to adequately distract the humeral head to allow ample working room when performing the anterior capsular plication (Fig. 5). The decision to perform a capsular plication is based on the presence of a patulous capsule and a positive drive-through sign, and no evidence of a Bankart lesion or other contributing labral abnormality. Associated lesions, such as fraying of the posterior rotator cuff and superior labral tears, are documented and treated appropriately (Figs. 6 and 7).

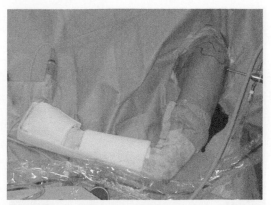

Fig. 4. A patient in the beach chair position with the McConnell arm holder.

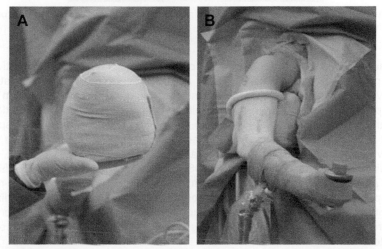

Fig. 5. (*A*, *B*) An axillary bolster composed of 3 sterile cotton rolls wrapped in a triangular shape with an Ace bandage, which is used to distract the arm laterally.

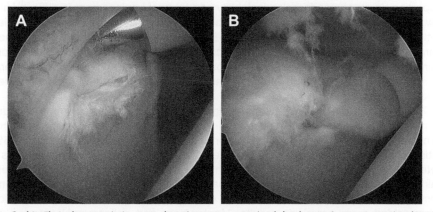

Fig. 6. (*A*, *B*) Arthroscopic images showing an a superior labral anterior to posterior (SLAP) lesion, a common finding in internal impingement, which was fixed using a knotless technique.

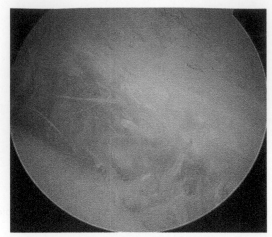

Fig. 7. An arthroscopic image revealing fraying of the posterior rotator cuff, a common finding in the overhead athlete.

The authors prefer to perform arthroscopic suture plication with the operative extremity positioned in approximately 70° of abduction and 45° of external rotation to avoid overtensioning of the capsuloligamentous structures. Capsule-to-labrum plication is performed, because it is technically simple and provides a foundation for capsular tightening. Initially, the capsule is abraded to stimulate a healing response. At least 20% of the anterior capsule that seems to be the most attenuated is penetrated with a 45° Spectrum MVP Suture Passer (ConMed Linvatec, Largo, FL, USA). A shuttling suture, consisting of No. 0 PDS (Ethicon, Somerville, NJ, USA), is used to pass a nonabsorbable No. 2 braided suture and is then tied to advance the redundant capsule. The amount of observed capsular redundancy in each patient dictates the number of sutures and the amount of capsular tightening; in general, additional sutures are placed until capsular tension is restored and the drive-through sign is eliminated.

TREATMENT OUTCOMES

Reporting on outcomes for microinstability and internal impingement is difficult for a few reasons. First, the clinical entity is still being characterized and the exact interplay between laxity and instability is still being delineated. Second, a paucity of published literature has reported on the clinical outcomes for arthroscopic capsular plication. Third, commonly occurring concomitant pathologic lesions, such as superior labral tears and partial rotator cuff tears, present potential confounding variables when reporting outcomes.

Older studies examining the outcomes in overheard athletes after simple debridement of rotator cuff and posterior labral tears reported poor outcomes and rates of return to sport. Payne and colleagues[41] reported a 25% rate of return to sport and 38% satisfactory results in 43 overhead athletes, and Sonnery-Cottet and colleagues[42] noted a 50% rate of return to sport, with 91% of 28 athletes reporting persistent pain, both after isolated debridement of partial articular-sided rotator cuff tears and posterior labral tears. More recent studies examining arthroscopic capsular plication have yielded more promising results. Montgomery and colleagues[43] reported an average postoperative American Shoulder and Elbow score of 78 and an 80% rate of return to sport in 15 competitive swimmers after arthroscopic capsular plication at a mean follow-up of 29 months. Levitz and colleagues[44] compared the clinical outcomes in 2 groups of baseball players who underwent either arthroscopic debridement alone or arthroscopic debridement with thermal capsulorrhaphy. They reported a 90% rate of return to sport in athletes who underwent the additional capsulorrhaphy compared with 67% in those who underwent isolated debridement. However, the athletes who were treated with capsulorrhaphy had a mean loss of 7° of external rotation at a mean follow-up of 30 months.[44]

Recently, the authors reported the outcomes for 20 overhead athletes who underwent isolated arthroscopic capsular plication at their institution. At a mean follow-up of 3.6 years, 90% of patients returned to their sports with an average Kerlan-Jobe Orthopaedic Clinic score of 82 and no complications.[45] No appreciable loss of external rotation was seen when objectively measured and compared with the contralateral extremity. These findings suggest that suture plication may be a more precise technique than thermal shrinkage; this is the authors' preferred technique, because any loss of external rotation in these overhead athletes could compromise performance and must be avoided.

BRIEF SUMMARY

- A complex interplay exists between the static and dynamic shoulder stabilizers in athletes who need enough hypermobility to perform overhead activity yet sufficient stability to prevent joint subluxation.
- Microinstability and internal impingement are diagnosed based on patient history, physical examination, EUA, and pathologic findings during arthroscopy.
- Exercises focused on rotator cuff and scapular stabilizer strengthening combined with posterior capsule stretching should be performed before any surgical intervention.
- If surgical intervention is needed, arthroscopic suture plication combined with treatment of other concomitant lesions has produced the best clinical outcomes.

REFERENCES

1. Jobe FW, Kvitne RS, Giangarra CE. Shoulder pain in the overhand or throwing athlete. The relationship of anterior instability and rotator cuff impingement. Orthop Rev 1989;18:963–75.
2. Wilk KE, Arrigo C. Current concepts in the rehabilitation of the athletic shoulder. J Orthop Sports Phys Ther 1993;18(1):365–78.
3. Kisner C, Colby LA. Therapeutic exercise: foundations and techniques. 4th edition. Philadelphia: F.A. Davis; 1990.
4. Wilk KE, Reinold MM, Andrews JR. The athlete's shoulder. 2nd edition. Philadelphia: Churchill Livingstone/Elsevier; 2009.
5. Walch G, Boileau C, Noel E. Impingement of the deep surface of the supraspinatus tendon on the posterior superior glenoid rim: an arthroscopic study. J Shoulder Elbow Surg 1992;1:238–45.
6. Walch G, Liotard JP, Boileau P, et al. Postero-superior glenoid impingement. Another shoulder impingement. Rev Chir Orthop Reparatrice Appar Mot 1991; 77(8):571–4 [in French].
7. Chung CB, Steinbach LS. MRI of the upper extremity: shoulder, elbow, wrist and hand. Philadelphia: Wolters Kluwer Health/Lippincott Williams & Wilkins; 2010.
8. McGinty JB, Burkhart SS. Operative arthroscopy. 3rd edition. Philadelphia: Lippincott Williams & Wilkins; 2003.

9. Jobe FW, Giangarra CE, Kvitne RS, et al. Anterior capsulolabral reconstruction of the shoulder in athletes in overhand sports. Am J Sports Med 1991;19:428–34.
10. Kvitne RS, Jobe FW. The diagnosis and treatment of anterior instability in the throwing athlete. Clin Orthop Relat Res 1993;(291):107–23.
11. Fleisig GS, Dillman CJ, Andrews JR. Biomechanics of the shoulder during throwing. In: Andrews JR, Wilk KE, editors. The athlete's shoulder. New York: Churchill Livingstone; 1994. p. 360–5.
12. Malicky DM, Kuhn JE, Frisancho JC, et al. Nonrecoverable strain fields of the anteroinferior glenohumeral capsule under subluxation. J Shoulder Elbow Surg 2002;11:529–40.
13. Jobe CM. Posterior superior glenoid impingement: expanded spectrum. Arthroscopy 1995;11(5):530–6.
14. Jobe CM, Pink MM, Jobe FW, et al. Anterior shoulder instability, impingement, and rotator cuff tear: theories and concepts. In: Jobe FW, editor. Operative techniques in upper extremity sports injuries. St Louis (MO): Mosby; 1996. p. 164–76.
15. Wilk KE, Arrigo CA, Andrews JR. Current concepts: the stabilizing structures of the glenohumeral joint. J Orthop Sports Phys Ther 1997;25(6):364–79.
16. Burkhart SS, Morgan CD. The peel-back mechanism: its role in producing and extending posterior type II SLAP lesions and its effect on SLAP repair rehabilitation. Arthroscopy 1998;14:637–40.
17. Laudner KG, Myers JB, Pasquale MR, et al. Scapular dysfunction in throwers with pathologic internal impingement. J Orthop Sports Phys Ther 2006;36(7):485–94.
18. Crockett HC, Gross LB, Wilk K, et al. Osseous adaptation and range of motion at the glenohumeral joint in professional baseball players. Am J Sports Med 2002;30(1):20–6.
19. Osbahr DC, Cannon DL, Speer KP. Retroversion of the humerus in the throwing shoulder of college baseball pitchers. Am J Sports Med 2002;30(3):347–53.
20. Reagan KM, Meister K, Horodyski MB, et al. Humeral retroversion and its relationship to glenohumeral rotation in the shoulder of college baseball players. Am J Sports Med 2002;30(3):354–60.
21. Myers JB, Oyama S, Clarke JP. Ultrasonographic assessment of humeral retrotorsion in baseball players: a validation study. Am J Sports Med 2012;40(5):1155–60.
22. Pieper HG. Humeral torsion in the throwing arm of handball players. Am J Sports Med 1998;26(2):247–53.
23. Budoff JE, Nirschl RP, Ilahi OA, et al. Internal impingement in the etiology of rotator cuff tendinosis revisited. Arthroscopy 2003;19:810–4.
24. Halbrecht JL, Tirman P, Atkin D. Internal impingement of the shoulder: comparison of findings between the throwing and nonthrowing shoulders of college baseball players. Arthroscopy 1999;15:253–8.
25. Kaplan LD, McMahon PJ, Towers J, et al. Internal impingement: findings on magnetic resonance imaging and arthroscopic evaluation. Arthroscopy 2004;20:701–4.
26. Struhl S. Anterior internal impingement: an arthroscopic observation. Arthroscopy 2002;18:2–7.
27. Braun S, Kokmeyer D, Millett PJ. Shoulder injuries in the throwing athlete. J Bone Joint Surg Am 2009;91:966–78.
28. Kirchhoff C, Imhoff AB. Posterosuperior and anterosuperior impingement of the shoulder in overhead athletes – evolving concepts. Int Orthop 2012;34(7):1049–58.

29. Oyama S, Myers JB, Wassinger CA, et al. Asymmetric resting scapular posture in healthy overhead athletes. J Athl Train 2008;43(6):565–70.
30. Ruotolo C, Price E, Panchal A. Loss of total arc of motion in collegiate baseball players. J Shoulder Elbow Surg 2006;15:67–71.
31. Myers JB, Oyama S, Wassinger CA, et al. Reliability, precision, accuracy, and validity of posterior shoulder tightness assessment in overhead athletes. Am J Sports Med 2007;35(11):1922–30.
32. Meister K. Internal impingement in the shoulder of the overhand athlete: pathophysiology, diagnosis, and treatment. Am J Orthop 2000;29:433–8.
33. Meister K, Buckley B, Batts J. The posterior impingement sign: diagnosis of rotator cuff and posterior labral tears secondary to internal impingement in overhand athletes. Am J Orthop (Belle Mead NJ) 2004;33(8):412–5.
34. Altchek DW, Warren RF, Skyhar MJ, et al. T-plasty modification of the Bankart procedure for multidirectional instability of the anterior and inferior types. J Bone Joint Surg Am 1991;73(1):105–12.
35. Bennett GE. Elbow and shoulder lesions of baseball players. Am J Surg 1959;98:484–92.
36. Gusmer PB, Potter HG, Schatz JA, et al. Labral injuries: accuracy of detection with unenhanced MR imaging of the shoulder. Radiology 1996;200:519–24.
37. Giaroli EL, Major NM, Higgins LD. MRI of internal impingement of the shoulder. AJR Am J Roentgenol 2005;185(4):925–9.
38. Singh H, Osbahr DC, Holovacs TF, et al. The efficacy of continuous cryotherapy on the postoperative shoulder: a prospective, randomised investigation. J Shoulder Elbow Surg 2001;10:522–5.
39. Burkhart SS, Morgan CD, Kibler WB. The disabled throwing shoulder: spectrum of pathology: part I. Pathoanatomy and biomechanics. Arthroscopy 2003;19:404–20.
40. Castagna A, Garofalo R, Cesari E, et al. Posterior superior internal impingement: an evidence-based review [corrected]. Br J Sports Med 2010;44(5):382–8.
41. Payne LZ, Altchek DW, Craig EV, et al. Arthroscopic treatment of partial rotator cuff tears in young athletes. Am J Sports Med 1997;25(3):299–305.
42. Sonnery-Cottet B, Edwards TB, Noel E, et al. Results of arthroscopic treatment of posterosuperior glenoid impingement in tennis players. Am J Sports Med 2002;30:227–32.
43. Montgomery SR, Chen NC, Rodeo SA. Arthroscopic capsular plication in the treatment of shoulder pain in competitive swimmers. HSS J 2010;6(2):145–9.
44. Levitz CL, Dugas J, Andrews JR. The use of arthroscopic thermal capsulorrhaphy to treat internal impingement in baseball players. Arthroscopy 2001;17:573–7.
45. Jones KJ, Kahlenberg CA, Dodson CC, et al. Arthroscopic capsular plication for microtraumatic anterior shoulder instability in overhead athletes. Am J Sports Med 2012;40(9):2009–14.

Arthroscopic Management of the Contact Athlete with Instability

Joshua D. Harris, MD[a],*, Anthony A. Romeo, MD[b]

KEYWORDS

- Shoulder • Instability • Dislocation • Athlete • Arthroscopy

KEY POINTS

- The shoulder is the most commonly dislocated joint in the body, with a greater incidence of instability in contact and collision athletes.
- In contact and collision athletes that have failed nonoperative treatment, the most important factors to consider when planning surgery are amount of bone loss (glenoid, humeral head) and patient age.
- Clinical outcomes, instability recurrence rate, and return to sport rate are not significantly different between arthroscopic suture anchor and open techniques.
- Lateral decubitus positioning with distraction and four portal (including seven-degree and 5-o'clock positions) techniques allow for 360-degree access to the glenoid rim, with at least three anchors below 3 o'clock.
- In patients with significant glenoid bone loss (>20%–25%, "inverted pear" glenoid), open bone augmentation techniques are indicated and arthroscopic techniques are contraindicated.
- Three-dimensional computed tomography is the most accurate imaging modality for evaluation of glenoid bone loss.

Funding Sources: None.
Conflicts of Interest: Dr J.D. Harris: None. Dr A.A. Romeo: Arthrex (royalties, speakers bureau, paid consultant, research support), DJO Surgical (research support, material support); Smith & Nephew (research support); Ossur (research support); Saunders/Mosby Elsevier (royalties, financial, or material support from publishers); Medical publications editorial/governing board (Journal of Shoulder & Elbow Surgery, SLACK Inc, Sports Health); Board member (American Orthopedic Society for Sports Medicine, American Shoulder & Elbow Surgeons, Arthroscopy Association of North America, Techniques in Shoulder & Elbow Surgery).
[a] The Methodist Center for Sports Medicine, Division of Sports Medicine, Department of Orthopaedic Surgery, 6560 Fannin Street, Scurlock Tower, Suite 400, Houston, TX 77030, USA; [b] Shoulder and Elbow Fellowship, Shoulder and Elbow Surgery, Division of Sports Medicine, Department of Orthopedic Surgery, Midwest Orthopaedics at Rush, Rush Medical College, Rush University Medical Center, Rush University, 1611 West Harrison Street, Suite 300, Chicago, IL 60612, USA
* Corresponding author. Midwest Orthopaedics at Rush, Rush University Medical Center, 1611 West Harrison Street, Suite 300, Chicago, IL 60612.
E-mail address: joshuaharrismd@gmail.com

Clin Sports Med 32 (2013) 709–730
http://dx.doi.org/10.1016/j.csm.2013.07.007
0278-5919/13/$ – see front matter © 2013 Elsevier Inc. All rights reserved.

ANATOMY

The glenohumeral joint is remarkable in the amount of attainable motion across six degrees of freedom (**Table 1**). It is this superiority in motion, however, that also gives it the propensity for instability when any one of several static or dynamic structures involved in maintenance of stability is disrupted. Static restraints to glenohumeral subluxation or dislocation include the humeral head, proximal humerus, glenoid, labrum, and capsule. The inferior glenohumeral ligament's anterior band is the thickest and strongest within the shoulder capsule. As such, it is the primary restraint to anterior shoulder instability in the provocative abducted and externally rotated position. The articular surface of the glenoid and labrum create a shallow (9-mm deep in superior-inferior direction; 5-mm deep in anterior-posterior direction) socket on which the humeral head may translate and rotate.[1] Although the labrum has been described to contribute 10% to 20% of stability to the glenohumeral joint,[2–4] its loss reduces the force required to translate the shoulder anteriorly by 50%.[5] The radii of curvature of the glenoid are unique in the superior-inferior (30 mm) and anterior-posterior (25 mm) dimensions.[6] This, in essence, reflects a relatively flat surface articulation with minimal articular conformity-based constraint (25%–30% of humeral head contacts glenoid at any given anatomic position).[7,8] Thus, joint stability is enhanced by adhesion and cohesion, finite joint volume, and dynamic muscular control imposed by the rotator cuff muscles.

The normal "pear-shaped" glenoid is wider (anterior to posterior) inferiorly than superiorly.[9] Anterior-to-posterior dimensions (at the midpoint of each half of the "pear") are 23 mm superiorly and 24 to 29 mm inferiorly.[9,10] The ratio of the lower to upper half of the glenoid is consistently 1:0.8 ($\pm$0.01).[10] Knowledge of these dimensions is important because critical evaluation of bone loss is necessary in patients with instability given the higher rate of recurrence with isolated soft tissue repair in patients with anterior-inferior glenoid insufficiency greater than 19% to 25%.[11–14] Visual appearance of an "inverted pear glenoid" in patients with anterior instability is associated with significantly greater anterior bone loss (mean, 8.6 mm; 36% of inferior glenoid width) than those without an inverted pear.[15] In cadavers, conversion to an inverted pear glenoid requires a 6.5- to 9-mm defect (mean, 7.5 mm; 28.8% of inferior glenoid

Table 1	
Pearls of shoulder anatomy and pathoanatomy in instability	
Key Shoulder Anatomy	**Key Shoulder Pathoanatomy in Instability**
Glenohumeral joint has largest range of motion in body	Glenohumeral joint is most commonly dislocated joint in the body
Most important passive soft tissue stabilizers are inferior glenohumeral ligament complex and glenoid labrum, especially in abduction and external rotation	Shoulder laxity (asymptomatic) is normal; instability is pathologic (symptomatic)
Glenoid is wider inferiorly than superiorly, "pear-shaped"	Bankart (anterior-inferior labral tear) and Hill-Sachs (posterior-lateral humeral head) lesions and anterior-inferior capsular stretch are frequently associated with anterior shoulder instability
Glenoid "socket" is only 5 mm deep in anterior-posterior direction (minimal articular conformity-based constraint)	Do not miss less common causes of instability: HAGL, ALPSA, GLAD, SLAP
25%–30% of humeral head contacts glenoid at any range of motion	"Inverted pear" glenoid is indicative of significant glenoid bone loss (>20%–25%)

Abbreviations: ALPSA, anterior labroligamentous periosteal sleeve avulsion; GLAD, glenoid-labral articular disruptions; HAGL, humeral avulsion of glenohumeral ligaments; SLAP, superior labrum anterior-to-posterior.

width).[15] The critical size of bony loss is probably only 20% to 25% of the anterior-inferior glenoid (6–8 mm).[16] The glenoid "bare spot," devoid of articular cartilage, is an anatomic structure that may be used to quantify glenoid bone loss in the setting of instability.[17] The bare spot may approximate the center of the inferior half of the glenoid.[9] Measurements from the bare spot to the articular margins (anterior, inferior, and posterior) are comparable.[9,17] Although the frequency of bare spot identification during arthroscopy (<50%) has recently precluded reliability and consistency in bone loss measurement, it is still commonly used by shoulder surgeons.[18,19] Using the bare spot as a reference point, evaluation of bone loss preoperatively is most accurate and reliable using three-dimensional computed tomography.[20,21]

Pathoanatomy

The Bankart lesion was believed to occur in 100% of all shoulder dislocations, the so-called "lesion of necessity" (**Fig. 1**).[22] More contemporary studies have demonstrated arthroscopic evidence of closer to 90% incidence of Bankart lesions.[23] Described nearly 100 years ago, the Bankart lesion is an anterior labroligamentous avulsion of the inferior glenohumeral ligament's anterior band from the anterior glenoid rim.[22] However, the Bankart lesion alone is not sufficient to produce pathologic translation necessary for anterior dislocation.[24] Additionally, the capsule stretches and becomes insufficient and the anterior periosteum tears off the scapula, resulting in anterior-medial displacement of the capsulolabral-ligamentous complex, inhibiting its role in anterior stability.[23] Even in patients with anterior glenohumeral subluxation events, Bankart lesions are present in 96% of shoulders.[25] Anterior dislocations may also cause anterior-inferior glenoid fracture, the so-called "bony Bankart" (**Fig. 2**). The incidence of bony Bankart lesions ranges from 4% to 70% in patients with anterior dislocations.[23,26] Whether the mechanism is a single instability event or chronic recurrent events leading to repetitive attrition, significant loss of articular congruence from the anterior-inferior glenoid may occur, leading to anterior instability with little provocation. Other lesions that may be present in anterior shoulder instability include humeral avulsion of glenohumeral ligaments (**Fig. 3**),[27] anterior labroligamentous periosteal

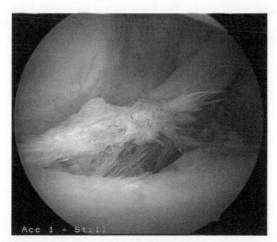

Fig. 1. Arthroscopic photograph in right shoulder, viewing from posterior portal. Thirty-degree arthroscope with lens aiming inferiorly. The anterior-inferior labrum is torn (Bankart lesion). The attachment of the anterior band of the inferior glenohumeral ligament complex can be seen attaching anterior to the torn labrum.

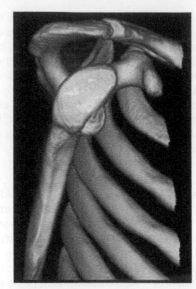

Fig. 2. Three-dimensional computed tomography (CT) with humerus digitally subtracted of right shoulder. Bony Bankart lesion visible off of anterior-inferior glenoid.

sleeve avulsion,[28] Perthes lesions,[29] glenoid-labral articular disruptions,[30] superior labrum anterior-to-posterior tears,[31] and multidirectional instability/capsular insufficiency.[32]

In addition to glenoid-sided pathology, Hill-Sachs defects of the posterolateral humeral head are frequently encountered in anterior shoulder instability.[33] The incidence of Hill-Sachs lesions may be up to 67% and 84% in first-time and recurrent dislocations, respectively.[29] In first-time anterior glenohumeral subluxation, the incidence of Hill-Sachs lesions has been demonstrated to be even higher (93%).[25] It is important to differentiate the pathologic Hill-Sachs defect from the normal posterolateral "bare area" during shoulder arthroscopy. The bare area is just medial adjacent to the infraspinatus footprint on the greater tuberosity and is composed of dense subchondral bone. The bare area appears as an impaction fracture, with signs of acute or chronic

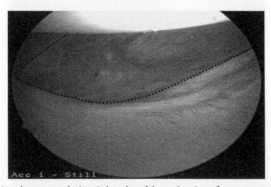

Fig. 3. Arthroscopic photograph in right shoulder, viewing from posterior portal. Thirty-degree arthroscope with lens aiming anteroinferiorly into the axillary pouch, under the humeral head. There is evidence of a humeral avulsion of glenohumeral ligaments lesion (*dotted black line*) outlining the torn retracted capsule.

injury, with bleeding, hemorrhagic bone, or covering fibrocartilage. Dynamic arthroscopic examination of the glenohumeral joint can reveal engagement of the Hill-Sachs lesion over the anterior rim of the glenoid. This "engaging Hill-Sachs lesion" is a predictor for recurrence of instability after arthroscopic stabilization.[13] Among all Hill-Sachs defects, the prevalence of engaging lesions is 7%.[34] Engaging lesions are significantly larger and more horizontally positioned relative to the humeral shaft than nonengaging lesions.[35]

Several patient-specific factors are also predictive of the pathology encountered in shoulder instability. Age at the time of dislocation plays a significant role in the rate of recurrent instability and the incidence of concomitant rotator cuff tear. In patients younger than 20 years of age, the chance of recurrence is greater than 90%.[36–40] The rate of recurrent dislocation decreases with increasing age, with a 56% recurrence rate in those 23 to 29 years of age,[41] 27% rate in those older than the age of 30 years,[41] and 14% to 22% rate of recurrence in those older than 60 years.[42] In young patients with acute (mean age, 22 years) and recurrent (mean age, 27 years) anterior instability, the rate of full-thickness cuff tear is 8.7% and 12%, respectively.[43] However, in patients older than the age of 40, the rate of rotator cuff tear significantly increases.[44–46] In patients aged 40 to 55 years, the rate of rotator cuff tear with shoulder dislocation was 41%, versus 71% for those aged 56 to 70 years, and 100% for those older than 70 years.[47] Although the risk of rotator cuff tear increases in older patients (>40 years), the risk of capsulolabral injury (eg, Bankart lesion) decreases. In patients with first-time primary and chronic recurrent anterior instability, the incidence of a Bankart lesion is 50% and 70%, respectively, in those aged 41 to 50 years; 40% and 52%, respectively, in those aged 51 to 60 years; 15% and 40%, respectively, in those aged 61 to 70 years; and 0% and 20%, respectively, in those older than 70 years.[48] As the rate of capsulolabral injury decreases with increasing age, so does the rate of recurrent dislocation. However, beyond the age of 40 years, concomitant factors significantly affect redislocation rates (bony Bankart lesion,[49] greater tuberosity fracture,[50] axillary nerve palsy,[50] subscapularis tear,[45] and full-thickness supraspinatus tear[50]).

INCIDENCE OF INSTABILITY IN CONTACT ATHLETES

An important patient-specific factor that plays a significant role in instability incidence and recurrence is type of sport played. The glenohumeral joint is the most commonly dislocated articulation in the body. The overall incidence of dislocation is 2.39 per 1000 person-years in the general population presenting to emergency departments[51] and 1.69 per 1000 person-years in a military population.[52] During a 5-year period in US high schools, the largest number of shoulder dislocations occurred in contact sports, specifically football and wrestling.[53] In a level-one evidence prognostic study of 131 subjects with a first-time dislocation reporting 4 years follow-up, 86% (37 of 43) of patients with a recurrent dislocation were contact or collision athletes.[54] In football, the most common mechanism of shoulder dislocation is contact with another player (70%) or contact with the playing surface (21%).[53] In wrestling, the most common mechanisms of dislocation are contact with another player (47%) and the playing surface (41%).[53] Forty-seven percent of dislocations in wrestling occur during takedowns.[53] In rugby, 97% of all shoulder injuries occur because of contact with either another player or the playing surface.[55] In rugby, shoulder dislocations are the most severe shoulder injuries sustained, with the highest rate of recurrence (62%), and account for the most days lost because of injury (mean, 81 days).[55] Most dislocations in rugby occurred during tackling (62%), ruck or maul (10%), and scrum (10%).[55]

In South African rugby, the incidence of dislocation is significantly greater than that in American football[13] and Australian Rules football.[55] Additionally, the incidence of inverted pear glenoid is significantly greater in rugby versus football.[13] The typical mechanism of injury explains the latter: in rugby, the "stiff-arm" extended elbow, abducted and extended shoulder axially loads the anterior-inferior glenoid rim; in football, the ball carrier holds the arm adducted and rotational or torsional moments peel the glenohumeral ligaments from the glenoid.[13] At the NFL Combine, anterior instability was the second most common prior injury (21% of all shoulder injuries), occurring in 14% of all players, with greater incidence in defensive players.[56] In elite Swedish hockey, the incidence of shoulder dislocation was 8% and the rate of recurrence was 76% (90% if <20 years of age).[57] However, even without surgery, a recurrent dislocation in ice hockey did not preclude one-third of the players from playing competitively.[57]

PATIENT EVALUATION
History

Evaluation of the patient's history, physical examination, and imaging allows the clinician to make an appropriate diagnosis (**Table 2**). The history is especially important in the setting of shoulder instability in the contact athlete, because the timing and possibility of recurrence play a large role in selection of treatment. Furthermore, the wide range of shoulder motion makes it difficult to clearly determine the differences between normal motion, asymptomatic hypermobility or laxity, or symptomatic pathologic instability. It requires not only asking specific questions pertinent to the chief complaint, but also actively listening. This allows characterization of ill-defined subjective complaints, such as looseness, apprehension, and subluxation. The clinician must also recognize that abnormal findings on imaging (radiographs, magnetic resonance imaging, arthroscopic photographs) may not always be symptomatic. Therefore, the history and physical examination are the only ways to determine if the subjective complaints correspond to the imaging ("treat the patient and not the magnetic resonance image").

The history of present illness may often be sufficient to make the diagnosis in the setting of shoulder instability. In these patients, assess the chief complaint (eg,

Table 2
Pearls of history and physical examination in shoulder instability

Key History Items	Key Physical Examination Items
Age at time of first dislocation	Inspection: atrophy, prominence/fullness of
Exact injury situation description (mechanism,	humeral head, ecchymosis, winging
arm position, nerve symptoms)	Palpation: glenohumeral joint line,
Number of dislocations	acromioclavicular joint, cervical spine,
Sports played, timing in relation to season,	periscapular, upper extremity
desire to return to sport, career length	Motion: active and passive; forward
Other joints dislocated (hypermobility	elevation, internal and external rotation
syndromes)	Strength: deltoid, rotator cuff, biceps and
Prior treatments (eg, immobilization, surgery)	triceps brachii
	Special: identify correct direction of instability
	(anterior, posterior, inferior)
	Apprehension, relocation, load-and-shift
	Posterior jerk test, load-and-shift
	Sulcus sign, Beighton's criteria

instability or pain). Seven entities should be described in the categorization of the chief complaint:

1. Location and direction (location of pain, direction of dislocation)
2. Quality
3. Severity (could they finish the practice or game)
4. Timing (age at first dislocation, number of dislocations and subluxations, recent frequency)
5. Setting (practice, games, activities of daily living, while asleep, in-season, off-season, playoffs)
6. Exacerbating or relieving factors (mechanism of injury, arm position, immobilization)
7. Associated manifestations (arm dominance, night pain, weakness, numbness, tingling, stiffness, other loose joints or dislocations, necessity of reduction with or without sedation or muscle relaxation)

An exact situational description of the dislocation may often be difficult to ascertain, although is very helpful. An abducted, externally rotated shoulder with the arm in extension may precipitate anterior instability. An axial load to an outstretched forward-flexed arm (lineman's blocking position) may induce posterior instability. A thorough past medical and surgical history is essential to document prior treatments including shoulder reduction; rest (duration and use and type of immobilization [eg, simple sling, external rotation brace, immobilizer or stabilization brace]); activity modification; physical therapy; injections; and arthroscopic or open surgeries. If instability is relatively atraumatic, the clinician must evaluate for potential underlying connective tissue disease, such as Marfan or Ehlers-Danlos syndromes. Unique to athletes is the relationship of the injury and treatment to contract, scholarship, bonus, timing within the season, expected or desired length of career, and opinions from other medical and nonmedical sources (coaches, trainers, owners, managers, teammates, family, and friends).

Physical Examination

The physical examination for the unstable shoulder, as with all shoulders, should be comprehensive and systematic. This permits consistency and reproducibility. Once there is evidence from the history suggestive of instability, the examination techniques performed should focus on these subjective symptoms. Physical assessment of any joint mandates visual inspection (males disrobed and females with modesty-retained gowns that permit visualization); palpation; motion; strength; and special testing (eg, apprehension, relocation, load-and-shift, translation). To understand if pathology exists in the involved shoulder, the contralateral shoulder also should be thoroughly evaluated. Extensions of the unstable shoulder physical examination include assessment of the cervical spine, elbow, wrist, and hand, and neurovascular evaluation.

Inspection should include assessment for cutaneous abnormalities (eg, ecchymosis, erythema, atrophy, humeral head position if dislocated anteriorly, acromioclavicular separation "bump"). Palpation should be complete and assess the whole upper extremity, periscapular areas, and cervical spine. Active and passive motion should be measured in forward elevation in the scapular plane, external rotation in the adducted and abducted arm, internal rotation in the abducted arm, and internal rotation behind the back. Strength testing should, at a minimum, assess the deltoid, rotator cuff, biceps and triceps brachii, and brachialis. Evaluation for scapular dyskinesis (scapular assist test, winging) is also performed. Apprehension testing for anterior instability relies on the patient feeling "apprehension" or fear of dislocation rather than pain. Although this test may be performed standing or sitting, the authors prefer supine positioning. The arm is brought into abduction, external rotation, and extension until apprehension is experienced for test positivity. This test is highly sensitive (72%) and specific (96%), with 93% accuracy and has a positive likelihood ratio of 20.[58] The relocation test is performed next: application of a posteriorly directed force to reposition the humeral head back onto the glenoid. Apprehension relief is a positive test and is 81% sensitive, 92% specific, 91% accurate, and has a positive likelihood ratio of 10.[58] Load-and-shift testing is easiest performed supine because the scapula is stabilized by the examination table. The examiner abducts and externally rotates the arm, applies an axial load to the arm, and then shifts the humeral head anteriorly or posterior to assess degree of translation relative to the glenoid rim and amount of spontaneous reduction. Assessment of the amount of translation allows for grading with use of the Hawkins scale: grade 1 (humeral head does not translate to the glenoid rim); grade 2 (humeral head translates over glenoid rim but spontaneously reduces); and grade 3 (humeral head translates over glenoid rim, does not reduce spontaneously).[59] Observation of a sulcus sign may indicate multidirectional instability. Sulcus reduction with external rotation indicates competence of the rotator interval. If concern for excessive laxity or multidirectional instability exists, Beighton score is a helpful tool (elbow hyperextension, knee hyperextension, thumb-to-forearm, small finger metacarpophalangeal joint greater than 90-degree extension, and placing hands flat on floor with straight legs while standing).[60]

Posterior instability is more difficult to reliably diagnose on physical examination than anterior instability. Pain is more of an issue rather than frank instability. The posterior apprehension test may be performed standing or sitting, with application of a posteriorly directed force to the forward elevated (~90 degrees) and adducted arm. This test has a sensitivity of 42% and specificity of 92%.[61] The jerk test may be performed standing or sitting, with the arm adducted across the body and then horizontally extended until the humeral head "jerks" back onto the glenoid face.[62] This test has a sensitivity of 73% and a specificity of 98%.[62] Posterior load-and-shift testing is performed and graded similarly to anterior, with the difference being the direction of applied force.

Classification

Shoulder instability may be classified by four criteria: (1) degree (dislocation, subluxation, apprehension); (2) frequency (acute, primary, chronic, recurrent); (3) origin (traumatic, atraumatic); and (4) direction (unidirectional [anterior, posterior, inferior], multidirectional).[63] Additionally, instability may be broadly grouped using the mnemonics TUBS (traumatic, unilateral, Bankart, surgery) and AMBRI (atraumatic, multidirectional, bilateral, rehabilitation, inferior capsular shift).[64]

TREATMENT ALGORITHM

Management of shoulder instability is multifactorial. Nonoperative treatment may allow return to sport, even at high levels, at a much faster rate than operative treatment. This strategy may be useful for the in-season athlete looking to complete the season and then undergo off-season stabilization. It may also be the most appropriate option in lower-demand patients that do not want surgery, with multidirectional instability, and without a traumatic cause. In patients that fail nonoperative measures that elect surgery, arthroscopic shoulder stabilization is a successful option. Even after a first-time dislocation, "consequence" athletes or patients (military servicemen and women, overhead/contact/collision professional athletes, those whose job safety relies on stable shoulder) are indicated for stabilization.

The highest priority for selection of surgical technique in the contact or collision athlete is accurate determination of the amount of glenoid bone loss (**Fig. 4**). This factor has been incorporated into the shoulder instability severity index score (ISIS), which was developed by Boileau to identify patients at risk for recurrence after arthroscopic Bankart repair.[65] The ISIS is a six-item, 10-point maximum questionnaire. Illustrative of the importance of contact sports, three points are devoted to competitive contact or collision athletes. Some authors believe that contact and collision athletes are at such high risk for recurrence that they have reported their outcomes of open Latarjet stabilization in contact athletes without significant bone loss.[66] In the latter, 27% of rugby players had no glenoid bony deficiency and in those that did, the amount was not quantified. There were no recurrent instability events during the mean 12 years follow-up.[66] However, the rate of complications and reoperations after open glenoid

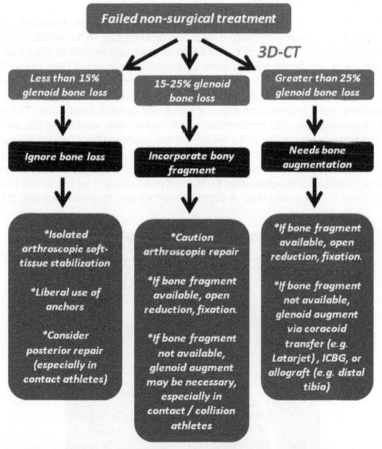

Fig. 4. Surgical technique decision-making algorithm. If patient has failed nonoperative management, then selection of surgical technique is based on assessment of glenoid bone loss. 3D-CT, three-dimensional computed tomography; ICBG, iliac crest bone graft. (*Adapted from* Bhatia S, Ghodadra NS, Romeo AA, et al. The importance of the recognition and treatment of glenoid bone loss in an athletic population. Sports Health 2011;3(5):435–40; with permission.)

bone augmentation stabilization is 30% and 7%, respectively.[67] In addition to sport participation, the other items on ISIS are age (less or greater than 20 years); presence of shoulder hyperlaxity; Hill-Sachs lesion on anterior-posterior radiograph; and glenoid loss of contour on anterior-posterior radiograph.[65] Patients with ISIS greater than or equal to six have at least a 70% risk of recurrence with arthroscopic Bankart repair and therefore should undergo bony stabilization. Regardless of approach (open vs arthroscopic), operative goals should be to fully define the pathologic lesion, establish healing potential, anatomically repair the pathology with secure fixation and appropriate ligament tensioning, and avoid complications. The authors believe and have shown[68,69] that, even in high-level contact or collision athletes without significant bone loss, excellent outcomes with low recurrence rates may be achieved (and should be expected) using arthroscopic techniques that are equivalent to that of open techniques.[68,69]

ARTHROSCOPIC MANAGEMENT

The ideal candidate for arthroscopic stabilization is a patient with traumatic etiology, Bankart lesion, no glenoid rim fracture, with few recurrences, in the nondominant arm, in a noncollision, noncontact sport, and capsular laxity symmetric to the other shoulder. Presence of significant glenoid bone loss (>20%) or inverted pear shape (**Fig. 5**), with multiple recurrences, no Bankart lesion, poor-quality tissue, and abnormal capsular laxity are contraindications to arthroscopic treatment (**Table 3**).

The authors prefer interscalene regional block and general anesthesia. The surgical procedure commences with examination under anesthesia, evaluating the amount of translation anterior, posterior, and inferior and the spontaneity of reduction once over the glenoid rim. The authors prefer the lateral decubitus position with a bean-bag positioner for arthroscopic treatment of instability with use of less than 10 lb of longitudinal and lateral overhead distraction (**Fig. 6**). Patient positioning is an extremely important step that must not be overlooked. A slight posterior body tilt (~30 degrees) (**Fig. 7**) is

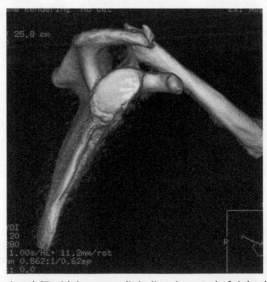

Fig. 5. Three-dimensional CT with humerus digitally subtracted of right shoulder with significant glenoid bone loss (>20%–25%) with "inverted pear" glenoid.

Table 3
Pearls and pitfalls for arthroscopic shoulder stabilization

Pearls	Pitfalls
Successful interscalene regional block anesthesia	Poor patient positioning and visualization, with body tilted straight upright or leaning forward
Lateral decubitus position, with slight (~30 degrees) posterior body tilt	Poor portal placement, avoid iatrogenic articular cartilage damage
Longitudinal and overhead lateral traction	
Accurate and precise portal placement (including seven-degree and 5-o'clock portals)	Failure to recognize significant glenoid bone loss (>20%–25%), "inverted pear"
At least three anchors below 3 o'clock	Failure to identify other pathology: HAGL, ALPSA, SLAP, GLAD, rotator cuff tear
Recognition of concomitant hypermobility and tissue quality, thus allowing individualized greater degrees of capsular plication as necessary	Failure to completely mobilize the capsulolabral Bankart/inferior glenohumeral ligament complex off the glenoid neck
Appropriate ligament tensioning	Inability to access four degrees to 8 o'clock on glenoid
Appropriate rehabilitation (know your physical therapist)	Fewer than three suture anchors

Abbreviations: ALPSA, anterior labroligamentous periosteal sleeve avulsion; GLAD, glenoid-labral articular disruptions; HAGL, humeral avulsion of glenohumeral ligaments; SLAP, superior labrum anterior-to-posterior.

helpful for arthroscopic visualization. If the patient's body continues to fall forward, visualization is difficult throughout the entirety of the case, especially anterior-inferior. Sufficient bony prominence padding avoids nerve injury.

Atraumatic portal placement should avoid iatrogenic osteochondral damage. The first portal established is the posterior portal, placed 2-cm distal to the posterolateral edge of the acromion (**Fig. 8**). Diagnostic arthroscopy ensues with an evaluation of all intra-articular structures. All pathologic lesions are identified and arthroscopic photographs taken to document the injury. The arthroscopist should always ensure that any bone loss is not greater than 20%. Without bone loss, the decision to proceed with capsulolabral repair is made. The surgeon should also identify the presence or absence of humeral avulsion of glenohumeral ligaments, anterior labroligamentous periosteal sleeve avulsion, and engaging Hill-Sachs lesions.

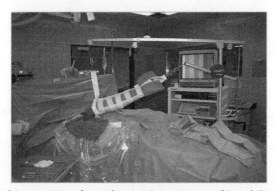

Fig. 6. Lateral decubitus position for arthroscopic treatment of instability. Longitudinal and overhead lateral distraction are used with less than 10-lb weight.

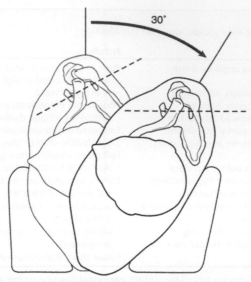

Fig. 7. Posterior tilt of the body is advantageous for arthroscopic visualization. The most important area to visualize is between the four-degree to 8-o'clock position inferiorly. If the body continues to fall forward during the procedure, this area is very difficult to access and see.

Two anterior portals are made using spinal needle localization (see **Fig. 8**). The first portal is high, adjacent to the long head biceps tendon anteriorly in the rotator interval, just adjacent to the anterolateral tip of the acromion on the surface. The second portal, the mid-glenoid portal, may be placed just superior to the subscapularis or transsubscapularis at the 5-o'clock position. A 7-o'clock portal may be placed by spinal needle localization approximately 4-cm lateral from the posterolateral corner of the acromion (**Fig. 9**).[70] The latter portal should follow the trajectory of the posterior border of the clavicle laterally, nearly perpendicular to the floor. The posterolateral portal gives approximately 180-degree access to the inferior half of the glenoid (**Fig. 10**). The

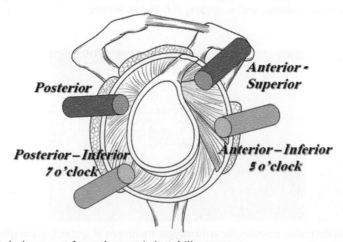

Fig. 8. Portal placement for arthroscopic instability surgery.

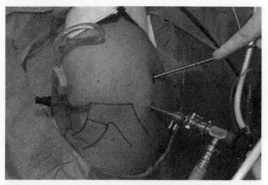

Fig. 9. Photograph of location of 7-o'clock portal placement. This is superior view, looking down onto shoulder, illustrating posterior and posterolateral 7-o'clock portal.

authors have found that these four arthroscopic portals allow for easy 360-degree navigation of the glenohumeral joint by "four-quadrant approach" without any undue risk to nearby neurovascular structures.[70,71]

Placement of the arthroscope in the anterior-superior portal then provides a bird's-eye view looking down the anterior glenoid, permitting identification and preparation of the Bankart capsulolabral injury. A tissue liberator is used from the 5-o'clock portal to fully prepare the glenoid and labrum, such that the capsule/labrum is peeled off the glenoid neck, the medialized position is eliminated, and the underlying subscapularis muscle fibers are visualized. Then, the bony surface is decorticated using a rasp or bur (**Fig. 11**). The surgeon must be prudent to avoid iatrogenic damage to the labrum and avoid overly aggressive bony debridement. A percutaneous drill guide is placed via the posterolateral portal to achieve a position low on the glenoid that matches the extent of the labral injury. Firm pressure or even taps with a mallet permit stable placement of

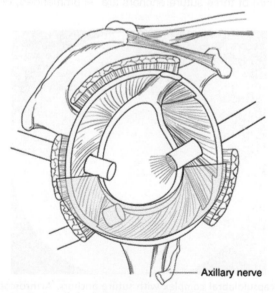

Axillary nerve

Fig. 10. A 180-degree access of the inferior glenoid afforded by the 7-o'clock portal in a right shoulder.

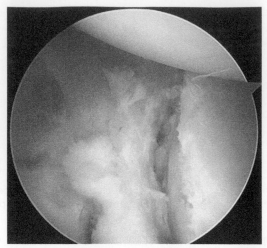

Fig. 11. Elevated mobilized capsulolabral complex. Arthroscopic photograph in right shoulder, viewing from anterosuperior portal. Thirty-degree arthroscope with lens aiming inferiorly down the anterior aspect of the glenoid.

the guide 1 to 2 mm onto the glenoid face. Drilling and subsequent anchor placement is then performed. Posterior portal cannulation allows for proper suture management and passage of the tissue penetrator–suture passer. Depending on the patient's capsulolabral injury and the desired amount of plication (illustrating importance of examination under anesthesia), the surgeon may pass the penetrator-passer once or twice ("pinch-tuck" maneuver) to bring the anterior and inferior capsule back up to the labral anchor. After the simple sutures are passed, arthroscopic knot-tying techniques are used ensuring that the knot is as far off the glenoid articular surface as possible (**Fig. 12**). A minimum of three suture anchors are recommended, given that the rate

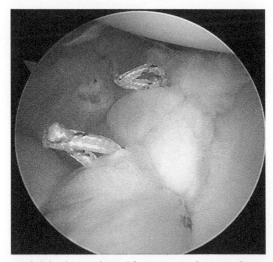

Fig. 12. Repaired capsulolabral complex with suture anchors. Arthroscopic photograph in right shoulder, viewing from anterosuperior portal. Thirty-degree arthroscope with lens aiming inferiorly down the anterior aspect of the glenoid.

of recurrence after arthroscopic stabilization is significantly increased with fewer than three.[12,72] In fact, the authors recommend at least three anchors below 3 o'clock for a reliable repair, with motion recovery, and reliable results. Once completed, usually 180 degrees of the glenoid circumference has an anchor placed (**Fig. 13**).

Postoperatively, the patient is placed in a padded pillow abduction sling, which is kept on at all times for 4 weeks, except while putting a shirt on, during bathing, during physical therapy, and during home elbow/wrist/hand exercises. Motion (passive advanced to active) is restricted to 90 degrees of forward elevation, 20 degrees external rotation, internal rotation to the abdomen, and 45 degrees abduction. Cross-body adduction is avoided for 6 weeks after surgery. Motion is progressed over Weeks 4 to 8. Strengthening is progressed from isometrics (beyond Week 1); scapular stabilizers and light bands (beyond Week 4); and light bands and weights for deltoid, rotator cuff, and periscapular muscles (beyond Week 8). Sport-specific rehabilitation is commenced at 3 months.

OUTCOMES

Clinical outcomes after arthroscopic shoulder stabilization are successful (**Table 4**). A recent systematic review of long-term outcomes after open or arthroscopic Bankart shoulder stabilization analyzed 26 studies and nearly 2000 patients.[68] Although 92% of studies in the latter were either level III or IV evidence, the mean length of follow-up was 11 years with validated clinical outcomes. There was no significant difference in recurrence of instability between arthroscopic suture anchor (8.5%) and open (8%) techniques ($P = .82$). There was no significant difference in rate of return

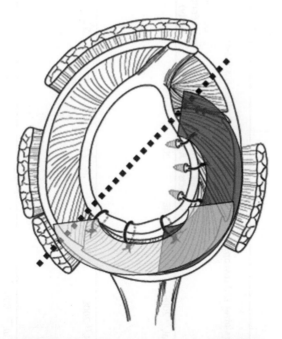

Fig. 13. Completed positions of anchor placement, covering 180 degrees of the glenoid circumference. The *yellow* radius is based on access by posterolateral portal. The *red* radius is based on access by anterior-inferior portal. The *orange* radius is based on access by either posterior-lateral or anterior-inferior portal.

Table 4
Outcomes after arthroscopic stabilization in contact or collision athletes

Study	Level of Evidence	Number Subjects	Mean Age (y)	Population	Length of Follow-up (y)	Outcomes
Rhee et al,[76] 2006	IV	46	20	Collision	6	VAS, Rowe, Constant significantly improved after both open and arthroscopic repair No significant difference between open and arthroscopic groups (VAS, Rowe, Constant) Greater number of recurrent dislocations in arthroscopic group (19% vs 9.4%; $P = .04$)
Cho et al,[77] 2006	III	29	21	Collision vs noncollision	5.2	Significantly ($P<.05$) improved Rowe, Constant, VAS after arthroscopic suture anchor repair Greater recurrence rate (29%; 4 of 14) in collision group vs noncollision group (7%; 1 of 15) 57% (8 of 14) return to sport in collision vs noncollision group (73%; 11 of 15)
Calvo et al,[78] 2005	IV	61	27.5	Contact	3.7	Significantly ($P<.05$) improved Rowe scores after arthroscopic transglenoid suture repair Overall, 20% rate of recurrence (recurrence mean 23 y of age; no recurrence mean 29) 58% rate of recurrence in contact athletes (7 of 12) vs 11% recurrence in noncontact (4 of 38)

Study	Level	N		Sport		Findings
Mazzocca et al,[69] 2005	IV	18	17	Collision and contact	3.1	11% rate of recurrence (0% contact, 15% collision) after arthroscopic suture anchor repair / Significant improvements (P<.05) in ASES, SST, VAS, Rowe, and SF-12 PCS / 100% return to sport at previous level of play (mean, 5.7 mo) by 10 mo after surgery
Ide et al,[79] 2004	II	55	19.5	Collision and contact	3.5	Significantly (P<.05) improved Rowe scores after arthroscopic suture anchor repair / No difference (P>.05) in recurrence rate between contact (10%) and noncontact (6%) athletes / 80% return to sport at previous level of play (44 of 55) at mean 5.8 mo
Hubbell et al,[80] 2004	III	50	25.5	Collision	5.7	Significantly (P<.05) greater rate of recurrent dislocation in arthroscopic vs open (44% vs 0%) / 100% return to sport at previous level (9 of 9) in arthroscopic group
Burkhart & De Beer,[13] 2000	IV	194	28	Collision and contact	2.3	Following arthroscopic suture anchor repair: / 6.5% recurrence rate in contact athletes without significant bone loss (inverted pear glenoid) / 89% recurrence rate in contact athletes with significant bone loss
O'Neill,[81] 1999	IV	41	20	Collision	4.3	12% rate of recurrent subluxation (2 of 17) after arthroscopic transglenoid suture repair
Bacilla et al,[82] 1997	IV	40	18	Collision and contact	2.5	7.5% rate of recurrent instability (3 of 40) after arthroscopic transglenoid suture repair / 90% return to sport at previous level of play in high school or college (26 of 29)

Abbreviations: ASES, american shoulder and elbow surgeons score; SF-12, short-form; PCS, physical component score; SST, simple shoulder test; VAS, visual analog scale.

to sport between arthroscopic suture anchor (87%) and open (89%) techniques (*P* = .43). There was no significant difference in the rate of postoperative osteoarthritis between arthroscopic suture anchor (26%) and open (33%) techniques (*P* = .06). Despite smaller study and subject numbers, a separate recent meta-analysis had similar conclusions, with no significant difference in rates of recurrent instability or reoperation.[73] The difference between the latter two reviews and multiple older systematic reviews and meta-analyses lies in that prior reviews[74,75] were analyzing and comparing older arthroscopic techniques, rather than more modern suture anchor-based repairs.

SUMMARY

The shoulder is the most commonly dislocated joint in the body, with a greater incidence of instability in contact and collision athletes. In contact and collision athletes that have failed nonoperative treatment, the most important factors to consider when planning surgery are amount of bone loss (glenoid, humeral head); patient age; and shoulder hyperlaxity. Clinical outcomes, instability recurrence rate, and return to sport rate are not significantly different between arthroscopic suture anchor and open techniques. Lateral decubitus positioning with distraction and four portal (including seven-degree and 5-o'clock positions) techniques allow for 360-degree access to the glenoid rim, with placement of at least three sutures anchors below 3 o'clock for optimal results. In patients with significant glenoid bone loss (>20%–25%, inverted pear glenoid), open bone augmentation techniques are indicated and arthroscopic techniques are contraindicated.

REFERENCES

1. Ghodadra N, Gupta A, Romeo AA, et al. Normalization of glenohumeral articular contact pressures after Latarjet or iliac crest bone-grafting. J Bone Joint Surg Am 2010;92(6):1478–89.
2. Lippitt S, Matsen F. Mechanisms of glenohumeral joint stability. Clin Orthop Relat Res 1993;(291):20–8.
3. Lazarus MD, Sidles JA, Harryman DT 2nd, et al. Effect of a chondral-labral defect on glenoid concavity and glenohumeral stability. A cadaveric model. J Bone Joint Surg Am 1996;78(1):94–102.
4. Halder AM, Kuhl SG, Zobitz ME, et al. Effects of the glenoid labrum and glenohumeral abduction on stability of the shoulder joint through concavity-compression: an in vitro study. J Bone Joint Surg Am 2001;83-A(7):1062–9.
5. Matsen FA 3rd, Harryman DT 2nd, Sidles JA. Mechanics of glenohumeral instability. Clin Sports Med 1991;10(4):783–8.
6. Dehaan A, Munch J, Durkan M, et al. Reconstruction of a bony Bankart lesion: best fit based on radius of curvature. Am J Sports Med 2013;41(5):1140–5.
7. Bost F, Inman V. The pathological changes in recurrent dislocation of the shoulder: a report of Bankart's operative procedure. J Bone Joint Surg Am 1942;23: 596–613.
8. Codman E. The shoulder. Boston: Thomas Todd; 1934.
9. Huysmans PE, Haen PS, Kidd M, et al. The shape of the inferior part of the glenoid: a cadaveric study. J Shoulder Elbow Surg 2006;15(6):759–63.
10. Iannotti JP, Gabriel JP, Schneck SL, et al. The normal glenohumeral relationships. An anatomical study of one hundred and forty shoulders. J Bone Joint Surg Am 1992;74(4):491–500.

11. Yamamoto N, Muraki T, Sperling JW, et al. Stabilizing mechanism in bone-grafting of a large glenoid defect. J Bone Joint Surg Am 2010;92(11):2059–66.
12. Boileau P, Villalba M, Hery JY, et al. Risk factors for recurrence of shoulder instability after arthroscopic Bankart repair. J Bone Joint Surg Am 2006;88(8): 1755–63.
13. Burkhart SS, De Beer JF. Traumatic glenohumeral bone defects and their relationship to failure of arthroscopic Bankart repairs: significance of the inverted-pear glenoid and the humeral engaging Hill-Sachs lesion. Arthroscopy 2000; 16(7):677–94.
14. Tauber M, Resch H, Forstner R, et al. Reasons for failure after surgical repair of anterior shoulder instability. J Shoulder Elbow Surg 2004;13(3):279–85.
15. Lo IK, Parten PM, Burkhart SS. The inverted pear glenoid: an indicator of significant glenoid bone loss. Arthroscopy 2004;20(2):169–74.
16. Bhatia S, Ghodadra NS, Romeo AA, et al. The importance of the recognition and treatment of glenoid bone loss in an athletic population. Sports Health 2011; 3(5):435–40.
17. Burkhart SS, DeBeer JF, Tehrany AM, et al. Quantifying glenoid bone loss arthroscopically in shoulder instability. Arthroscopy 2002;18(5):488–91.
18. Kralinger F, Aigner F, Longato S, et al. Is the bare spot a consistent landmark for shoulder arthroscopy? A study of 20 embalmed glenoids with 3-dimensional computed tomographic reconstruction. Arthroscopy 2006;22(4):428–32.
19. Saintmard B, Lecouvet F, Rubini A, et al. Is the bare spot a valid landmark for glenoid evaluation in arthroscopic Bankart surgery? Acta Orthop Belg 2009; 75(6):736–42.
20. Rerko MA, Pan X, Donaldson C, et al. Comparison of various imaging techniques to quantify glenoid bone loss in shoulder instability. J Shoulder Elbow Surg 2013;22(4):528–34.
21. Bishop JY, Jones GL, Rerko MA, et al. 3-D CT is the most reliable imaging modality when quantifying glenoid bone loss. Clin Orthop Relat Res 2013;471(4): 1251–6.
22. Bankart AS. Recurrent or habitual dislocation of the shoulder-joint. Br Med J 1923;2(3285):1132–3.
23. Hintermann B, Gachter A. Arthroscopic findings after shoulder dislocation. Am J Sports Med 1995;23(5):545–51.
24. Speer KP, Deng X, Borrero S, et al. Biomechanical evaluation of a simulated Bankart lesion. J Bone Joint Surg Am 1994;76(12):1819–26.
25. Owens BD, Nelson BJ, Duffey ML, et al. Pathoanatomy of first-time, traumatic, anterior glenohumeral subluxation events. J Bone Joint Surg Am 2010;92(7): 1605–11.
26. Porcellini G, Paladini P, Campi F, et al. Long-term outcome of acute versus chronic bony Bankart lesions managed arthroscopically. Am J Sports Med 2007;35(12):2067–72.
27. George MS, Khazzam M, Kuhn JE. Humeral avulsion of glenohumeral ligaments. J Am Acad Orthop Surg 2011;19(3):127–33.
28. Tischer T, Vogt S, Kreuz PC, et al. Arthroscopic anatomy, variants, and pathologic findings in shoulder instability. Arthroscopy 2011;27(10):1434–43.
29. Spatschil A, Landsiedl F, Anderl W, et al. Posttraumatic anterior-inferior instability of the shoulder: arthroscopic findings and clinical correlations. Arch Orthop Trauma Surg 2006;126(4):217–22.
30. Neviaser TJ. The GLAD lesion: another cause of anterior shoulder pain. Arthroscopy 1993;9(1):22–3.

31. Virk MS, Arciero RA. Superior labrum anterior to posterior tears and glenohumeral instability. Instr Course Lect 2013;62:501–14.
32. Lo IK, Bishop JY, Miniaci A, et al. Multidirectional instability: surgical decision making. Instr Course Lect 2004;53:565–72.
33. Hill H, Sachs R. The grooved defect of the humeral head: a frequently unrecognized complication of dislocations of the shoulder joint. Radiology 1940;35: 690–700.
34. Kurokawa D, Yamamoto N, Nagamoto H, et al. The prevalence of a large Hill-Sachs lesion that needs to be treated. J Shoulder Elbow Surg March 1, 2013 [Epub ahead of print]. http://www.ncbi.nlm.nih.gov/pubmed/23466174.
35. Cho SH, Cho NS, Rhee YG. Preoperative analysis of the Hill-Sachs lesion in anterior shoulder instability: how to predict engagement of the lesion. Am J Sports Med 2011;39(11):2389–95.
36. Postacchini F, Gumina S, Cinotti G. Anterior shoulder dislocation in adolescents. J Shoulder Elbow Surg 2000;9(6):470–4.
37. Marans HJ, Angel KR, Schemitsch EH, et al. The fate of traumatic anterior dislocation of the shoulder in children. J Bone Joint Surg Am 1992;74(8):1242–4.
38. Hovelius L, Erikksson K, Fredin H, et al. Recurrences after initial dislocation of the shoulder. Results of a prospective study of treatment. J Bone Joint Surg Am 1983;65(3):343–9.
39. Hovelius L. Anterior dislocation of the shoulder in teen-agers and young adults. Five-year prognosis. J Bone Joint Surg Am 1987;69(3):393–9.
40. Hovelius L. The natural history of primary anterior dislocation of the shoulder in the young. J Orthop Sci 1999;4(4):307–17.
41. Hovelius L, Olofsson A, Sandstrom B, et al. Nonoperative treatment of primary anterior shoulder dislocation in patients forty years of age and younger. A prospective twenty-five-year follow-up. J Bone Joint Surg Am 2008;90(5): 945–52.
42. Gumina S, Postacchini F. Anterior dislocation of the shoulder in elderly patients. J Bone Joint Surg Br 1997;79(4):540–3.
43. Yiannakopoulos CK, Mataragas E, Antonogiannakis E. A comparison of the spectrum of intra-articular lesions in acute and chronic anterior shoulder instability. Arthroscopy 2007;23(9):985–90.
44. Hawkins RJ, Bell RH, Hawkins RH, et al. Anterior dislocation of the shoulder in the older patient. Clin Orthop Relat Res 1986;(206):192–5.
45. Neviaser RJ, Neviaser TJ. Recurrent instability of the shoulder after age 40. J Shoulder Elbow Surg 1995;4(6):416–8.
46. Neviaser RJ, Neviaser TJ, Neviaser JS. Concurrent rupture of the rotator cuff and anterior dislocation of the shoulder in the older patient. J Bone Joint Surg Am 1988;70(9):1308–11.
47. Simank HG, Dauer G, Schneider S, et al. Incidence of rotator cuff tears in shoulder dislocations and results of therapy in older patients. Arch Orthop Trauma Surg 2006;126(4):235–40.
48. Loew M, Thomsen M, Rickert M, et al. Injury pattern in shoulder dislocation in the elderly patient. Unfallchirurg 2001;104(2):115–8.
49. Habermeyer P, Jung D, Ebert T. Treatment strategy in first traumatic anterior dislocation of the shoulder. Plea for a multi-stage concept of preventive initial management. Unfallchirurg 1998;101(5):328–41 [discussion: 327].
50. Robinson CM, Kelly M, Wakefield AE. Redislocation of the shoulder during the first six weeks after a primary anterior dislocation: risk factors and results of treatment. J Bone Joint Surg Am 2002;84-A(9):1552–9.

51. Zacchilli MA, Owens BD. Epidemiology of shoulder dislocations presenting to emergency departments in the United States. J Bone Joint Surg Am 2010; 92(3):542–9.
52. Owens BD, DeBerardino TM, Nelson BJ, et al. Incidence of shoulder dislocation in the United States military: demographic considerations from a high-risk population. J Bone Joint Surg Am 2009;91(4):791–6.
53. Kerr ZY, Collins CL, Pommering TL, et al. Dislocation/separation injuries among US high school athletes in 9 selected sports: 2005-2009. Clin J Sport Med 2011; 21(2):101–8.
54. Sachs RA, Lin D, Stone ML, et al. Can the need for future surgery for acute traumatic anterior shoulder dislocation be predicted? J Bone Joint Surg Am 2007; 89(8):1665–74.
55. Headey J, Brooks JH, Kemp SP. The epidemiology of shoulder injuries in English professional rugby union. Am J Sports Med 2007;35(9):1537–43.
56. Kaplan LD, Flanigan DC, Norwig J, et al. Prevalence and variance of shoulder injuries in elite collegiate football players. Am J Sports Med 2005;33(8):1142–6.
57. Hovelius L. Shoulder dislocation in Swedish ice hockey players. Am J Sports Med 1978;6(6):373–7.
58. Farber AJ, Castillo R, Clough M, et al. Clinical assessment of three common tests for traumatic anterior shoulder instability. J Bone Joint Surg Am 2006; 88(7):1467–74.
59. McFarland EG, Torpey BM, Curl LA. Evaluation of shoulder laxity. Sports Med 1996;22(4):264–72.
60. Beighton P, Horan F. Orthopaedic aspects of the Ehlers-Danlos syndrome. J Bone Joint Surg Br 1969;51(3):444–53.
61. McFarland E, Kim T. Examination of the shoulder: the complete guide, vol. 1. New York: Thieme; 2006.
62. Kim SH, Park JS, Jeong WK, et al. The Kim test: a novel test for posteroinferior labral lesion of the shoulder–a comparison to the jerk test. Am J Sports Med 2005;33(8):1188–92.
63. Cole BJ, Warner JJ. Arthroscopic versus open Bankart repair for traumatic anterior shoulder instability. Clin Sports Med 2000;19(1):19–48.
64. Thomas SC, Matsen FA 3rd. An approach to the repair of avulsion of the glenohumeral ligaments in the management of traumatic anterior glenohumeral instability. J Bone Joint Surg Am 1989;71(4):506–13.
65. Balg F, Boileau P. The instability severity index score. A simple pre-operative score to select patients for arthroscopic or open shoulder stabilisation. J Bone Joint Surg Br 2007;89(11):1470–7.
66. Neyton L, Young A, Dawidziak B, et al. Surgical treatment of anterior instability in rugby union players: clinical and radiographic results of the Latarjet-Patte procedure with minimum 5-year follow-up. J Shoulder Elbow Surg 2012;21(12):1721–7.
67. Griesser MJ, Harris JD, McCoy BW, et al. Complications and re-operations after Bristow-Latarjet shoulder stabilization: a systematic review. J Shoulder Elbow Surg 2013;22(2):286–92.
68. Harris JD, Gupta AK, Mall NA, et al. Long-term outcomes after Bankart shoulder stabilization. Arthroscopy 2013;29(5):920–33.
69. Mazzocca AD, Brown FM Jr, Carreira DS, et al. Arthroscopic anterior shoulder stabilization of collision and contact athletes. Am J Sports Med 2005;33(1): 52–60.
70. Davidson PA, Rivenburgh DW. The 7-o'clock posteroinferior portal for shoulder arthroscopy. Am J Sports Med 2002;30(5):693–6.

71. Seroyer ST, Nho SJ, Provencher MT, et al. Four-quadrant approach to capsulo-labral repair: an arthroscopic road map to the glenoid. Arthroscopy 2010;26(4):555–62.
72. Randelli P, Ragone V, Carminati S, et al. Risk factors for recurrence after Bankart repair a systematic review. Knee Surg Sports Traumatol Arthrosc 2012;20(11):2129–38.
73. Petrera M, Patella V, Patella S, et al. A meta-analysis of open versus arthroscopic Bankart repair using suture anchors. Knee Surg Sports Traumatol Arthrosc 2010;18(12):1742–7.
74. Lenters TR, Franta AK, Wolf FM, et al. Arthroscopic compared with open repairs for recurrent anterior shoulder instability. A systematic review and meta-analysis of the literature. J Bone Joint Surg Am 2007;89(2):244–54.
75. Freedman KB, Smith AP, Romeo AA, et al. Open Bankart repair versus arthro-scopic repair with transglenoid sutures or bioabsorbable tacks for recurrent anterior instability of the shoulder: a meta-analysis. Am J Sports Med 2004;32(6):1520–7.
76. Rhee YG, Ha JH, Cho NS. Anterior shoulder stabilization in collision athletes: arthroscopic versus open Bankart repair. Am J Sports Med 2006;34(6):979–85.
77. Cho NS, Lubis AM, Ha JH, et al. Clinical results of arthroscopic bankart repair with knot-tying and knotless suture anchors. Arthroscopy 2006;22(12):1276–82.
78. Calvo A, Martinez AA, Domingo J, et al. Rotator interval closure after arthro-scopic capsulolabral repair: a technical variation. Arthroscopy 2005;21(6):765.
79. Ide J, Maeda S, Takagi K. Arthroscopic Bankart repair using suture anchors in athletes: patient selection and postoperative sports activity. Am J Sports Med 2004;32(8):1899–905.
80. Hubbell JD, Ahmad S, Bezenoff LS, et al. Comparison of shoulder stabilization using arthroscopic transglenoid sutures versus open capsulolabral repairs: a 5-year minimum follow-up. Am J Sports Med 2004;32(3):650–4.
81. O'Neill DB. Arthroscopic Bankart repair of anterior detachments of the glenoid labrum. A prospective study. J Bone Joint Surg Am. 1999;81(10):1357–66.
82. Bacilla P, Field LD, Savoie FH 3rd. Arthroscopic Bankart repair in a high demand patient population. Arthroscopy 1997;13(1):51–60.

The Latarjet-Patte Procedure for Recurrent Anterior Shoulder Instability in Contact Athletes

Mithun A. Joshi, MBBS[a],
Allan A. Young, MBBS, MSpMed, PhD, FRACS (Orth)[a,*],
Jean-Christian Balestro, MD[a], Gilles Walch, MD[b]

KEYWORDS

• Shoulder instability • Athlete • Latarjet-Patte • Dislocation

KEY POINTS

• Bone loss is common with recurrent anterior shoulder instability in contact athletes.
• The failure rate in these situations with a soft tissue procedure alone is high.
• The Latarjet-Patte procedure addresses both bony and soft tissue deficiencies with its "triple-blocking" effect.
• The Latarjet-Patte procedure has few complications and allows early return to contact sports without recurrence.
• The Latarjet-Patte technique is the authors' preferred management for recurrent instability in contact athletes.

RECURRENT ANTERIOR SHOULDER INSTABILITY IN CONTACT ATHLETES
Contact Athletes Are a High-risk Group

Glenohumeral dislocation and anterior shoulder instability are most common in young athletes involved in contact sports.[1] Ongoing sports participation in this population is associated with a high recurrence rate.[2] Recurrent instability has physical and psychological consequences for the athlete, with more severe soft tissue and bony pathologic abnormality,[3] greater time away from sports participation,[4] and a negative impact on quality of life.[5] Surgery is therefore generally recommended in contact athletes experiencing recurrent anterior shoulder instability.[3]

Disclosure: The authors listed below have identified no professional or financial affiliations for themselves or their spouse/partners relevant to this article: Allan A. Young, MBBS, FRACS (Orth), Mithun A. Joshi, MBBS, Jean-Christian Balestro, MD, Gilles Walch, MD.
[a] Sydney Shoulder Specialists, Suite 201, 156 Pacific Highway, St Leonards, Sydney, New South Wales 2065, Australia; [b] Centre Orthopédique Santy, 24 Avenue Paul Santy, Lyon 69008, France
* Corresponding author.
E-mail address: allanyoung@sydneyshoulder.com.au

Clin Sports Med 32 (2013) 731–739
http://dx.doi.org/10.1016/j.csm.2013.07.009
0278-5919/13/$ – see front matter © 2013 Elsevier Inc. All rights reserved.

Open or Arthroscopic Techniques for Soft Tissue Pathology

The operative management of recurrent instability has evolved since its first description by Bankart in 1923.[6] Following the introduction of arthroscopic surgery, debate centered over whether open or arthroscopic repairs best addressed the Bankart lesion,[6] a soft tissue pathologic abnormality characterized by capsulolabral detachment from the anteroinferior aspect of the glenoid. Open Bankart stabilization has traditionally been considered the gold standard with early studies demonstrating better outcomes compared with arthroscopic stabilization.[7–9] Arthroscopic techniques and equipment have however continued to evolve and arthroscopic repairs using suture anchors now achieve similar results to open surgery in the treatment of such soft tissue lesions.[10,11]

Soft Tissue or Bony Procedures for Recurrent Instability

With improved understanding of the pathoanatomic changes associated with recurrent instability, more recently debate has shifted focus to soft tissue versus bony surgical stabilization procedures. Shoulders with recurrent instability are associated with a high incidence of bone loss.[12] Glenoid and/or humeral bone lesions have been shown to be present in 90% to 95% of shoulders with recurrent instability.[13,14] Failure to address these bone defects can result in a poor outcome. A glenoid defect approaching 21% of its length has been shown to compromise shoulder stability.[15,16] Burkhart and De Beer[17] observed a 67% recurrence rate in patients with an "inverted pear" glenoid configuration if they only underwent a soft tissue procedure. The recurrence rate was 4.9% in these patients with an open Latarjet technique.[18] This evidence has led some authors to favor a bony procedure for recurrent anterior shoulder instability associated with bone loss.[19]

Open Bony Procedures Best for Contact Athletes

Contact athletes are more prone to bone loss because of the high-energy injuries they sustain.[17,20] Successful treatment in this group must provide a stable reconstruction with a pain-free, mobile, and strong shoulder, thereby allowing early return to sports participation without recurrence. Higher failure rates have been reported in contact athletes with recurrent instability following arthroscopic soft tissue stabilization.[17,21–24] An open bony procedure seems to give better results in this group.[18,25] Balg and Boileau[26] have proposed the Instability Severity Index Score to determine which patients would in fact benefit from an open bony reconstruction. Contact athletes by definition have many of their proposed risk factors and would score high on the Instability Severity Index Score, resulting in the Latarjet procedure being recommended.

For all of the reasons mentioned above, the authors' preferred management of the contact athlete is therefore the Latarjet procedure.

THE LATARJET-PATTE PROCEDURE

Michel Latarjet[27] described his technique for shoulder stabilization in 1954, whereby the horizontal limb of the coracoid process was transposed to the anteroinferior glenoid rim through a window in the subscapularis and fixed with a single screw. The Latarjet-Patte procedure is a modification of this involving the use of 2 screws and including repair of the anterior capsule to the stump of the coracoacromial ligament.[28]

Proposed Mechanism of Action

The Latarjet-Patte procedure has been proposed to address both bony and soft tissue deficiencies with a "triple-blocking" effect (**Fig. 1**).[28] The coracoid graft provides a

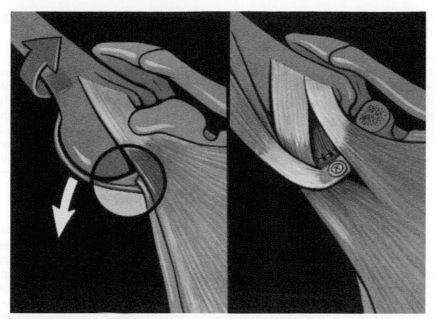

Fig. 1. Demonstration of the triple-blocking effect as described by Patte. (*Data from* Patte D, Debeyre J. Luxations recidivantes de l'épaule. Encycl Med Chir Paris-Technique chirurgicale Orthopédie 1980;44265:44–52.)

"bony effect" by restoring the anteroposterior diameter of the glenoid, thereby increasing stability and preventing an otherwise engaging Hill-Sachs lesion from levering on a deficient anteroinferior glenoid rim.[18,29] The most important stabilizing mechanism of the Latarjet-Patte procedure is however the interaction between the conjoint tendon and lower subscapularis with the arm in abduction and external rotation.[30] In this position, the conjoint tendon reinforces the inferior subscapularis fibers and anteroinferior joint capsule to provide a so-called "sling effect." It also counteracts the ligament laxity seen with recurrent instability through a tensioning effect on the lower subscapularis as it passes through a split in the muscle.[29,31] Essentially, the lower subscapularis fills the potential space into where the humeral head would otherwise dislocate. The further the arm moves into the at-risk position of abduction and external rotation, the tighter the sling effect becomes. Finally, repair of the anterior capsule to the stump of the coracoacromial ligament completes the triple-blocking effect.[31] This mechanism is most important in abduction and neutral rotation.[30]

Technique

Patient position
The patient is placed in a beach chair position with the lateral most aspect of the acromion level with the edge of the operating table. A small towel is placed between the scapula and table to stabilize and flatten the scapula. The arm is draped free to allow intraoperative abduction and external rotation.

Surgical approach
A limited deltopectoral approach is used. The skin incision is 4 to 5 cm long and extends vertically downward from the coracoid tip. Branching vessels from the cephalic vein are ligated. A self-retaining retractor between the deltoid and pectoralis

major is used to maintain exposure. A Hohmann retractor is placed over the top of the coracoid.

Coracoid harvesting

The coracoacromial ligament (CAL) is incised 1 cm lateral to its coracoid attachment. The CAL is released. The pectoralis minor tendon is released from the coracoid. Care should be taken not to release past the coracoid tip because the blood supply to the graft enters just medial to the conjoint tendon insertion. The inferior aspect of the "knee" of the coracoid (ie, the junction between its horizontal and vertical parts) is now exposed and is the site of the osteotomy. A coracoid graft greater than 25 mm in length can routinely be harvested without damaging the coracoclavicular ligaments using this technique.[32] The inferior coracoid surface is decorticated. Two central drill holes are made in the coracoid about 1 cm apart.

Glenoid exposure and preparation

The subscapularis is split at the junction of its superior two-thirds and inferior one-third. The underlying capsule is exposed and a vertical incision is made at the level of the joint line. An intra-articular retractor is placed. The anterior labrum and periosteum are excised. An osteotome is used to decorticate the anterior glenoid surface with the aim of creating a flat surface of bleeding cancellous bone. The inferior hole in the glenoid is drilled at a position between 4 and 5 o'clock in the right shoulder. The hole must be sufficiently medial to avoid lateral coracoid overhang from the glenoid and the recommended distance is typically 7 mm from the glenoid margin.[32,33] Drilling is parallel to the glenoid articular surface and passes through the posterior glenoid cortex.

Graft fixation

The coracoid graft is fixed with a 35-mm-long 4.5-mm partially threaded malleolar screw. The screw is fully inserted into the inferior hole of the graft (ie, the conjoint tendon end). Although this is typically the correct length, it can later be exchanged after placement of the superior screw. The screw is placed in the already drilled hole in the glenoid and tightened, correcting rotation of the graft to ensure the lateral margin of the coracoid is flush with the glenoid articular margin (**Fig. 2**). Although this is the ideal position for the graft, a slightly medial position (1–2 mm) is acceptable. The drill is used to create a second hole in the glenoid through the superior hole in the graft. A depth gauge is used to measure the length of the malleolar screw (typically 35 mm, usual range 30–40 mm). Both screws are tightened using a 2-finger technique. Aggressive over-tightening should be avoided to prevent fracture of the graft. The position of the coracoid is rechecked. If any lateral overhang is noticed, it should be removed with bone rongeurs or a high-speed burr. Alternatively, the graft can be repositioned and the glenoid drilled in a slightly different direction by removing one screw and loosening the other.

The CAL stump is repaired to the capsule using sutures. This repair must be performed with the shoulder in full external rotation to enable immediate postoperative full range of motion and prevent stiffness in external rotation. The authors do not repair the split in the subscapularis muscle.

Rehabilitation and return to sport

Patients wear a simple sling for 15 days to encourage rest and reduce the risk of a postoperative hematoma. Self-directed full range-of-motion exercises in elevation and external rotation are initiated immediately. At 15 days, usual activities of daily living are allowed. Patients progressively resume athletic conditioning (jogging,

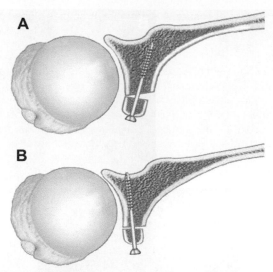

Fig. 2. Incorrect (*A*) and correct (*B*) screw positioning during coracoid graft fixation to the glenoid. Inserting screws parallel to the articular surface reduces risk of lateral overhang and nonunion of the graft.

cycling) without any upper limb strengthening at 1 month. Plain radiographs (true anteroposterior, scapular lateral, and Bernageau[34] views) are obtained at 3 months to assess graft healing (**Fig. 3**). If graft healing is satisfactory, progressive sport-specific training is started with noncontact training for 2 weeks followed by contact training for 2 weeks. Contact and collision athletes can return to competition by 4 months.[35]

DISCUSSION

The goal of surgical treatment of recurrent instability in contact athletes is to achieve a stable shoulder, allowing early return to sports participation without recurrence and with minimal risk of complications.

The presence of bony lesions in contact athletes with instability puts them at a higher risk of recurrence.[17,20] Rugby players who underwent the Latarjet-Patte procedure showed no recurrence of dislocation or subluxation at a mean follow-up of 12 years.[20] Similar results have been reported with variations of the technique.[17,36–39] This is better than the 89% and 38% recurrence rates for arthroscopic and open Bankart reconstruction, respectively, in contact athletes.[17,24]

The coracoid bone block procedure according to Latarjet-Patte also allows contact athletes to return to full competition at a faster rate compared with arthroscopic and open Bankart procedures.[20,22,23,25] Of the professional level rugby players in the authors' series, almost all returned to full competition by 4 months. Mean return to full training was 6 months, with 7 months for return to competitive sport in the entire cohort. Only one player of 34 did not return to playing rugby because of the operated shoulder.

High satisfaction rates have been reported with the Latarjet procedure.[38,39] The authors observed similar rates (mean Rowe score of 93, subjective satisfaction rate of 94%) in rugby players who underwent the Latarjet-Patte reconstruction.[20] Outcome

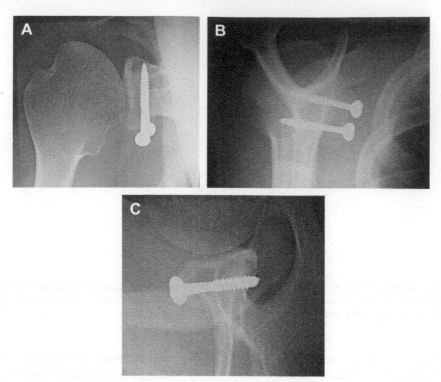

Fig. 3. Postoperative radiographs showing satisfactory graft position and healing at 3 months: anteroposterior (*A*), lateral (*B*), and Bernageau view (*C*).

scores after a bony procedure seem to be comparable to results following arthroscopic and open soft tissue reconstruction in contact athletes.[22,23,25,40]

In addition to this, complications with the Latarjet-Patte procedure are rare with a meticulous surgical technique. Although a 62% glenohumeral arthritis rate has previously been reported with the Latarjet procedure,[38] only 30% of the rugby players in the authors' study showed arthritis at 12-year follow-up.[20] All these patients had mild (Samilson and Prieto[41] grade 1) arthritis, which has been shown to have no effect on shoulder function.[38]

The precise cause of degenerative joint disease following a Latarjet procedure is unknown. Hovelius and Saebö[42] suggest that it may be related to pre-existing factors (increased age at first dislocation, recurrent dislocation, increased age at surgery, and presence of arthritis before surgery), because no significant difference in postoperative arthritis is seen following soft tissue and bony stabilization procedures.[43] The authors think the main preventable factor at the time of the Latarjet procedure surgery is lateral coracoid overhang. Allain and colleagues[38] showed functionally significant (Samilson and Prieto[41] grade 2 or higher) arthropathy only in grafts that were too lateral. In the authors' operative technique, they repeatedly check the position of the graft with both visual inspection and palpation and never accept any lateral overhang. They also confirm the position of the graft on follow-up imaging, including a Bernageau[34] view.

Shoulder stiffness and loss of external rotation is another complication reported following the Latarjet procedure. A loss of up to 21 of external rotation was observed following subscapularis tenotomy for glenoid exposure.[38] The transection causes dense scar formation leading to tendon shortening and decreased excursion.[44] The authors use a subscapularis-splitting approach for glenoid exposure. A horizontal split preserves the continuity of the muscle fibers and allows immediate unrestricted postoperative range-of-motion exercises, including external rotation. The authors think it is also important to repair the capsule to the CAL stump with the arm positioned in maximal external rotation to avoid external rotation deficits. The authors have not observed significant loss of external rotation in their Latarjet-Patte patients using this method.[35]

SUMMARY

The Latarjet-Patte procedure satisfies all of the requirements for treating recurrent anterior instability in contact athletes and is therefore their preferred management in this patient group.

REFERENCES

1. Owens B, Agel J, Mountcastle S, et al. Incidence of glenohumeral instability in collegiate athletics. Am J Sports Med 2009;37(9):1750–4.
2. Sachs R, Lin D, Stone M, et al. Can the need for future surgery for acute traumatic anterior shoulder dislocation be predicted? J Bone Joint Surg Am 2007;89(8): 1665–74.
3. Owens B, Dickens J, Kilcoyne K, et al. Management of mid-season traumatic anterior shoulder instability in athletes. J Am Acad Orthop Surg 2012;20(8): 518–26.
4. Headey J, Brooks J, Kemp S. The epidemiology of shoulder injuries in English professional rugby players. Am J Sports Med 2007;35(9):1537–43.
5. Meller R, Krettek C, Gösling T, et al. Recurrent shoulder instability among athletes: changes in quality of life, sports activity, and muscle function following open repair. Knee Surg Sports Traumatol Arthrosc 2007;15(3):295–304.
6. Bankart A. Recurrent or habitual dislocation of the shoulder-joint. Br Med J 1923; 2(3285):1132–3.
7. Freedman K, Smith A, Romeo A, et al. Open Bankart repair versus arthroscopic repair with transglenoid sutures or bioabsorbable tacks for recurrent anterior instability of the shoulder: a meta-analysis. Am J Sports Med 2004;32(6):1520–7.
8. Mohtadi N, Bitar I, Sasyniuk T, et al. Arthroscopic versus open repair for traumatic anterior shoulder instability: a meta-analysis. Arthroscopy 2005;21(6):652–8.
9. Lenters T, Franta A, Wolf F, et al. Arthroscopic compared with open repairs for recurrent anterior shoulder instability: a systematic review and meta-analysis of the literature. J Bone Joint Surg Am 2007;89(2):244–54.
10. Hobby J, Griffin D, Dunbar M, et al. Is arthroscopic surgery for stabilization of chronic shoulder instability as effective as open surgery? A systematic review and meta-analysis of 62 studies including 3044 arthroscopic operations. J Bone Joint Surg Br 2007;89(9):1188–96.
11. Brophy R, Marx R. The treatment of traumatic anterior instability of the shoulder: nonoperative and surgical treatment. Arthroscopy 2009;25(3):298–304.
12. Yiannakopoulos C, Mataragas E, Antonogiannakis E. A comparison of the spectrum of intra-articular lesions in acute and chronic anterior shoulder instability. Arthroscopy 2007;23(9):985–90.
13. Sugaya H, Moriishi J, Dohi M, et al. Glenoid rim morphology in recurrent anterior glenohumeral instability. J Bone Joint Surg Am 2003;85(5):878–84.

14. Edwards T, Boulahia A, Walch G. Radiographic analysis of bone defects in chronic anterior shoulder instability. Arthroscopy 2003;19(7):732–9.
15. Itoi E, Lee SB, Berglund L, et al. The effect of a glenoid defect on anteroinferior stability of the shoulder after Bankart repair: a cadaveric study. J Bone Joint Surg Am 2000;82(1):35–46.
16. Yamamoto N, Itoi E, Abe H, et al. Effect of an anterior glenoid defect on anterior shoulder instability: a cadaveric study. Am J Sports Med 2009;37(5):949–54.
17. Burkhart S, De Beer J. Traumatic glenohumeral bone defects and their relationship to failure of arthroscopic Bankart repairs: significance of the inverted-pear glenoid and the humeral engaging Hill-Sachs lesion. Arthroscopy 2000;16(7): 677–94.
18. Burkhart S, De Beer J, Barth J, et al. Results of modified Latarjet reconstruction in patients with anteroinferior instability and significant bone loss. Arthroscopy 2007;23(10):1033–41.
19. Boileau P, Villalba M, Héry J, et al. Risk factors for recurrence of shoulder instability after arthroscopic Bankart repair. J Bone Joint Surg Am 2006;88(8): 1755–63.
20. Neyton L, Young A, Dawidziak B, et al. Surgical treatment of anterior instability in rugby union players: clinical and radiographic results of the Latarjet-Patte procedure with minimum 5-year follow-up. J Shoulder Elbow Surg 2012;21(12): 1721–7.
21. Bonnevialle N, Mansat P, Bellumore Y, et al. Surgical treatment of anterior shoulder instability in rugby players: clinical and radiographic results with minimum five-year follow-up. Rev Chir Orthop Reparatrice Appar Mot 2008;94(7):635–42 [in French].
22. Cho N, Hwang J, Rhee Y. Arthroscopic stabilization in anterior shoulder instability: collision athletes versus noncollision athletes. Arthroscopy 2006;22(9):947–53.
23. Pagnani M, Dome D. Surgical treatment of traumatic anterior shoulder instability in American football players. J Bone Joint Surg Am 2002;84(5):711–5.
24. Roberts S, Taylor D, Brown J, et al. Open and arthroscopic techniques for the treatment of traumatic anterior shoulder instability in Australian rules football players. J Shoulder Elbow Surg 1999;8(5):403–9.
25. Larrain M, Montenegro H, Mauas D, et al. Arthroscopic management of traumatic anterior shoulder instability in collision athletes: analysis of 204 cases with a 4- to 9-year follow-up and results with the suture anchor technique. Arthroscopy 2006; 22(12):1283–9.
26. Balg F, Boileau P. The instability severity index score: a simple pre-operative score to select patients for arthroscopic or open shoulder stabilization. J Bone Joint Surg Am 2007;89(11):1470–7.
27. Latarjet M. Treatment of recurrent dislocation of the shoulder. Lyon Chir 1954;49: 994–1003 [in French].
28. Patte D, Debeyre J. Luxations recidivantes de l'épaule. Encycl Med Chir Paris-Technique chirurgicale Orthopédie 1980;44265:44–52.
29. Lafosse L, Boyle S. Arthroscopic Latarjet procedure. J Shoulder Elbow Surg 2010;19(2):2–12.
30. Wellmann M, de Ferrari H, Smith T, et al. Biomechanical investigation of the stabilization principle of the Latarjet procedure. Arch Orthop Trauma Surg 2012; 132(3):377–86.
31. de Beer J, Roberts C. Glenoid bone defects- open Latarjet with congruent arc modification. Orthop Clin North Am 2010;41(3):407–15.

32. Young A, Baba M, Neyton L, et al. Coracoid graft dimensions after harvesting for the open Latarjet procedure. J Shoulder Elbow Surg 2013;22(4):485–8.
33. Butt U, Charalambous C. Complications associated with open coracoid transfer procedures for shoulder instability. J Shoulder Elbow Surg 2012;21(8):1110–9.
34. Bernageau J, Patte D, Bebeyre J. Value of the glenoid profil in recurrent luxations of the shoulder. Rev Chir Orthop Reparatrice Appar Mot 1976;62:142–7 [in French].
35. Young A, Maia R, Berhouet J, et al. Open Latarjet for management of bone loss in anterior instability of the glenohumeral joint. J Shoulder Elbow Surg 2011;20: S61–9.
36. Walch G. La luxation récidivante antérieure de l'épaule. Rev Chir Orthop Reparatrice Appar Mot 1991;77:177–91.
37. Walch G, Boileau P. Latarjet-Bristow procedure for recurrent anterior instability. Tech Shoulder Elbow Surg 2000;1:256–61.
38. Allain J, Goutallier D, Glorion C. Long-term results of the Latarjet procedure for the treatment of anterior instability of the shoulder. J Bone Joint Surg Am 1998; 80(6):841–52.
39. Hovelius L, Sandström B, Sundgren K, et al. One hundred eighteen Bristow-Latarjet repairs for recurrent anterior dislocation of the shoulder prospectively followed for fifteen years: study I- clinical results. J Shoulder Elbow Surg 2004; 13(5):509–16.
40. Mazzocca A, Brown F, Carreira D, et al. Arthroscopic anterior shoulder stabilization of collision and contact athletes. Am J Sports Med 2005;33(1):52–60.
41. Samilson R, Prieto V. Dislocation arthropathy of the shoulder. J Bone Joint Surg Am 1983;65(4):456–60.
42. Hovelius L, Saebö M. Neer Award 2008: arthropathy after primary anterior shoulder dislocation- 223 shoulders prospectively followed up for twenty-five years. J Shoulder Elbow Surg 2009;18(3):339–47.
43. Buscayret F, Edwards T, Szabö I, et al. Glenohumeral arthrosis in anterior instability before and after surgical treatment: incidence and contributing factors. Am J Sports Med 2004;32(5):1165–72.
44. Chen A, Hunt S, Hawkins R, et al. Management of bone loss associated with recurrent anterior glenohumeral instability. Am J Sports Med 2005;33(6):912–25.

Shoulder Instability with Concomitant Bone Loss in the Athlete

Justin W. Griffin, MD, Stephen F. Brockmeier, MD*

KEYWORDS

• Glenoid insufficiency • Bony Bankart • Shoulder instability • Dislocation

KEY POINTS

• The prevalence of clinically relevant bone loss is likely underestimated, with critical bone deficiency present in a high percentage of patients with multiple recurrent dislocations or prior failed stabilization surgery.

• Of the several options for the imaging quantification of bone loss, 3-dimensional computed tomography reconstruction is the current gold standard.

• As little as 6 mm of bone loss can translate into approximately 20% to 25% of the native glenoid surface; when glenoid bone loss exceeds 20%, glenoid bone augmentation is the currently accepted form of surgical management.

• Adopting an algorithmic approach to the athlete with glenohumeral instability and associated bone deficiency will help achieve the most predictable outcomes with regard to stability and return to activities.

INTRODUCTION

Shoulder instability is common in athletes, often resulting from an initial traumatic dislocation event. Glenohumeral dislocations and subluxations, especially those occurring at a young age, can lead to recurrent instability events, which can jeopardize performance in elite athletes. Following initial traumatic dislocation, repeated trauma to the glenoid can result in glenoid rim fractures, attritional bone loss, and soft-tissue injury. Over time this may lead to glenoid, humeral, or dual-sided bony deficiency and a change in the overall architecture of the shoulder. Previous failed fixation of bony Bankart and labral abnormality may also lead to insufficiency, prompting consideration of further options.

Thorough evaluation of the athlete with persistent shoulder instability and appropriate use of imaging modalities can help quantify the severity of bony deficiency.

Department of Orthopaedic Surgery, University of Virginia, Charlottesville, VA, USA
* Corresponding author. Department of Orthopaedic Surgery, University of Virginia, 400 Ray C. Hunt Drive, Suite 330, Charlottesville, Virginia 22908, USA
E-mail address: sfb2e@virginia.edu

Clin Sports Med 32 (2013) 741–760
http://dx.doi.org/10.1016/j.csm.2013.07.008
0278-5919/13/$ – see front matter © 2013 Elsevier Inc. All rights reserved.

Based on obtained imaging and examination, surgical and nonsurgical methods can be considered. In many situations both the humeral-sided and glenoid-sided bone loss must be addressed. Depending on the extent of bone loss, athletic demands, and surgeon experience, arthroscopic or open surgical options can provide shoulder stability and return athletes to their prior level of activity.

NATURAL HISTORY OF BONE LOSS

The ability to counsel athletes presenting with varying degrees of bone loss depends on a proper understanding of the natural history of glenoid and humeral bone defects. The unconstrained nature of the glenohumeral joint in terms of osseous stability imparts a predisposition for recurrent joint instability. Young athletes and those who participate in contact sports are most prone to developing recurrent dislocation or subluxation events after an initial traumatic dislocation.[1,2] These events most commonly result in anterior inferior "Bankart" labral tears, occurring in approximately 97% of dislocations.[3,4]

Age has long been regarded as the most important factor for recurrence.[1,5] Sachs and colleagues[6] reported on predictive factors for recurrence and identified young age and contact sports as primary risk factors for recurrence. Glenoid fractures and Hill-Sachs lesions can be present from the initial dislocation event as well, and may go unrecognized; this can alter the necessary bony constraint within the glenohumeral joint.[7] Burkhart and De Beer[8] identified that failure to address the bony aspect of injury, including Hill-Sachs lesions, may lead to failed instability surgery.[7,8] This finding has led to recent discussion regarding proper treatment of first-time dislocators.[9] Even if there is not an initial bony lesion, repeated dislocation events over time will often lead to glenoid erosion and development of a characteristic pattern of bone loss, known as the "inverted pear" glenoid.[8]

Some athletes may be predisposed to glenohumeral instability based on their native glenoid architecture and glenoid version. Some amount of bony deficiency is present in approximately 22% of patients after initial dislocation. The incidence climbs to nearly 90% after failed prior stabilization surgery.[8] Most of these defects are located on the anterior inferior glenoid between 2 and 6 o'clock, consistent with the common direction of instability events.[10] Posterior glenoid fractures and insufficiency do occur, though much less commonly.

The type of sport may also influence the morphology of the glenoid lesion depending on the mixture of direction of axial and shear force applied to the joint at the time of injury, as demonstrated by Burkhart and De Beer.[8] Smooth-appearing lesions without a clear fracture fragment may be found in the setting of lower-energy chronic dislocations presenting over a longer term, whereas glenoid rim fractures are more common among football players presenting more acutely.[8] In the setting of recurrent dislocations persistent for longer than 6 months, the glenoid may remodel completely.[7,11]

The Hill-Sachs lesion is a compression defect of the humeral head that is associated with shoulder instability. This lesion occurs in approximately 40% to 90% of athletic shoulder instability and generally occurs in the abducted, externally rotated position.[12] Those humeral-sided lesions that do not engage are typically not parallel to the glenoid face when the shoulder is in abduction and external rotation. Reverse Hill-Sachs lesions (anterosuperomedial humerus lesion) occur in posterior shoulder instability.

The humeral head defect may also remodel, and the progression on the humeral side combined with attritional glenoid-sided loss can combine to lead to an "engaging" Hill-Sachs lesion (**Fig. 1**). These bipolar lesions need to be assessed by

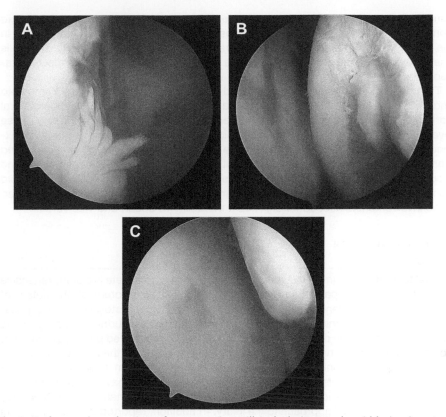

Fig. 1. Arthroscopic evaluation of an engaging Hill-Sachs lesion. A glenoid lesion is noted (*A*) in addition to an engaging Hill-Sachs humeral head defect (*B, C*).

quantification of both the glenoid and humeral involvement, and treatment in this setting can be challenging. In the setting of isolated humeral-sided bone loss with engagement, which is less common than isolated glenoid-sided loss, a specific subset of surgical options can be considered.

BIOMECHANICAL EFFECTS OF BONE LOSS

The stability of the native glenohumeral joint depends on both static and dynamic restraints. Provencher and colleagues[13] identify 3 key contributors to joint stability: concavity-compression and the bony architecture, the glenohumeral capsuloligamentous structures (static stabilizers), and the coordinated contraction of the rotator cuff and periscapular musculature (dynamic stabilizers).

Bone loss on the glenoid and/or humeral sides can lead to a well-described cascade of events. Loss on the glenoid side can create a discrepancy in the articular area.[11,14] The concave surface of the glenoid provides a point on which the humerus can be compressed, assisted by the labrum, which deepens the concavity of the glenoid and serves as a site of ligament attachment. Lack of the labral buttress and disruption of bony architecture can lead to instability events, which can contribute to a cycle whereby both the glenoid-sided and humeral-sided lesions increase in size, compounding the problem. The cancellous architecture of the posterolateral humerus is prone to continued compression injury, with the cortical anterior glenoid bone as the assailant. In addition, the capsule has been demonstrated to stretch in the setting of recurrent instability.[15] Restoration of the proper glenoid articular arc is one method to help restore stability that is affected by these numerous disadvantageous factors.[16]

The concept of glenoid track is influenced by bone loss. As described by Yamamoto and colleagues,[17] the glenoid contact area shifts from inferomedial to superolateral portion of the posterior aspect of the humeral head, termed the glenoid track. These investigators reported that a Hill-Sachs lesion is at higher risk of engagement if it extends medially over the medial margin of the glenoid track.[17] For the athlete, increased glenoid bone loss decreases the size of this glenoid track, making engagement and recurrent instability more common. In the setting of more substantial loss of glenoid bone, the bipolar nature of these lesions makes it possible that less humeral-sided bone involvement is needed for significant instability to occur, and vice versa.

CLINICAL EVALUATION
History

Crucial to treating recurrent instability with bone loss in the athlete is a comprehensive understanding of the patient's history of instability. First and foremost, the details of the initial instability event should be identified. Patients with a history of shoulder instability have been determined to have a 5-fold increased risk of further instability.[18] The direction of dislocation can be helpful in determining the expected pathology (anterior, posterior, multidirectional). The mechanism of injury, including the position of the arm at the time of both the initial dislocation, is important to ascertain. In addition, the point at which the patient feels initial subluxation and apprehension may provide information on the degree of bone loss. The method by which the patient has been reduced may also assist in the initial approach to the injury. In addition, reported dislocation events that occur during low-energy activity such as sleeping and reaching for an object are concerning for more severe pathoanatomy associated with recurrent instability, especially concomitant bone loss on one or both sides of the joint.

Understanding the patient's prior treatment to date is also critical in creating a plan moving forward. An initial period of attempted nonsurgical management may or may not be advised depending on the patient's presentation, time in season, and the existing soft-tissue and bony abnormality.

An expanding volume of literature is available on the significance of instability following previous stabilization attempts.[8] These prior attempts may increase the likelihood of bony insufficiency. Every effort should be made to obtain prior arthroscopic photos and imaging to assist in formulating an appropriate strategy for each individualized patient.

Physical Examination

The approach to physical examination of the patient with suspected glenohumeral instability should be both comprehensive and standardized. The patient should be examined with both shoulder girdles well visualized. Examination should always begin with examination of the unaffected side to provide a framework within which to compare the pathologic side. Observation of the active shoulder motion from behind the patient may reveal scapular dyskinesis, scapular winging, or muscular atrophy. Joint range of motion, both active and passive, should be measured and compared with the unaffected side, looking for both laxity and adaptive loss of motion such as internal rotation deficit, which can be seen in the overhead athlete.

Separate from general range of motion testing is evaluation of stability in specific planes. Provocative maneuvers include the load and shift test (**Fig. 2**), which may be used to evaluate translation of the humeral head over the glenoid rim. The apprehension sign is a useful test to evaluate shoulder instability.[14] This test is best performed with the patient lying flat on the examination table. In the case of bone loss, nearly all patients will exhibit a positive apprehension test at 90° abduction and maximal external rotation of the involved shoulder. Of note, patients with critical bone loss will frequently demonstrate apprehension in a lower position of abduction (20°–60°), likely indicating engagement at this position.[10] Inferior shoulder laxity can be tested by the sulcus sign, which is achieved with inferior traction on the humerus and measurement of the distance from the lateral acromion to the humerus, and comparison with the contralateral side. Position of subluxation or engagement of a Hill-Sachs lesion is often better quantified under anesthesia.

Side-to-side comparison of strength testing should be performed next. Although structural injury to the rotator cuff with a dislocation event is more common in older individuals, rotator cuff strength should also be closely evaluated in the younger athlete. Subscapularis function, as delineated by strength testing of internal rotation as well as the lift-off and belly-press tests, should be documented, especially in patients who have had previous anterior open procedures. Knowledge of the management of subscapularis should be obtained in the referral situation.

Imaging Analysis

On initial presentation plain radiographs are helpful in confirming reduction, and may show a bony Bankart fragment, best detected on a variation of the axillary lateral. Hill-Sachs lesions can be visualized best on an anteroposterior variant called the Stryker Notch view. This internal-rotation view of the humerus brings the posterior and lateral aspect of the humerus, the typical Hill-Sachs area, into view. Certain radiographs provide more accurate assessment of the glenoid articular surface, including the West Point view and Garth apical oblique view.

Advanced imaging, which should be considered in the further workup of glenohumeral instability in most patients, may often include magnetic resonance (MR) imaging

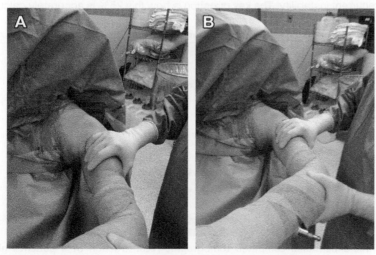

Fig. 2. (A, B) Load and shift examination performed under anesthesia.

or MR arthrography, which best evaluates the soft-tissue structures such as the labrum, joint capsule, rotator cuff, and cartilage. When there is suspicion for bone loss, the optimal study is currently a computed tomography (CT) scan.

Glenoid rim fragments and attritional bone loss can be best characterized by CT scan with 3-dimensional (3D) reconstruction. Two-dimensional (2D) CT depends on orienting the beam perpendicular to the glenoid face, which thereby depends on the version. If not entirely perpendicular, the bone loss may be either overestimated or underestimated. The surgeon must also understand the role of the slice distance to quantify bone loss.

Sugaya and colleagues[11] evaluated 100 shoulders with recurrent instability using en-face 3D reconstructed CT. Fifty osseous Bankart fragments of varying sizes were identified, with large fragments occupying 26% of the glenoid fossa. In addition, 90% of those evaluated had a glenoid-rim lesion of some type.[11]

DEFICIENCY MEASUREMENT AND CLASSIFICATION

Preoperative quantification of bone loss is crucial for surgical decision making. CT has been shown to be superior to plain radiography when evaluating the glenoid, as it provides an en-face oblique view.[19] 3D CT with digital subtraction of the humerus is now considered the gold standard, and allows reliable surgical planning and quantification of glenoid defects (**Fig. 3**). The humerus can also be included and later subtracted to allow for evaluation of Hill-Sachs defects.

Bigliani and colleagues[7] defined 3 types of glenoid lesions based on plain radiographs, with type I being an avulsion fracture, type II a medially displaced fragment, and type III an erosion of the glenoid. Typically the critical value of 25% of total glenoid surface (or 6–8 mm defect in most glenoids) is used when discussing the need for open techniques and augmentation procedures, because of the known failure of standard Bankart repairs in this subset of patients.[20]

Itoi and colleagues[21] performed a biomechanical study testing shoulder instability with progressive bone loss, in which they osteotomized the glenoid sequentially and identified a critical drop-off in glenohumeral stability when 21% of the glenoid was removed. Patients with glenoid bone loss and inferior hyperlaxity are particularly at risk for recurrent instability, according to Boileau and colleagues'[20] analysis of risk factors for recurrent instability. The key question is how this 25% is accurately calculated.

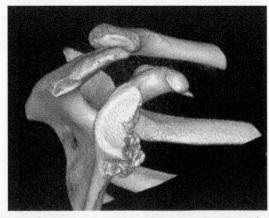

Fig. 3. Three-dimensional computed tomographic reconstruction of a patient's glenoid, demonstrating significant glenoid bone loss.

There are several methods to determine bone loss by imaging and arthroscopy (**Fig. 4**). One technique involves measuring the distance from the bare spot to the posterior or unaffected rim, and then from the bare spot to the edge of the area of bony deficiency. The percentage of attritional loss is then calculated using the following formula: $([B - A]/2B) \times 100\%$. Another method involves using the en-face view of the glenoid on 2D CT imaging and measuring the width-to-length ratio and glenoid bone defect length calculations which, when compared with glenoid diameter, are predictive of recurrent instability.

As discussed previously, glenoid bone loss can also be perhaps most accurately assessed using CT with multiplanar reconstructions and digital subtraction of the humeral head. Once the en-face view is obtained, the defect can be measured directly. In addition, a true best-fit circle around the inferior glenoid can be drawn with the center at the approximate bare area (**Fig. 5**).[22,23] Once the circle is drawn, the amount of bone loss can be calculated relative to this by dividing the surface area of the bony defect by the area of the circle. Measuring the length of the glenoid defect alone has also been shown to provide prognostic information regarding recurrent instability.

Arthroscopy also can be used to qualify and quantify glenoid bone loss. The glenoid bare-spot method can be used, although this may overestimate bone loss depending on the location of the bony defect in relation to the bare spot, which may be difficult to identify in all shoulders. The bare-spot method has been scrutinized and found to be unreliable by some surgeons. It is best at estimating those defects that occur parallel to the long axis of the glenoid.[24,25]

Classification of humeral-sided lesions has also been described. Most of these descriptions use either CT-scan quantification based on the humeral defect as a percentage of the circumference of the humeral head, or direct visualization of the humeral-sided defect.[12] To date, no consensus has been reached on the clinical utility of these classifications in guiding treatment. Some classifications focus on significance, whereas others focus on size or grade of injury.[26]

Finally, it is important to consider the athlete who has undergone multiple attempts at stabilization. Inflammatory reaction to retained devices may provide a larger relative zone of damaged bone.[27] Glenoid rim fractures that propagate through prior anchor

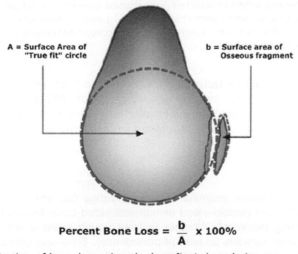

$$\text{Percent Bone Loss} = \frac{b}{A} \times 100\%$$

Fig. 4. Quantification of bone loss using the best-fit circle technique.

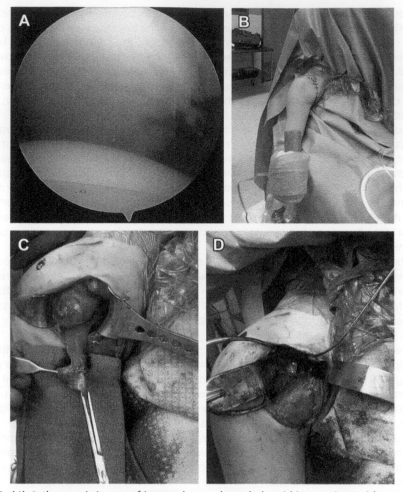

Fig. 5. (*A*) Arthroscopic image of inverted pear–shaped glenoid in a patient with recurrent instability. (*B*) Preparation with beach-chair positioning and mechanical arm holder. (*C*) The coracoid process is harvested with preservation of the conjoined tendon. (*D*) The coracoid is fixed in the appropriate position.

sites can occur and can be technically challenging to treat. Previous arthroscopic images coupled with current imaging consisting of both MR arthrography and 3D CT can demonstrate expected bone loss after debridement of the glenoid edge. It is clear that even 1 to 2 mm of bone can make a large difference for the athlete in terms of stability.

NONSURGICAL CARE

Following history, physical examination, and imaging quantification of both soft-tissue abnormality and glenoid-sided or humeral-sided bone loss, a decision must be made regarding treatment. Whether to treat young athletes with surgery after first-time dislocation remains an area of controversy. Buss and colleagues[28] evaluated 30 athletes with shoulder instability over a 2-year period. Although nearly all returned to play, 37% had recurrent instability when treated nonoperatively. Another recent study demonstrated that primary arthroscopic stabilization may in fact be more cost effective than nonoperative management for first-time dislocation.[29] Risk factors for recurrence after arthroscopic stabilization include bone loss, fewer than 4 anchor points, and shoulder hyperlaxity.[20] Given that bone loss is a risk factor for recurrent instability, there is little room for nonoperative care in the athlete presenting with bone loss.

The options for nonsurgical management in the athlete with recurrent instability include rest, physical therapy/rehabilitation with an emphasis on rotator cuff and periscapular strengthening and dynamic stability, and bracing for competition. In-season bracing has been evaluated by Buss and colleagues[28] and is an option for some athletes, primarily based on their sport and position. In a cohort of 30 patients who were managed in season with a shoulder brace or harness for anterior instability, 26 were able to return to sports. Of these, 10 reported at least 1 episode of recurrence in the brace and 16 eventually required surgical stabilization at the completion of the season.

If immobilization and physical therapy is pursued, some evidence has suggested that doing so in external rotation can decrease recurrence rates.[30] Although the initial data on this approach offered some promise, the timeliness required to institute this intervention combined with difficulties with patient compliance have led to inferior results in duplicated studies of external-rotation bracing.

SURGICAL OPTIONS: GLENOID

Once the extent of bone loss has been quantified, the surgeon can help the athlete with an informed decision regarding treatment. Athletes with persistent instability and glenoid bone loss are in most situations indicated for surgery. The timing of this surgery is predicated on the athlete's sport, timing of injury within the season, and severity of bone loss. A discussion of expectations, risks, and benefits of various surgical options should happen after quantifying the degree of bone loss. Return to play can be variable and depends on the sport, as well as the procedure and associated rehabilitation.

On the glenoid side, patients can be generally grouped into those with less than 20% bone loss, those with 20% to 25% bone loss, and those with more than 25% bone loss who have taken on an inverted pear–shaped glenoid (see **Fig. 5**A). The latter group is largely thought to require bony augmentation procedures.

Arthroscopic Repair

Athletes presenting with isolated labral or glenoid rim injuries without prior stabilization attempts may be amenable to primary arthroscopic procedures. Generally speaking, those with 0% to 20% bone loss can undergo initial arthroscopic attempts at stabilization. Athletes with small, nonengaging Hill-Sachs lesions may also be managed arthroscopically. Arthroscopic procedures do offer the advantage of lack of violation of the subscapularis. Timing to surgery is important in these patients, as fragments can resorb.

Before incision, an examination under anesthesia is crucial to delineate the severity and direction of instability, followed by diagnostic arthroscopy. Portal placement should be carefully executed, typically including a standard posterior viewing portal and a low-placed anterior portal just over the superior border of the subscapularis tendon. An additional anterior portal can be used for suture passage, shuttling, and management. Some advocate for a trans-subscapularis portal to allow for anchor placement low on the anteroinferior glenoid, but in the authors' experience this is frequently not necessary. A variety of arthroscopic repair techniques have been described, including various suture constructs (single- vs double-loaded anchors, simple vs mattress suture configurations, tied vs knotless techniques) and order of repair (suture first, anchor first and so forth). These technical factors are likely predicated on surgeon preference, although it is generally accepted that a minimum of 3 anchors should be used for a standard anteroinferior repair, with additional anchors used as delineated by associated abnormalities and bone involvement.

Regardless of suture passer design, suture anchor type, or final repair construct, all must work to incorporate the bone fragment if one is present. When a bone fragment has been identified, proper preparation of the bony edge of the glenoid and anatomic reduction are critical factors in achieving successful healing.[7,20,31] Failures following arthroscopic Bankart repair are commonly a result of lack of appreciation of bony-defect reduction as well as excess capsular laxity.[8] In a recent level I study, Ahmed and colleagues[32] demonstrated that an engaging Hill-Sachs lesion, bone loss, and age at time of surgery were independent predictors of recurrence. In their study, Cole and colleagues[33] found no difference in the outcome of 63 patients treated with either open or arthroscopic repair, with all cases of recurrence noted in reinjury in contact sport or from a fall.

Techniques for addressing bony defects arthroscopically have been described, and can be useful in the management of an acute or chronic bony Bankart injury with a reparable fragment. In a recent study, Millet and colleagues[34] describe a novel arthroscopic approach to bony Bankart repair with dual-row anchor fixation that they term the bony Bankart bridge. These investigators followed a series of 15 patients longitudinally using their technique. Anchor placement was medial to the fracture site with sutures shuttled around the bony piece and subsequently secured with loadable anchors at the level of the joint surface. The investigators highlight the importance of placing an anchor inferior to the bony glenoid fragment to secure the inferior glenohumeral ligament complex, and advancing the capsuloligamentous repair in concert with reduction of the bony fragment.

Open Repair

Open Bankart repair with associated capsulorrhaphy, with bony Bankart fragment fixation if present, has long been considered the gold standard for management of shoulder instability, especially in the athletic population. Open stabilization is performed through a deltopectoral approach with subscapularis tenotomy and subsequent repair, or through a subscapularis split.

Open fixation of large bony fragments reaching 25% to 30% of the glenoid has achieved good results when performed acutely. Athletes with large bony defects, including large Hill-Sachs lesions, humeral avulsions of the glenohumeral ligament, and capsular deficiency may have lower recurrence rates if managed in an open fashion.

In addition, collision athletes have higher recurrence rates than other athletes, and may be better managed with open techniques.[35,36] Care must be taken with open procedures when performing an anatomic repair to avoid overtensioning of the anterior soft tissues. Boileau and colleagues[37] describe their results using the Neer modification (inclusion of a superoinferior capsular shift) of open Bankart repair in 64 patients, noting an increase in postoperative osteoarthritis at 25 months postoperatively as well as an average of 13° loss of external rotation.

Latarjet Coracoid Transfer

When isolated soft-tissue reconstruction is not a viable or predictable option, a bony augmentation procedure should be considered. In many settings, transfer of the coracoid process with the conjoint tendon, called the Latarjet procedure, has become the workhorse of bony augmentation procedures for patients presenting with bone loss greater than 20% to 25% (see **Fig. 5**B–D; **Fig. 6**). First developed by anatomist Michel Latarjet, many variations of this elegant procedure have evolved, including isolated coracoid transfer without soft tissue, and procedures leaving the soft-tissue attachments.

Carried out most commonly in the "beach-chair" position, a standard axillary incision and deltopectoral interval approach exposes the anterior aspect of the glenohumeral joint and coracoid process. The coracoid is osteotomized using a 90° oscillating saw at the intersection of the vertical and horizontal aspects to yield a graft of approximately 2.5 cm with the conjoint tendon attached. The pectoralis minor is released from the medial aspect of the harvested coracoids, and care is taken to localize and protect the musculocutaneous nerve and other neurovascular structures in the area. Fixation of the graft is best accomplished through a subscapularis split between the upper and lower halves of the muscle, with screw and washer fixation parallel to the glenoid face using 2 4.0-mm or 4.5-mm screws. Commercially available systems can be useful for graft harvest, preparation, and positioning, but attention must be paid to positioning the graft either flush with the glenoid joint line or slightly medial to it. Lateral overlap of the graft can lead to increased mechanical forces on the graft and potential failure of the transfer, as well as impingement of the humerus on the graft or hardware and associated pain. The graft can be positioned flat, with the posterior surface of the transferred coracoid adjacent to the anterior glenoid neck, or alternatively can be flipped 90° so that the posterior surface of the coracoid is parallel to the joint surface. This modification has been dubbed the "congruent arc" by De Beer, and may be a better option for grafts positioned intra-articularly or for larger bone defects. Once the graft has been secured, the anterior capsule is fixed to the transferred remnant of coracoacromial ligament, although some surgeons

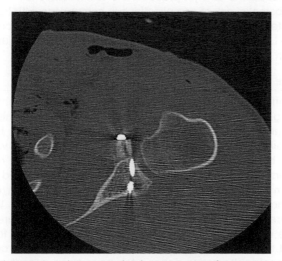

Fig. 6. Postoperative computed tomography demonstrating the trajectory of the screws parallel to the glenoid face.

prefer to use suture anchors for the capsular repair, thus rendering the graft completely extra-articular.

The Bristow procedure is analogous to the Latarjet transfer, although in the Bristow procedure the harvested coracoid fragment is smaller, is oriented differently, and is fixed using a solitary screw. In addition, some investigators have described arthroscopic techniques for Latarjet transfer, with some potential benefits.[38,39] Some proposed limitations to the arthroscopic Latarjet include technical complexity, the requirement for specific instrumentation, and increased surgical time and potential morbidity during the associated learning curve.

The Latarjet procedure has been proposed to confer stability in the setting of both glenoid, humeral, and combined bony deficiency, owing to 3 additional factors. First, the locally transferred coracoid autograft functions to extend the anterior face of the glenoid, providing greater surface area for contact. Additional dynamic stability can be provided by the so-called sling effect, created as the transferred conjoint tendon acts as a sling over the inferior portion of the subscapularis when the arm abducts and externally rotates. Finally, the repair of the anterior capsular tissue that can be affected by suturing the residual lateral anterior capsule to the retained stump of coracoacromial ligament adds additional static stability to the joint.

There are numerous studies demonstrating good to excellent clinical outcomes of the Latarjet procedure in the setting of bone loss. Burkhart and colleagues[40] reported a series of 47 modified Latarjet reconstructions with only a 4.9% recurrence rate noted. In their case series of 49 patients undergoing revision after failed instability surgery, Schmid and colleagues[41] reported no recurrent dislocations and 1 reported subluxation, with optimal graft placement related to better outcomes. In particular, grafts placed lateral to the rim had inferior outcomes in this series. In their prospective study, Hovelius and colleagues[42] reported long-term 15-year outcomes of 118 patients following Bristow-Latarjet, with a reported satisfaction rate of 98%, although these patients did demonstrate moderate to severe joint arthropathy with longer-term follow-up. These findings are reinforced by good to excellent results in another long-term study, compounding the evidence in favor of the Latarjet for extensive glenoid bone loss.[43]

Despite its success, the Latarjet procedure is technically challenging and carries with it a more substantial risk of complications in comparison with traditional arthroscopic or open stabilization. Recently, one center reported a 25% complication rate when performing Latarjet transfer, including infection, neurologic injury, and delayed union or nonunion of the transferred fragment.[44]

Autogenous Bone Graft

An alternative option to coracoid transfer for glenoid bone augmentation is autogenous iliac crest grafting. Called the Eden-Hybenette procedure, this option can be more useful in the management of larger glenoid-sided defects because of the increased availability of a more sizeable tricortical graft combined with the contour of the iliac crest bone graft (ICBG) and the biological properties of an autograft. Just as the undersurface of the coracoid is oriented to the glenoid face, the inner table of the ilium can also function as an extension of the rim of the glenoid. Intra-articular and extra-articular grafts have been described. Whereas some studies demonstrated significant arthrosis related to this procedure and recurrent instability, others have noted significant satisfaction at long-term follow-up.[16,45] It should be noted that while iliac crest is the most common source for structural grafts for the glenoid, alternative donor sites have been described, such as the distal clavicle.

Osteochondral Allograft

An alternative to the autogenous graft is a fresh or fresh-frozen osteochondral allo-graft. Allograft reconstruction carries the advantage of decreased surgical time, blood loss, and morbidity associated with autogenous graft harvest and coracoid transfer. In addition, despite all of the previously stated advantages, the Latarjet procedure results in a nonanatomic repair of the glenoid defect, nonanatomic capsular repair, and a lack of a traditional chondral surface in the region of the transferred coracoid graft.[24] By contrast, fresh osteochondral allograft confers the benefit of introduction of potentially viable cartilage matrix and chondrocytes into the area of glenoid bone loss. Osteo-chondral graft can be shaped from various described donor sites including fresh-frozen glenoid, humerus, and the distal tibial plafond. Proposed disadvantages associated with fresh osteochondral allografting include a potential increase in risk of infection and pathogen transmission, increased expense, limited graft availability, and less predictable graft healing and incorporation.

Distal tibia osteochondral allograft, in particular, has been the subject of recent in-terest and research (**Fig. 7**).[46,47] The architecture of the lateral aspect of the distal tibial plafond provides a reproducible articular surface for glenoid augmentation with sur-prisingly consistent congruence. Biomechanical studies have demonstrated that the dense subchondral bone in the weight-bearing distal tibia has characteristics superior to those of other commonly used grafts.[47]

The technique for distal tibia osteochondral graft augmentation is carried out in a fashion similar to that of a Latarjet procedure or autogenous ICBG. The anterior gle-noid is exposed through either a subscapularis split or tenotomy, the graft is con-toured to match the area of bone loss, and is subsequently fixed using 2 screws. It should be noted that this graft can also be used in patients with posterior glenoid defi-ciency.[48] Although this technique has been well described, there are currently no

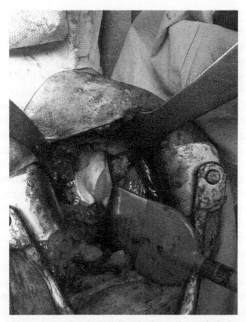

Fig. 7. Intraoperative photo demonstrating distal tibia allograft fashioned for glenoid bone augmentation.

published, peer-reviewed clinical outcomes available regarding the use of fresh osteochondral grafting.

SURGICAL OPTIONS: HUMERUS

Most cases of shoulder instability with bone loss can be successfully managed with a glenoid-based procedure. However, in certain situations humeral-sided procedures may be considered to provide reliable shoulder stability. The method by which glenoid-based procedures prevent engagement in the setting of advanced humeral-sided bone deficiency has been proposed to be secondary to the restoration of a more native glenoid diameter and normalization of the glenoid track.

Surgical options available for the management of humeral-sided bone loss include Hill-Sachs remplissage, autogenous or allograft resurfacing of a Hill-Sachs lesion, and Hill-Sachs disimpaction. Previously rotational osteotomy was advocated to rotate the defect outside of the range wherein engagement may occur, but this is no longer favored and certainly would be less optimal in the contact athlete. Reverse Hill-Sachs lesions can be managed similarly with inclusion of the modified McLaughlin procedure, with transfer of the lesser tuberosity and subscapularis insertion in this setting.

Regardless of the surgical technique, all procedures attempt to fill the humeral-sided defect. Of the clinical studies of patients with humeral head defects, more than 25% have been reported in small case series with improvement in clinical symptoms. There is currently no consensus on the critical size at which point humeral-sided reconstruction becomes necessary. In fact, Sekiya and colleagues[49] reported that defects as small as 12.5% of the humeral head may cause glenohumeral instability. Although it remains an option for humeral head bone loss in instability, complete and partial resurfacing of the humeral head is not generally an option for the athlete.

Humeral Head Bone Grafting

In certain scenarios, humeral-sided bone loss may be the sole lesion in recurrent instability without significant concomitant glenoid bone loss, although this is clearly a much less common occurrence. However, in this situation bone grafting of the humeral head has been described to restore the normal head architecture and prevent engagement. This decision depends on the location and size of the lesion. Typically, defects between 20% and 40% are needed to justify humeral-sided bone grafting.

Autograft options include ICBG, which can be fashioned to match the contour of the humeral head in the area of involvement. Fresh-frozen osteochondral allograft options including humeral head and other similarly shaped grafts can be used to fill measured defects. For the more common posterior lesion, the procedure is most commonly carried out using an open anterior deltopectoral approach. Exposure requires tenotomy of the upper half or entire subscapularis and extensive release of the capsule to expose the area of involvement. A posterior approach can be used as an alternative. Bulk grafts can be fixed with screws placed outside of the articular region or by using headless screws buried to the level of the subchondral bone. Alternatively, osteochondral plugs can be placed using a mosaicplasty technique.

Miniaci and Gish[50] demonstrated that patients with recurrent anterior instability or mechanical symptoms with an engaging Hill-Sachs lesion may be candidates for reconstruction. Diklic and colleagues[51] reported that 12 of 13 patients in their series had stable shoulders after undergoing fresh-frozen femoral head allograft for humeral head defects at more than 4 years postoperatively. Recently, Giles and colleagues[52] compared remplissage, allograft reconstruction, and partial resurfacing in a biomechanical study and demonstrated improved stability with all 3 techniques, with reduction in range of motion noted in the remplissage group. Reported complications include recurrent dislocation, graft collapse, and osteonecrosis.

Remplissage

Remplissage, translated from French as "to fill," is an arthroscopic procedure that has been advocated as an option for the management of moderately sized humeral defects. The procedure is an arthroscopic capsulotenodesis whereby the posterior capsule and overlying infraspinatus tendon is secured into a moderately sized Hill-Sachs lesion using 1 or multiple suture anchors. It can be coupled with Bankart repair when there is little glenoid-sided bone loss.

The technique is totally arthroscopic, and can be carried out in the beach-chair or lateral decubitus position. After management of the glenoid labral abnormality, the Hill-Sachs lesion is visualized and debrided to stimulate a healing response. One or more suture anchors are then placed through a posterior portal into the center or, ideally, medial aspect of the lesion. Sutures are passed through the posterior capsule and infraspinatus tendon using a bird-beak or suture shuttling device, and the repair is completed by securing the sutures in the subacromial space, thus filling the defect (**Fig. 8**).

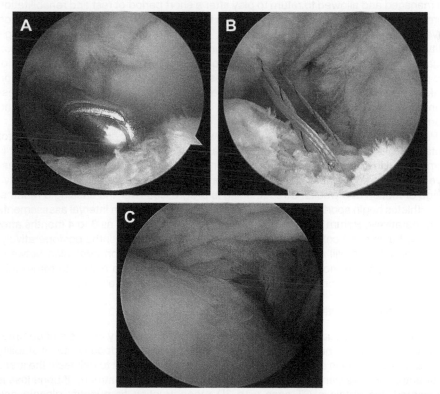

Fig. 8. Arthroscopic images demonstrate a large humeral head defect in a patient with an engaging Hill-Sachs lesion undergoing initial debridement (*A*), which is followed by anchor placement into the defect (*B*). The sutures are passed through the posterior capsule and infraspinatus to then "fill" the defect in the humeral head (*C*).

The effect of the remplissage procedure has been described as a check rein whereby the humeral lesion is obscured by both the interposed soft tissue and the translation anteriorly, and subsequent engagement is prevented because of the capsulotenodesis effect. Advantages of this procedure include limited morbidity associated with an all-arthroscopic procedure, ability to simultaneously manage concomitant glenoid-based abnormality, technical ease, and short surgical time. Several clinical studies have demonstrated that this technique does enhance stability in the setting of medium and large humeral defects. However, range of motion, particularly external rotation, can be potentially diminished after using this technique, which may be of concern for certain athletes.[52] Boileau and colleagues[53] performed a retrospective study of 459 patients undergoing Bankart repair plus remplissage for recurrent shoulder instability with a 2-year follow-up, and found a 7° to 8° loss of external rotation. In particular they noted that of 41 athletes in the group, 37 returned to their sport following the procedure. Franceschi and colleagues[54] performed a comparative study between two cohorts of patients, one undergoing arthroscopic Bankart repair and remplissage and the other isolated Bankart repair. New posttraumatic dislocations occurred in 5 patients, all in the Bankart-only group.

RETURN TO PLAY

As previously described, in-season athletes with acute shoulder instability can often be managed and allowed to return to play after a short period of rest and rehabilitation combined with the use of a shoulder harness if amenable. Such treatment depends on several factors including patient symptoms, pathology, sport, position, year of eligibility in collegiate athletes, and timing during the season. A pointed discussion regarding expectations should be carried out with the player, with involvement of the player's family, training staff, and coaches for a multifaceted approach to decision making. There are currently no studies that delineate the level of risk for injury progression or worsening severity with continued play, but this is of clear concern and warrants emphasis.

Published guidelines on return to play following arthroscopic or open procedures for instability with or without bone involvement are limited. In most centers, the patient is immobilized in a shoulder-abduction sling for the first 4 to 6 weeks after surgery. Passive motion is encouraged initially, being progressed to active assisted and active range of motion at 6 weeks. Strengthening is progressed over the ensuing 3 months, and athletes begin sport-specific exercises based on findings on interval assessments postoperatively. Return to play for some sports can be as early as 3 to 4 months after surgery, but in most collision athletes release is at around 6 months postoperatively. Overhead athletes will advance through a throwing progression beginning between the third and fourth month, and will often require 6 months to a year to return fully to sports, depending on their sport, position, and overall progression.

THE AUTHORS' PREFERRED APPROACH

The initial patient evaluation in the setting of traumatic instability consists of comprehensive history, examination, and plain films. In most cases of documented instability in an athlete, we obtain an MR image with intra-articular contrast to delineate the areas of structural involvement to most appropriately recommend treatment. If bone loss is suspected, we obtain a CT scan with 3D reconstruction to quantify glenoid and humeral involvement.

The management algorithm in the setting of glenohumeral instability with bone loss is well delineated in the literature, and we use a similar approach to the treatment of our patients. In the setting of limited bony involvement (isolated glenoid bone loss of <20%, no engaging humeral lesion), we routinely manage patients with an arthroscopic Bankart procedure using a minimum of 4 anchors. In patients with an acute or chronic reparable bony Bankart lesion, an open or, more commonly, arthroscopic stabilization is favored, using a dual-row suture anchor construct or screw fixation for larger fragments. In patients with advanced bone loss (glenoid loss >20%, combined glenoid and humeral involvement, or an engaging Hill-Sachs), we favor a Latarjet procedure in most circumstances. Fresh distal tibia osteochondral graft can be used as a primary option for larger defects with chondral involvement, or for scenarios when coracoid transfer is not an option, such as a concomitant coracoid fracture or revision for failed prior Latarjet. In patients with primary humeral bone loss, we most commonly use remplissage in concert with arthroscopic Bankart repair. In larger humeral defects, consideration is given to fresh allograft resurfacing or, in the older patient, prosthetic resurfacing or replacement.

REFERENCES

1. Hovelius L, Augustini BG, Fredin H, et al. Primary anterior dislocation of the shoulder in young patients. A ten-year prospective study. J Bone Joint Surg Am 1996;78(11):1677–84.
2. Owens BD, Agel J, Mountcastle SB, et al. Incidence of glenohumeral instability in collegiate athletics. Am J Sports Med 2009;37(9):1750–4.
3. Owens BD, Nelson BJ, Duffey ML, et al. Pathoanatomy of first-time, traumatic, anterior glenohumeral subluxation events. J Bone Joint Surg Am 2010;92(7): 1605–11.
4. Wang RY, Arciero RA. Treating the athlete with anterior shoulder instability. Clin Sports Med 2008;27(4):631–48.
5. Hovelius L, Saeboe M. Neer Award 2008: arthropathy after primary anterior shoulder dislocation—223 shoulders prospectively followed up for twenty-five years. J Shoulder Elbow Surg 2009;18(3):339–47.
6. Sachs RA, Lin D, Stone ML, et al. Can the need for future surgery for acute traumatic anterior shoulder dislocation be predicted? J Bone Joint Surg Am 2007; 89(8):1665–74.
7. Bigliani LU, Newton PM, Steinmann SP, et al. Glenoid rim lesions associated with recurrent anterior dislocation of the shoulder. Am J Sports Med 1998;26(1):41–5.
8. Burkhart SS, De Beer JF. Traumatic glenohumeral bone defects and their relationship to failure of arthroscopic Bankart repairs: significance of the inverted-pear glenoid and the humeral engaging Hill-Sachs lesion. Arthroscopy 2000; 16(7):677–94.
9. Cole BJ, Warner JJ. Arthroscopic versus open Bankart repair for traumatic anterior shoulder instability. Clin Sports Med 2000;19(1):19–48.
10. Piasecki DP, Verma NN, Romeo AA, et al. Glenoid bone deficiency in recurrent anterior shoulder instability: diagnosis and management. J Am Acad Orthop Surg 2009;17(8):482–93.
11. Sugaya H, Moriishi J, Dohi M, et al. Glenoid rim morphology in recurrent anterior glenohumeral instability. J Bone Joint Surg Am 2003;85(5):878–84.
12. Provencher MT, Frank RM, Leclere LE, et al. The Hill-Sachs lesion: diagnosis, classification, and management. J Am Acad Orthop Surg 2012;20(4):242–52.
13. Provencher MT, Ghodadra N, Romeo AA. Arthroscopic management of anterior instability: pearls, pitfalls, and lessons learned. Orthop Clin North Am 2010; 41(3):325–37.

14. Lo IK, Nonweiler B, Woolfrey M, et al. An evaluation of the apprehension, relocation, and surprise tests for anterior shoulder instability. Am J Sports Med 2004;32(2):301–7.

15. Urayama M, Itoi E, Sashi R, et al. Capsular elongation in shoulders with recurrent anterior dislocation. Quantitative assessment with magnetic resonance arthrography. Am J Sports Med 2003;31(1):64–7.

16. Warner JJ, Gill TJ, O'Hollerhan JD, et al. Anatomical glenoid reconstruction for recurrent anterior glenohumeral instability with glenoid deficiency using an autogenous tricortical iliac crest bone graft. Am J Sports Med 2006;34(2): 205–12.

17. Yamamoto N, Itoi E, Abe H, et al. Contact between the glenoid and the humeral head in abduction, external rotation, and horizontal extension: a new concept of glenoid track. J Shoulder Elbow Surg 2007;16(5):649–56.

18. Cameron KL, Mountcastle SB, Nelson BJ, et al. History of shoulder instability and subsequent injury during four years of follow-up: a survival analysis. J Bone Joint Surg Am 2013;95(5):439–45.

19. Stevens KJ, Preston BJ, Wallace WA, et al. CT imaging and three-dimensional reconstructions of shoulders with anterior glenohumeral instability. Clin Anat 1999;12(5):326–36.

20. Boileau P, Villalba M, Hery JY, et al. Risk factors for recurrence of shoulder instability after arthroscopic Bankart repair. J Bone Joint Surg Am 2006;88(8): 1755–63.

21. Itoi E, Lee SB, Berglund LJ, et al. The effect of a glenoid defect on anteroinferior stability of the shoulder after Bankart repair: a cadaveric study. J Bone Joint Surg Am 2000;82(1):35–46.

22. Huysmans PE, Haen PS, Kidd M, et al. The shape of the inferior part of the glenoid: a cadaveric study. J Shoulder Elbow Surg 2006;15(6):759–63.

23. Kwon YW, Powell KA, Yum JK, et al. Use of three-dimensional computed tomography for the analysis of the glenoid anatomy. J Shoulder Elbow Surg 2005; 14(1):85–90.

24. Provencher MT, Detterline AJ, Ghodadra N, et al. Measurement of glenoid bone loss: a comparison of measurement error between 45 degrees and 0 degrees bone loss models and with different posterior arthroscopy portal locations. Am J Sports Med 2008;36(6):1132–8.

25. Bois AJ, Fening SD, Polster J, et al. Quantifying glenoid bone loss in anterior shoulder instability: reliability and accuracy of 2-dimensional and 3-dimensional computed tomography measurement techniques. Am J Sports Med 2012; 40(11):2569–77.

26. Flatow EL, Miniaci A, Evans PJ, et al. Instability of the shoulder: complex problems and failed repairs: part II. Failed repairs. Instr Course Lect 1998;47: 113–25.

27. Freehill MQ, Harms DJ, Huber SM, et al. Poly-L-lactic acid tack synovitis after arthroscopic stabilization of the shoulder. Am J Sports Med 2003;31(5):643–7.

28. Buss DD, Lynch GP, Meyer CP, et al. Nonoperative management for in-season athletes with anterior shoulder instability. Am J Sports Med 2004;32(6):1430–3.

29. Crall TS, Bishop JA, Guttman D, et al. Cost-effectiveness analysis of primary arthroscopic stabilization versus nonoperative treatment for first-time anterior glenohumeral dislocations. Arthroscopy 2012;28(12):1755–65.

30. Itoi E, Hatakeyama Y, Sato T, et al. Immobilization in external rotation after shoulder dislocation reduces the risk of recurrence. A randomized controlled trial. J Bone Joint Surg Am 2007;89(10):2124–31.

31. Freedman KB, Smith AP, Romeo AA, et al. Open Bankart repair versus arthroscopic repair with transglenoid sutures or bioabsorbable tacks for recurrent anterior instability of the shoulder: a meta-analysis. Am J Sports Med 2004; 32(6):1520–7.

32. Ahmed I, Ashton F, Robinson CM. Arthroscopic Bankart repair and capsular shift for recurrent anterior shoulder instability: functional outcomes and identification of risk factors for recurrence. J Bone Joint Surg Am 2012;94(14): 1308–15.

33. Cole BJ, L'Insalata J, Irrgang J, et al. Comparison of arthroscopic and open anterior shoulder stabilization. A two to six-year follow-up study. J Bone Joint Surg Am 2000;82(8):1108–14.

34. Millett PJ, Horan MP, Martetschlager F. The "bony Bankart bridge" technique for restoration of anterior shoulder stability. Am J Sports Med 2013;41(3):608–14.

35. Rhee YG, Ha JH, Cho NS. Anterior shoulder stabilization in collision athletes: arthroscopic versus open Bankart repair. Am J Sports Med 2006;34(6):979–85.

36. Mazzocca AD, Brown FM Jr, Carreira DS, et al. Arthroscopic anterior shoulder stabilization of collision and contact athletes. Am J Sports Med 2005;33(1): 52–60.

37. Boileau P, Fourati E, Bicknell R. Neer modification of open Bankart procedure: what are the rates of recurrent instability, functional outcome, and arthritis? Clin Orthop Relat Res 2012;470(9):2554–60.

38. Lafosse L, Boyle S, Gutierrez-Aramberri M, et al. Arthroscopic Latarjet procedure. Orthop Clin North Am 2010;41(3):393–405.

39. Boileau P, Mercier N, Roussanne Y, et al. Arthroscopic Bankart-Bristow-Latarjet procedure: the development and early results of a safe and reproducible technique. Arthroscopy 2010;26(11):1434–50.

40. Burkhart SS, De Beer JF, Barth JR, et al. Results of modified Latarjet reconstruction in patients with anteroinferior instability and significant bone loss. Arthroscopy 2007;23(10):1033–41.

41. Schmid SL, Farshad M, Catanzaro S, et al. The Latarjet procedure for the treatment of recurrence of anterior instability of the shoulder after operative repair: a retrospective case series of forty-nine consecutive patients. J Bone Joint Surg Am 2012;94(11):e75.

42. Hovelius L, Sandstrom B, Sundgren K, et al. One hundred eighteen Bristow-Latarjet repairs for recurrent anterior dislocation of the shoulder prospectively followed for fifteen years: study I—clinical results. J Shoulder Elbow Surg 2004;13(5):509–16.

43. Schroder DT, Provencher MT, Mologne TS, et al. The modified Bristow procedure for anterior shoulder instability: 26-year outcomes in Naval Academy midshipmen. Am J Sports Med 2006;34(5):778–86.

44. Shah AA, Butler RB, Romanowski J, et al. Short-term complications of the Latarjet procedure. J Bone Joint Surg Am 2012;94(6):495–501.

45. Haaker RG, Eickhoff U, Klammer HL. Intraarticular autogenous bone grafting in recurrent shoulder dislocations. Mil Med 1993;158(3):164–9.

46. Provencher MT, LeClere LE, Ghodadra N, et al. Postsurgical glenohumeral anchor arthropathy treated with a fresh distal tibia allograft to the glenoid and a fresh allograft to the humeral head. J Shoulder Elbow Surg 2010; 19(6):e6–11.

47. Provencher MT, Ghodadra N, LeClere L, et al. Anatomic osteochondral glenoid reconstruction for recurrent glenohumeral instability with glenoid deficiency using a distal tibia allograft. Arthroscopy 2009;25(4):446–52.

48. Millett PJ, Schoenahl JY, Register B, et al. Reconstruction of posterior glenoid deficiency using distal tibial osteoarticular allograft. Knee Surg Sports Traumatol Arthrosc 2013;21(2):445–9.
49. Sekiya JK, Wickwire AC, Stehle JH, et al. Hill-Sachs defects and repair using osteoarticular allograft transplantation: biomechanical analysis using a joint compression model. Am J Sports Med 2009;37(12):2459–66.
50. Miniaci A, Gish M. Management of Anterior Glenohumeral Instability Associated with a Large Hill-Sachs Defect. Techniques in Shoulder and Elbow Surgery 2004;5(3):170–5.
51. Diklic ID, Ganic ZD, Blagojevic ZD, et al. Treatment of locked chronic posterior dislocation of the shoulder by reconstruction of the defect in the humeral head with an allograft. J Bone Joint Surg Br 2010;92(1):71–6.
52. Giles JW, Elkinson I, Ferreira LM, et al. Moderate to large engaging Hill-Sachs defects: an in vitro biomechanical comparison of the remplissage procedure, allograft humeral head reconstruction, and partial resurfacing arthroplasty. J Shoulder Elbow Surg 2012;21(9):1142–51.
53. Boileau P, O'Shea K, Vargas P, et al. Anatomical and functional results after arthroscopic Hill-Sachs remplissage. J Bone Joint Surg Am 2012;94(7):618–26.
54. Franceschi F, Papalia R, Rizzello G, et al. Remplissage repair—new frontiers in the prevention of recurrent shoulder instability: a 2-year follow-up comparative study. Am J Sports Med 2012;40(11):2462–9.

Pediatric and Adolescent Shoulder Instability

Matthew D. Milewski, MD[a,b,*], Carl W. Nissen, MD[a,b]

KEYWORDS

- Shoulder instability • Multidirectional instability • Arthroscopy • Pediatric
- Adolescent

KEY POINTS

- There is a high rate of recurrence after first-time shoulder instability in a young active population.
- Given the high risk of recurrent instability, young, active patients who seek to return to competitive contact sports should consider surgical stabilization after a first-time instability event.
- Multidirectional instability should be initially treated with conservative treatment.
- Traditional surgical options for shoulder instability utilized open techniques. Newer arthroscopic techniques may now approach the success rates of the traditional treatments options.

INTRODUCTION

Shoulder instability in young patients is a well-recognized spectrum of disease, from common traumatic anterior dislocations to recurrent multidirectional instability (MDI). In young adolescent or pediatric patients with open proximal humeral physes, shoulder instability was believed to be less common than physeal injury, but it may be more common than once believed.[1,2] Both traumatic and nontraumatic shoulder instability in young patients have been found to have a high rate of recurrence, and appropriate treatment is paramount in reducing the risk of recurrence and facilitating young patients' return to sports and other physical activities. The spectrum of shoulder instability seen in young athletes is discussed, including epidemiology, anatomy and biomechanical features, physical examination and imaging, and conservative and operative treatment strategies.

[a] Elite Sports Medicine, Connecticut Children's Medical Center, 399 Farmington Avenue, Farmington, CT 06032, USA; [b] University of Connecticut School of Medicine, Farmington, CT, USA
* Corresponding author. Elite Sports Medicine, Connecticut Children's Medical Center, 399 Farmington Avenue, Farmington, CT 06032.
E-mail address: mdmilewski@gmail.com

Clin Sports Med 32 (2013) 761–779
http://dx.doi.org/10.1016/j.csm.2013.07.010
0278-5919/13/$ – see front matter © 2013 Elsevier Inc. All rights reserved.

EPIDEMIOLOGY

Shoulder instability is common, with a rate of 11.2 per 100,000 person-years, as noted by Simonet and colleagues.[3] These investigators found younger male patients to be most frequently affected. In young ice hockey players, an incidence as high as 7% has been reported.[2,4] The classic study by Rowe[1] in 1956 reviewing 500 shoulder dislocations found that 20% of these dislocations occurred in patients between the ages of 10 and 20 years, but only 8 patients who were younger than 10 years had dislocations. Wagner and Lyne[5] found that 4.7% of the shoulder dislocations in their study occurred in children with open physes. More recent studies have estimated that up to 40% of shoulder instability events may occur in patients younger than 22 years.[2,6]

Perhaps more striking than the high incidence of first-time traumatic anterior shoulder stability is the high rate of recurrence of shoulder instability in young active patients. The rate of recurrence has been estimated to be between 60% and 100% in these patients.[1,4,5,7–10] Rowe[1] found the rate of recurrence in patients younger than 10 years to be 100%, and 94% if between 10 and 20 years of age. Wagner and Lyne[5] found an 80% rate of recurrence in 9 patients with open proximal humeral physes. Hovelius and colleagues[10] found a 60% recurrence rate in 12-year-old to 16-year-old patients. Deitch and colleagues[11] found a recurrence rate of 75% in 32 patients between the ages of 11 and 18 years. Lawton and colleagues[12] reviewed a cohort of 70 shoulders with instability, of which 67% received conservative treatment with physical therapy initially. These investigators found that 40% required surgical stabilization. Hovelius and colleagues[6,8] found 55% of patients younger than 22 years of age had 2 or more recurrences of instability at 5 year follow-up and 16% of these younger patients went on to have instability of the contralateral shoulder at 10 year follow-up. Postacchini and colleagues[13] found a recurrence rate of 92% in patients between the ages of 14 and 17 years after traumatic instability and a lower recurrence rate of 33% in patients 13 years old or younger, but their series had only 3 patients in this youngest age group.

The incidence and prevalence of MDI are difficult to estimate, given the spectrum of hyperlaxity and disease that might be present. Emery and Mullaji[14] examined 150 asymptomatic shoulders in patients between the ages of 13 and 18 years and found 57% of boys and 48% of girls had signs of shoulder instability using anterior drawer, posterior drawer, and sulcus tests. Although the incidence of MDI seems to be less than the incidence of traumatic anterior shoulder instability, MDI seems to have a higher incidence in overhead athletes, especially swimmers and gymnasts.[15,16]

ANATOMY AND BIOMECHANICS OF TRAUMATIC AND NONTRAUMATIC INSTABILITY IN YOUNG PATIENTS

The shoulder joint begins to form during the sixth week of gestation through different growth rates, known as the interzone.[17] At this early point, the glenoid lip is discernible and consists of dense fibrous and some elastic tissue, as opposed to fibrocartilaginous tissue of the knee meniscus. The shoulder capsule and the ligamentous thickenings are visible by the end of the eighth week, increasing in size only through development to adult proportions.[18] Variations in the final maturation of the glenoid and the capsulolabral tissues do exist but the effects on shoulder function and instability are not fully appreciated.

The anatomy of the shoulder and specifically the labrum and glenohumeral ligaments are well studied and variable. Although anatomists have documented the presence of the anterior ligamentous structures, it is the surgeons and arthroscopists who have refined these descriptions and allowed a better understanding in both the function and position of the capsular thickenings, which have led to modern concepts of treatment of shoulder instability. One such finding is the patulous inferior recess attached to the diminutive labrum seen in patients with significant joint laxity (**Fig. 1**). Although still present, the glenohumeral ligaments tighten only after significant rotation of the joint or translation of the humeral head has occurred. Often in these young, ligamentously lax patients, arthroscopic observation of the intra-articular space shows pristine, smooth articular cartilage, an endless-pool appearance of the labrum, and thin, almost translucent, shoulder capsules and the ability to sublux the humeral head over the anterior, inferior, and posterior labral edge. Addressing the diminutive labrum and the expansive capsule in these patients if multidirectional instability issues exist is visibly obvious and is discussed later. Although obvious, the need to create a labral bumper has not been established in the literature. The notion of creating a bumper to deepen the glenoid cavity and enhance the ability of glenohumeral compression to offer joint stability is mechanical founded. We believe from our experience that doing so is helpful and use this technique when treating patients with shoulder instability.

The presence of the inferior glenohumeral complex is also clearly shown arthroscopically. What is most apparent with regards to the inferior glenohumeral ligament (IGHL) is the reciprocal nature of the complex and its function as a hammock. The anterior portion fans out with external rotation and the posterior band of the IGHL becomes cordlike. When this appearance is lacking (or the opposite with internal rotation) during a diagnostic arthroscopy of patients with either unidirectional or multidirectional instability, addressing each of the aspects of a patient's disease is necessary.

HISTORY

Because there is such a wide spectrum of disease with shoulder instability in younger patients, the history and physical examination are paramount in understanding a particular young patient's disease and prognosis. Instability patterns are classically separated into either traumatic or atraumatic.

Traumatic dislocations occur after falls, altercations, motor or recreational vehicle accidents, or during sports events, particularly contact sports.[19] Owens and colleagues[20] found the highest rates of shoulder instability in football, wrestling, and

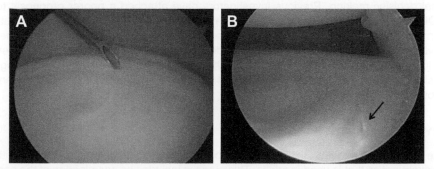

Fig. 1. (*A*) Arthroscopic image of inferior labrum viewed from posterior portal of diminutive labrum and patulous capsule in a patient with MDI. (*B*) Arthroscopic image of posterior labrum viewed from posterior portal with fraying (*arrow*) at labral-articular cartilage junction in a patient with MDI.

hockey. In the initial evaluation of the patient with shoulder instability, it is important to understand whether an underlying joint laxity was present before the first instability event or whether the instability issue followed a traumatic event. Also, it is important to note whether they required a formal reduction effort or not and where that occurred (eg, on the field or in the emergency department). Especially in younger patients, it can be difficult to understand the instability event if there was not a witnessed dislocation or necessary reduction. These younger patients may describe only intense shoulder pain, a dead arm feeling, or occasionally parasthesias in the distal upper extremity associated with subluxation or dislocation events.

Although anterior shoulder instability comprises 90% to 95% of shoulder instability, posterior shoulder instability can also be present. Posterior instability has been found in approximately 4% of all traumatic shoulder dislocations.[21] A good history can provide essential clues to the primary direction of instability. Pain in the abducted and externally rotated position, such as the overhead serving position for a racquet sport athlete or reaching overhead or with an outstretched arm for a pass in a basketball or football player, usually indicates anterior shoulder instability. Pain with internal rotation and pushing forward such as during a bench press maneuver, a football lineman in his blocking stance, or pushing open a heavy door may indicate posterior shoulder instability.

The symptoms of recurrent shoulder instability in the context of MDI in the young patient are even more vague. Atraumatic instability may occur during activities of daily living such as reaching overhead to get things from a shelf or during hair washing or grooming. Atraumatic instability can also occur during sporting events, particularly during noncontact sports such as overhead serving in racquet sports, during certain swimming strokes, or during weight-lifting activities. These patients describe occasional pain or mechanical symptoms, such as popping in the shoulder, which may be associated with particular overhead motions. A careful history for recurrent instability in other joints or in the family history may indicate a connective tissue disorder. History of connective tissue disorders such as Ehlers-Danlos syndrome changes the prognosis and potential treatment options for a young patient with recurrent shoulder instability.

Young patients with MDI usually do not require reduction maneuvers to reduce their shoulder dislocations. They may have pain with everyday activities, such as brushing their hair. Numbness in the hand while carrying heavier objects may indicate inferior shoulder subluxation.[22] Even in the setting of MDI, it is important to know which direction of subluxation seems to dominate, because this can affect surgical and nonsurgical decision making. Previous investigators have attached a poorer prognosis to MDI with a voluntary component.[23,24] These investigators have discussed poorer outcomes in patients with MDI secondary to seizure disorders, electrocution, and other psychological and medical conditions. Pediatric and adolescent patients have been included in these groups and collectively have been deemed to have poorer prognosis. However, the adolescent with MDI with or without a voluntary component should probably be viewed separately and, in our opinion, has a better prognosis.

PHYSICAL EXAMINATION

The physical examination for the younger patient with shoulder instability starts with an examination that is used in adults. This process includes an examination of the cervical spine and a scapular examination for signs of more central nerve causes of shoulder weakness and pain. Although cervical spine issues are less common in young healthy pediatric and adolescent patients, scapular winging is not uncommon in these patients and is caused by nerve dysfunction or injury along with muscle weakness, imbalance, and dyskinesia. Similarly, a careful neurovascular examination of the brachial plexus and specially the axillary nerve is important, because injury to this nerve is reported in 5% to 35% of fractures and dislocations.[25]

All patients with traumatic shoulder pain with presumed open physes should be evaluated for proximal humeral physeal injuries. Deformity of the shoulder girdle in this age group is not universally a dislocation. We recommend radiographic evaluation before any reduction maneuvers for shoulder instability, especially in prepubescent patients. Range of motion and strength should be tested bilaterally in all patients with a suspected traumatic shoulder injury. This strategy should include testing sensory perceptions and strength in axillary, musculocutaneous, ulnar, radial, and median nerve distributions. Proximally, the cervical spine should be examined for tenderness and range of motion. Spurling sign should also be assessed in patients able to comply with the test.

There are a variety of provocative maneuvers to test shoulder instability. These maneuvers include the anterior apprehension test, Jobe relocation test, anterior and posterior load-and-shift tests, Kim posterior jerk test, hyperabduction test, and the sulcus sign.[26] The anterior and posterior load-and-shift tests are generally performed with the patient supine to stabilize the scapula. The load-and-shift tests involve placing the arm in 20° of abduction and forward flexion, matching the plane of the scapular body and grading the amount of translation of the humeral head. Grade 1 translation is consistent with translation to the glenoid rim but not dislocating. Grade 2 translation is consistent with dislocation over the glenoid rim, but with spontaneous reduction when the force is removed. Grade 3 translation is consistent with dislocation either anteriorly or posteriorly without spontaneous reduction. The Kim posterior jerk test for posterior instability involves placing the affected arm at 90° of abduction, when the examiner holds the arm and elbow and applies an axial loading force. The arm is then elevated 45° while maintaining axial force that pushes the humeral head posteriorly and the result is considered positive if posterior pain or a palpable clunk is felt.[27] Hyperlaxity and inferior instability can be tested with the sulcus sign. Downward traction is applied to the arm, and if a dimple is seen or palpated between the lateral acromion and the humeral head, the test is considered positive. Humeral head displacement greater than 2 cm or the presence of the sulcus sign with the arm in 90° of abduction is considered to indicate a higher degree of inferior capsular laxity (**Figs. 2**A, B and **3**).[26,28,29] Gagey and Gagey[30] developed the hyperabduction test to evaluate for IGHL laxity. Passive glenohumeral abduction past 105° is considered to indicate inferior laxity.

All young patients with suspected glenohumeral instability should be evaluated for generalized hyperlaxity. The Beighton-Horan scale for joint hyperlaxity combines increased laxity at various joints, including the hand, elbow, knee, and trunk (**Table 1**). A score equal or greater than 4 on a 9-point scale is considered diagnostic for hyperlaxity. Borsa and colleagues[31] found that women are more likely to have hyperlaxity and anterior glenohumeral joint laxity than men.

IMAGING

Evaluation of a young patient with suspected shoulder instability includes a standard trauma series of radiographs with orthogonal views. This strategy is particularly important in the young patient with open physes, because of the risk of proximal humeral physeal fractures mimicking an anteriorly dislocated proximal humerus. A nontraumatic shoulder radiographic series includes an anterioposterior, scapular Y, and

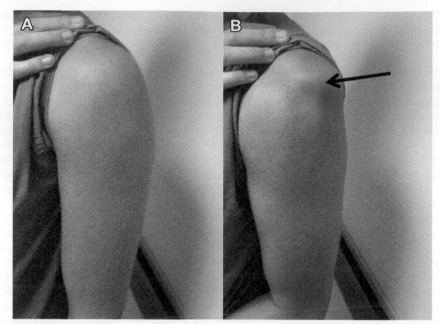

Fig. 2. Female with multidirectional instability. (*A*) Patient at rest. (*B*) Patient after voluntary anterior and inferior subluxation. Note anterior skin dimpling below the acromion (black arrow).

axillary view. If the young patient is too uncomfortable to comply with the arm positioning for a standard axillary view to confirm glenohumeral reduction, a Velpeau view may be performed. This view is typically performed with the arm at the side in a position of comfort with the patient leaning backwards over the radiograph plate and the beam angled straight downward. The West Point view is useful in suspected acute or recurrent shoulder instability, because it can best visualize the anterior glenoid rim.[32]

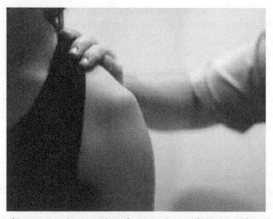

Fig. 3. Sulcus sign. (*From* Curtis RJ. Glenohumeral instability in the child. In: DeLee JC, Drez DJ, Miller MD, editors. Delee & Drez's orthopedic sports medicine. vol. 1. Philadelphia: Saunders/Elsevier; 2010; with permission.)

Table 1 Beighton-Horan joint hypermobility scoring system: a score of greater or equal to 4 out of a possible 9 points usually indicates generalized hypermobility		
Small finger	Dorsiflex the fifth metacarpophalangeal joint to at least 90°	1 point for each side (left/right)
Thumb	Oppose the thumb to volar aspect of the ipsilateral forearm	1 point for each side (left/right)
Elbow	Hyperextend the elbow to at least 10°	1 point for each side (left/right)
Knee	Hyperextend the knee to at least 10°	1 point for each side (left/right)
Trunk/hip	Place both hands flat on the floor with the knees fully extended	1 point

Data from Beighton P, Horan F. Orthopedic aspects of the Ehlers-Danlos syndrome. J Bone Joint Surg Br 1969;51(3):444–53.

Once a proximal humerus fracture is ruled out and glenohumeral reduction is confirmed, imaging of the young patient with suspected glenohumeral instability often includes magnetic resonance imaging (MRI). As in adults, the addition of intra-articular contrast is often recommended to improve the diagnostic ability of MRI in diagnosing labral disease. However, in the acute setting, intra-articular contrast is provided by the blood within the joint. Anterior instability in the young patient is often accompanied by a Bankart lesion or tear, an anterior labral periosteal sleeve avulsion lesion, or more infrequently, but important to identify on preoperative imaging, a humeral avulsion of the glenohumeral ligament (HAGL) lesion. Glenoid or humeral-sided bone loss or deformity (ie, bony Bankart lesions, glenoid fractures, inverted pear glenoid morphology, and Hill-Sachs deformities) can often be identified on radiographs or MRI but occasionally require evaluation by computed tomography (CT). Recent studies have shown that MRI can accurately assess glenoid bone loss when compared with CT scan with or without three-dimensional reconstructions.[33,34]

Imaging of the shoulder in patients with suspected MDI can be challenging to interpret, because the signs of instability that often accompany acute traumatic shoulder instability, such as labral, capsular, or ligamentous tears, are usually not present. Several imaging findings can be helpful in evaluating the patient with suspected MDI, although it is especially important in these patients to put the imaging findings in the appropriate clinical context with their history and physical examination findings. Dewing and colleagues[35] found a patulous capsule, increased glenohumeral volume, and labral abnormalities on MR arthrography in patients with MDI. Kim and colleagues[36] found increased rotator interval dimensions in patients with MDI. However, Provencher and colleagues[37] found no significant differences in MRI findings of patients with MDI when compared with adult controls, showing the importance of making the diagnosis of MDI based on history and physical examination findings.

TREATMENT AND OUTCOMES
Acute Management of a Shoulder Dislocation in a Young Athlete

Many providers of sports medicine are faced with the issue of a young patient with a suspected shoulder dislocation seen on the field of play. Although in older, skeletally mature patients, it is reasonable to consider on-field reduction maneuvers if the provider is comfortable and trained in these techniques, in the young patient with open physes, we recommend that the provider at a minimum should consider appropriate radiographic imaging before reduction attempts to evaluate for a proximal humeral physeal fracture.[38] Once a physeal fracture is ruled out or considered to be of low probability, several reduction maneuvers are possible. These maneuvers include traction-countertraction, Stimson maneuver, and abduction maneuvers.[38] Adequate sedation is recommended in the young patient both for patient comfort and also to reduce the amount of traction or force needed for reduction in this population in order to minimize further risk to the proximal humeral physis.

Nonoperative Conservative Treatment of Pediatric/Adolescent Anterior Shoulder Instability

Once glenohumeral reduction has been achieved, there are both conservative and operative treatment options for the management of the pediatric or adolescent patient with a first-time or recurrent traumatic anterior shoulder instability. Conservative treatment may include an initial period of sling or shoulder immobilizer use, followed by activity modification and physical therapy for range of motion and strengthening. Return to play is often allowed once painless full range of motion and normal, protective strength is achieved. Shoulder harness bracing is often used for young football players, or other contact athletes such as hockey and lacrosse players, who seek to return to play during the same season in which the instability has begun. The option to return to play with an unstable shoulder requires a full understanding by both the player and their parents; a player may also have to play in a position that can accommodate the restrictions of the brace (ie, limited overhead or abducted shoulder positioning). Physical therapy protocols designed for the rehabilitation of anterior shoulder instability treated nonoperatively focus primarily on scapular stabilization, with rotator cuff strengthening being added in the later stages of the process.

The main complication associated with conservative management of traumatic first-time anterior shoulder instability is the risk of recurrent instability. This risk is significant and although one study found this risk to be 21%,[39] most reports document this risk to be 60% or greater.[1,5,7,8,11,13,40]

Cordischi and colleagues[39] followed 14 patients between the ages of 10.9 and 13.1 years for an average of 3.4 years after a primary anterior shoulder dislocation and found 3 patients to have recurrent instability. Recurrent instability was associated with a HAGL lesion in all 3 cases and no patient had evidence of a discrete labral tear on MRI. Western Ontario Shoulder Instability Index scores were found to be better in the nonoperative group in this small series.

Other studies have found a higher rate of recurrent instability after conservative treatment of anterior shoulder instability in young patients. In 1956, Rowe[1] found a 100% risk of recurrent instability in children younger than 10 years. The risk was 94% in adolescents between 10 and 20 years of age. Wagner and Lyne[5] found an 80% recurrence rate in 10 adolescent shoulders between 12 and 16 years of age. Marans and colleagues[7] found a 100% recurrence rate with an average of 5 recurrent instability events in 21 pediatric and adolescent patients between 4 and 16 years of age. Postacchini and colleagues[13] found an 86% recurrence rate in adolescents between 12 and 17 years of age. The rate of recurrence was 92% for adolescents between 14 and 17 years of age but only 33% in patients younger than 13 years. Deitch and colleagues[11] found a 75% recurrence rate in 32 adolescents between the ages of 11 and 18 years. Echoing the findings of Postacchini and colleagues,[13] 8 of 15 patients (53%) with open humeral physes had recurrent instability, whereas 15 of 17 patients (88%) with closed humeral physes had recurrent instability. The high rate of recurrence in adolescents with shoulder instability is similar to the rates observed in late adolescents/collegiate-age athletes/military recruits seen in other studies.[4,41] It is still unclear whether the rate of recurrence is as high in younger adolescent and prepubescent children. If the rate of recurrence in this younger population is lower, as some investigators have suggested, it might be hypothesized that younger children and their families might be more willing to modify activities, especially avoiding contact sports. This hypothesis is similar to the findings by Postacchini and colleagues[13] that children younger than 13 years had a lower dislocation rate. However, that study had a small cohort of this youngest group of patients with traumatic dislocations. Further studies need to evaluate whether younger and older adolescents in larger cohorts have different rates of recurrence and seek to identify possible causes.

Nonoperative Conservative Treatment of Pediatric/Adolescent Multidirectional Shoulder Instability

One of the classic tenants of shoulder instability treatment is AMBRI, which refers to atraumatic, MDI, which is often bilateral, with treatment beginning with rehabilitation and if that fails, consideration for inferior capsular shift. Most sports medicine providers consider physical therapy and rehabilitation the first-line treatment of MDI. Burkhead and Rockwood[42] classically described good or excellent results with rehabilitation for 80% of patients with atraumatic instability. Takwale and colleagues[43] described 90% good results with specialized physical therapy for involuntary positional instability, which they described as "instability caused by an abnormal unbalanced muscle action which is involuntary and ingrained," which usually involves adolescent patients with posterior instability. Kuroda and colleagues[44] studied more than 300 patients with atraumatic shoulder instability and advocated following these patients for several years with conservative treatment. These investigators noted spontaneous recovery of stability in 50 of 450 shoulders (9%) and that spontaneous recovery was statistically more likely if patients were willing to switch to nonoverhead athletics. It is not clear if these patients still had symptoms but avoided frank instability because of activity modification. Misamore and colleagues[45] followed 64 patients with MDI with an average age of 16 years and found at 2 years follow-up that 34% had elected for surgery. Approximately half of the remaining patients had pain relief and graded their shoulders as having good or excellent stability. At mean 8-year follow-up, 78% of patients who had not undergone surgery reported persistent problems with their shoulders, and only 22% were symptom free. Conservative treatment of MDI can improve a patient's shoulder function and provide good or excellent results in many young patients. However, there are some patients for whom this treatment course may not fully restore stability or provide complete pain relief. In general, some investigators have recommended at least 6 months of physical therapy and conservative treatment of MDI of the shoulder in young athletes.

Operative Treatment of Pediatric/Adolescent Anterior Shoulder Instability

Operative intervention is advocated for recurrent instability after traumatic anterior shoulder dislocations in young patients. It has also been advocated for some young patients in high-risk sports or activities as the primary treatment after a first-time shoulder instability event. The classic studies by DeBernadino and colleagues[46] and Owens and colleagues[47] showed excellent subjective function and return to sport, with a redislocation rate of 14.3% at longest follow-up after arthroscopic Bankart repair after first-time traumatic instability in young active patients. However, these patients were collegiate-aged military academy students, and this patient population might be different than a younger adolescent population. A few studies have specifically examined the results of surgical stabilization for traumatic anterior shoulder instability in pediatric and adolescent patients.[5,7,11–13,48–51] Wagner and Lyne[5] reported on 7 shoulders in patients between 12 and 16 years of age who required surgical stabilization using open techniques between 1965 and 1979. These investigators reported no recurrence after surgery using older techniques such as Magnuson-Stack or Bristow procedures, which have since fallen out of favor for the treatment of primary shoulder instability. In 1992, Marans and colleagues[7] reported on 13 patients who were an average of 13 years old who underwent open anterior stabilization procedures, including Bankart repair, Putti-Platt procedure, capsular shift, and Bristow procedure. One recurrent instability event (8% recurrence) was reported after surgery in a patient who had a Bristow procedure, and this patient underwent a revision with a Putti-Platt procedure. Postacchini and colleagues[13] and Lawton and colleagues[12] reported on pediatric and adolescents treated with open surgical stabilization, and only 1 patient had recurrent instability after surgical stabilization. Deitch and colleagues[11] reported a higher rate (31%) of recurrence of instability after surgical stabilization but did not report on the specific surgical procedures performed in this cohort.

Newer studies have examined arthroscopic treatment of traumatic shoulder instability in pediatric and adolescent populations. Mazzocca and colleagues[48] examined a late adolescent population between 14 and 20 years of age who were contact and collision athletes and treated with arthroscopic anterior shoulder stabilization. These investigators reported a low recurrence rate of 11%, and all of their athletes were able to return to organized high-school or collegiate sports. Kraus and colleagues[50] reported on a series of 6 patients with an average age of 12 years old, in whom 5 of 6 cases were treated with arthroscopic stabilization. There were no recurrences at average 26-month follow-up and excellent Constant and Rowe scores. Jones and colleagues[49] reported on 32 anterior arthroscopic Bankart repairs in 30 patients treated at Children's Hospital of Philadelphia. Half of the patients had failed initial nonoperative management and half had primary surgical stabilization. The average age of the patients was 15 years, ranged between 11 and 18 years. Overall, there was a 15.6% rate of recurrence after surgery. Single Assessment Numeric Evaluation (SANE) scores were similar between groups treated with initial conservative treatment and initial surgical treatment at follow-up. Castagna and colleagues[51] reviewed their results of arthroscopic stabilization in adolescent athletes aged 13 to 18 years who played overhead or contact sports. These investigators found that 81% of their patients were able to return to their preinjury sport, and the remaining 19% were able to return to sport but at a lower level secondary to their shoulder. A recurrence rate of 21% was found overall, but this was significantly higher in athletes participating in water polo (40%) and rugby (33.3%).

Overall, arthroscopic stabilization for traumatic anterior shoulder instability seems to be an effective treatment in younger populations, with recurrence rates that approach the rates seen in collegiate-age populations. Primary surgical treatment after first-time traumatic anterior shoulder instability may be considered in adolescent patients, given the risk of recurrence in these younger populations, and if patients and their families are unable or unwilling to modify the child's activities and sports.

Operative Treatment of Pediatric/Adolescent Multidirectional Shoulder Instability

Operative treatment of MDI can be considered in young patients who have failed conservative treatment, including activity modification, physical therapy for strengthening, and scapular stabilization, and who continue to have pain and instability in their shoulders that interferes with their daily living or sports. Activity modification should be encouraged in this population as part of the initial conservative management. Operative intervention historically was considered a contraindication in patients with voluntary instability. We agree that these individuals require more intensive preoperative discussions and explanations as well as more structured postoperative management. However, we do not believe that this group should be viewed differently from other young patients with shoulder instability, apart from the issues mentioned. These issues are also important to consider before surgery in patients with connective tissue disorders and global ligamentous laxity.[52]

Traditional operative treatment of MDI of the shoulder involved open inferior capsular shift, as described by Neer and Foster.[28] These investigators reported satisfactory results in 39 of 40 patients. Other investigators have described good results with open inferior capsular shift for the treatment of MDI.[53–58] The rate of recurrent instability postoperatively varies from 4% to 26%. In Hamada and colleagues' series,[55] which had the highest recurrence rate of 26%, two-thirds of their recurrences occurred in patients with voluntary subluxation (50% of patients with voluntary subluxation recurred), and eliminating these patients brought their recurrence down to 14%.

Patients were able to return to sport postoperatively between 75% and 100% of the time, but Choi and Ogilvie-Harris[57] did note that only 17% of patients who underwent bilateral inferior capsular shifts were able to return to sport, and Altchek and colleagues[53] stated that throwing athletes noted decreased velocity postoperatively.

As improvements and closer examination of the success of older stabilization procedures occur, technique modifications to Neer and Foster's original description have been described. A subscapularis splitting technique has been described to eliminate the need to detach and reattach the subscapularis tendon.[58] In addition, a glenoid-based T-plasty modification has also been described by Altchek and colleagues.[53] Reduction in capsular volume has been considered crucial to the success of the procedure and is proportional to the amount of capsular shift.[59]

As the treatment of traumatic shoulder instability has gravitated toward arthroscopic techniques, so has the operative treatment of MDI. Advantages of arthroscopic treatment include the ability to address anterior, inferior, and particularly posterior disease at the same time and close the rotator interval if deemed necessary.[60,61] Initial investigations into arthroscopic treatment of MDI used thermal capsulorrhaphy and showed good results.[62,63] However, this technique has fallen out of favor and is no longer recommended given the concerns over thermal-induced chondrolysis.[64–66]

Multiple series have shown good results with arthroscopic treatment of MDI of the shoulder.[61,67–70] Recurrence rates are reported to be between 2% and 12%, and subjective outcome scores report satisfactory results after 88% to 97% of procedures. Baker and colleagues[70] reported that 86% of their patients were able to return to sports, with 65% returning to the same level as previously. The ability to tighten the capsule and attach it to a solid labrum or to fix the redundant capsular tissue to the glenoid rim via a suture anchor technique with newer techniques and equipment have greatly improved the ability to address all aspects of capsular laxity of patients with MDI. This improvement, as mentioned, allows the surgeon to not only reduce capsular volume but to do so selectively to reflect variations in that laxity.

One of the specific improvements in surgical technique that has occurred with the change to arthroscopic techniques is the ability to address the rotator cuff interval. Although the closure of the rotator interval remains a controversial portion of arthroscopic management of glenohumeral instability, the addition of a closure in selected patients is important and can improve outcomes. Harryman and colleagues[71] initially showed that in vitro imbrication to the rotator interval capsule resisted inferior and posterior translation. Others[72,73] have shown that rotator interval closure may not affect posterior stability but can affect anterior stability. However, not all unstable shoulders (traumatic or atraumatic) should have the rotator cuff interval closed routinely, because that closure may restrict external rotation.[72,74–76]

Outcomes after arthroscopic treatment of MDI seem to show equivalent results with open procedures in adolescent populations. In addition, although many series examining MDI operative treatment include adolescent patients, there are no series to our knowledge studying an exclusively pediatric or adolescent patient population treated with surgical intervention for MDI. As surgical techniques evolve to treat this complicated spectrum of shoulder disease, our subjective and objective outcomes measures also need to evolve. Although judging success based on recurrence rate is certainly an important component to the outcome after these procedures, further refinement of subjective outcomes aimed especially at pediatric or adolescent populations is needed.

OUR PREFERRED TECHNIQUES

Our preferred treatment of pediatric or adolescent patients who have failed conservative treatment of traumatic or MDI is arthroscopic labral repair and capsulorrhaphy using suture anchor fixation. We use lateral decubitus positioning with an adjustable arm holder (Spider arm positioner, Smith & Nephew, Memphis, TN) for arthroscopic shoulder instability surgery (**Figs. 4** and **5**). After examination under anesthesia and diagnostic arthroscopy to document the extent and directions of instability and labral/capsular disease, 4 portals are established (standard posterior viewing, posteroinferior, anterosuperior, and anteroinferior portals). The proper placement of these portals cannot be overemphasized. During the placement of each portal, the ability to maneuver within the joint to access all aspects of the joint is imperative and should be checked. Moving or creating additional portals is not common but should be performed if better accessibility is needed. We have found that slight modifications of the portal placement, especially posteriorly, make the procedure technically easier. The first of these changes is moving the posterosuperior portal more lateral. Traditionally, this portal has been placed inferior and medial to the posterolateral corner of the acromion. We believe that this is an appropriate portal for rotator cuff surgery and other procedures when performing surgery in the beach chair position. However, in the lateral decubitus position, this portal needs to be slightly inferior and as lateral

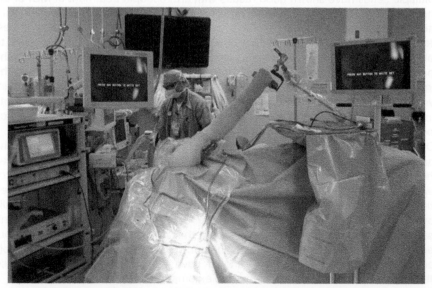

Fig. 4. Lateral decubitus positioning for right shoulder arthroscopy (side view). Note the use of Spider arm positioner (Smith & Nephew, Memphis, TN).

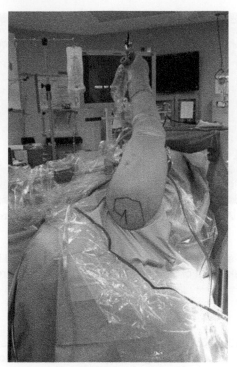

Fig. 5. Lateral decubitus positioning for right shoulder arthroscopy (overhead view). Note the use of Spider arm positioner (Smith & Nephew, Memphis, TN).

as possible when referenced to the posterolateral corner of the acromion. This strategy allows us to gain an angle down onto the posterosuperior labrum, making this a working portal as well as a viewing portal.

The next 3 portals are made under direct visualization with the use of an 18-gauge spinal locator needle. The anterosuperior portal is placed above the biceps initially. During the case, it is slipped below the biceps. This procedure gives us the greatest possible separation between the 2 anterior portals and allows more ease of functioning. The anteroinferior portal is placed just superior to the subscapularis tendon and is angled inferiorly. To be sure that this placement is achieved, when using the locator needle, after the needle is in place, we let go of the needle. If it remains directed inferior, then we believe that it is appropriately placed. However, if the needle direction shifts superiorly after we let go, we re-establish the skin surface position to allow a better untethered angle. The posteroinferior portal is placed as inferiorly as we can. This strategy establishes the greatest separation between the posterior portals, as performed anteriorly, and allows us to use this inferior portal for inferior suture anchor placement and inferior capsular plication (**Fig. 6**).

Adequate mobilization of labral and capsular tissue from the glenoid rim is necessary for appropriate tensioning and providing a bleeding base to allow for healing. For both anterior and posterior lesions or combined lesions, capsulorrhaphy, suture, and suture anchors are placed inferiorly first and capsulolabral tissue is advanced to the glenoid rim using a suture passer (Accu-Pass suture shuttles, Smith & Nephew, Memphis, TN) (**Fig. 7**). This step is repeated as the repair and capsulorrhaphy is

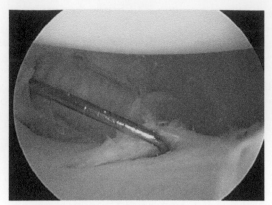

Fig. 6. Bankart lesion. Arthroscopic view of right shoulder from posterior portal.

advanced superiorly either anteriorly or posteriorly as the labral bumper is restored. The arm should be taken out of traction at the conclusion of the repair to test stability in all directions.

REHABILITATION

Rehabilitation after arthroscopic anterior stabilization for anterior shoulder instability or pancapsular capsulorrhaphy for MDI generally begins with a period of immobilization. We generally use an Ultra-sling (DonJoy, Vista, CA) for 6 weeks postoperatively or until normal range of motion is achieved, whichever comes last. Initial rehabilitation centers around maintaining finger, wrist, and elbow motion. Isometric periscapular muscle activation is also begun in the first weeks to assist the early discomfort and smoother transition to advancing stages of rehabilitation. Range of motion activities begins with physical therapy and home exercise programs, including pendulum exercises, table slides, and wall pulleys. Isometric shoulder exercises are begun in weeks 2 to 4 and are advanced to isotonic exercises in weeks 4 to 8. Rotator cuff and scapular strengthening is begun once the sling has been discontinued and range of motion has been restored. Stationary bicycle and elliptical use without use of the arms are allowed

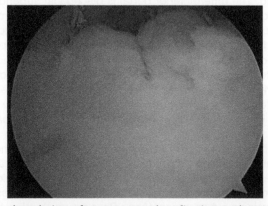

Fig. 7. Anterior Bankart lesion after suture anchor fixation and capsulorrhaphy. (Right shoulder viewed from posterior portal). Note restoration of bumper anteriorly.

before sling discontinuation. After the sling has been discontinued, jogging and running are allowed. At this point, rehabilitation shifts to more strengthening and plyometric exercises. After 3 months and once full range of motion as well as near normal strength have been achieved, we initiate sport-specific training. Isokinetic strength testing of shoulder internal and external rotators, along with endurance and power testing of the upper extremity is performed before return to sport, which is generally at the 4-month postoperative point. Return to sports is predicated by achieving these rehabilitative milestones as well as the specific sport that is being played. Noncontact, nonoverhead sports are possible often by the 4-month mark. Contact sports are generally not allowed before 6 months postoperatively. Overhead sports also are allowed at the 6-month mark, although we normally initiate a tossing or interval-throwing program at 4 months.

Rehabilitation after pancapsular procedures for MDI may be progressed more slowly given the extent of instability, amount of capsular shift needed, and often poor quality of soft tissue in these cases.

SUMMARY

Instability of the shoulder is a common issue faced by sports medicine providers caring for pediatric and adolescent patients. A thorough history and physical examination can help distinguish traumatic instability from multidirectional or voluntary instability. A systematic understanding of the relevant imaging characteristics and individual patient disease and goals can help guide initial treatment. Given the high risk of recurrent instability, young, active patients who seek to return to competitive contact sports should consider arthroscopic stabilization after a first-time instability event. MDI should be treated initially with conservative rehabilitation. Patients who fail extensive conservative treatment may benefit from surgical stabilization. Arthroscopic techniques may now approach the results found from traditional open capsular shift procedures. Future studies should be designed to examine the outcomes in solely pediatric and adolescent populations after both conservative and operative treatment of shoulder instability.

REFERENCES

1. Rowe CR. Prognosis in dislocations of the shoulder. J Bone Joint Surg Am 1956; 38(5):957–77.
2. Cleeman E, Flatow EL. Shoulder dislocations in the young patient. Orthop Clin North Am 2000;31(2):217–29.
3. Simonet WT, Melton LJ 3rd, Cofield RH, et al. Incidence of anterior shoulder dislocation in Olmsted County, Minnesota. Clin Orthop Relat Res 1984;(186): 186–91.
4. Hovelius L. Shoulder dislocation in Swedish ice hockey players. Am J Sports Med 1978;6(6):373–7.
5. Wagner KT Jr, Lyne ED. Adolescent traumatic dislocations of the shoulder with open epiphyses. J Pediatr Orthop 1983;3(1):61–2.
6. Hovelius L, Augustini BG, Fredin H, et al. Primary anterior dislocation of the shoulder in young patients. A ten-year prospective study. J Bone Joint Surg Am 1996;78(11):1677–84.
7. Marans HJ, Angel KR, Schemitsch EH, et al. The fate of traumatic anterior dislocation of the shoulder in children. J Bone Joint Surg Am 1992;74(8):1242–4.
8. Hovelius L. Anterior dislocation of the shoulder in teenagers and young adults. Five-year prognosis. J Bone Joint Surg Am 1987;69(3):393–9.

9. Robinson CM, Howes J, Murdoch H, et al. Functional outcome and risk of recurrent instability after primary traumatic anterior shoulder dislocation in young patients. J Bone Joint Surg Am 2006;88(11):2326–36.

10. Hovelius L, Olofsson A, Sandstrom B, et al. Nonoperative treatment of primary anterior shoulder dislocation in patients forty years of age and younger. A prospective twenty-five-year follow-up. J Bone Joint Surg Am 2008;90(5): 945–52.

11. Deitch J, Mehlman CT, Foad SL, et al. Traumatic anterior shoulder dislocation in adolescents. Am J Sports Med 2003;31(5):758–63.

12. Lawton RL, Choudhury S, Mansat P, et al. Pediatric shoulder instability: presentation, findings, treatment, and outcomes. J Pediatr Orthop 2002;22(1): 52–61.

13. Postacchini F, Gumina S, Cinotti G. Anterior shoulder dislocation in adolescents. J Shoulder Elbow Surg 2000;9(6):470–4.

14. Emery RJ, Mullaji AB. Glenohumeral joint instability in normal adolescents. Incidence and significance. J Bone Joint Surg Br 1991;73(3):406–8.

15. Bak K. Nontraumatic glenohumeral instability and coracoacromial impingement in swimmers. Scand J Med Sci Sports 1996;6(3):132–44.

16. Meeusen R, Borms J. Gymnastic injuries. Sports Med 1992;13(5):337–56.

17. Gardner E, Gray DJ. Prenatal development of the human shoulder and acromioclavicular joints. Am J Anat 1953;92(2):219–76.

18. O'Brien SJ, Arnoczky SP, Warren RF, et al. Developmental anatomy of the shoulder and anatomy of the glenohumeral joint. In: Rockwood CA Jr, Matsen FA 3rd, editors. The shoulder, vol. 1. Philadelphia: WB Saunders; 1990. p. 1–33.

19. Sachs RA, Lin D, Stone ML, et al. Can the need for future surgery for acute traumatic anterior shoulder dislocation be predicted? J Bone Joint Surg Am 2007; 89(8):1665–74.

20. Owens BD, Agel J, Mountcastle SB, et al. Incidence of glenohumeral instability in collegiate athletics. Am J Sports Med 2009;37(9):1750–4.

21. McLaughlin H. Posterior dislocation of the shoulder. J Bone Joint Surg Am 1952; 24(3):584–90.

22. Fabian LM, Levine WN. Shoulder instability in young athletes. In: Ahmad CS, editor. Pediatric adolescent sports injuries. Rosemont (IL): American Academy of Orthopaedic Surgeons; 2010. p. 57–69.

23. Keiser RP, Wilson CL. Bilateral recurrent dislocation of the shoulder (atraumatic) in a thirteen-year-old girl. Report of an unusual case. J Bone Joint Surg Am 1961;43:553–4.

24. Rowe CR, Pierce DS, Clark JG. Voluntary dislocation of the shoulder. A preliminary report on a clinical, electromyographic, and psychiatric study of twenty-six patients. J Bone Joint Surg Am 1973;55(3):445–60.

25. Curtis RJ, Dameron TB, Rockwood CA Jr. Fractures and dislocations of the shoulder in children. In: Rockwood CA Jr, Wilkins KE, King RE, editors. Fractures in children. Philadelphia: JB Lippincott; 1991. p. 829–919.

26. Gaskill TR, Taylor DC, Millett PJ. Management of multidirectional instability of the shoulder. J Am Acad Orthop Surg 2011;19(12):758–67.

27. Kim SH, Park JS, Jeong WK, et al. The Kim test: a novel test for posteroinferior labral lesion of the shoulder–a comparison to the jerk test. Am J Sports Med 2005;33(8):1188–92.

28. Neer CS 2nd, Foster CR. Inferior capsular shift for involuntary inferior and multidirectional instability of the shoulder. A preliminary report. J Bone Joint Surg Am 1980;62(6):897–908.

29. Warner JJ, Deng XH, Warren RF, et al. Static capsuloligamentous restraints to superior-inferior translation of the glenohumeral joint. Am J Sports Med 1992; 20(6):675–85.
30. Gagey OJ, Gagey N. The hyperabduction test. J Bone Joint Surg Br 2001;83(1): 69–74.
31. Borsa PA, Sauers EL, Herling DE. Patterns of glenohumeral joint laxity and stiffness in healthy men and women. Med Sci Sports Exerc 2000;32(10): 1685–90.
32. Pavlov H, Warren RF, Weiss CB Jr, et al. The roentgenographic evaluation of anterior shoulder instability. Clin Orthop Relat Res 1985;(194):153–8.
33. Huijsmans PE, Haen PS, Kidd M, et al. Quantification of a glenoid defect with three-dimensional computed tomography and magnetic resonance imaging: a cadaveric study. J Shoulder Elbow Surg 2007;16(6):803–9.
34. Gyftopoulos S, Hasan S, Bencardino J, et al. Diagnostic accuracy of MRI in the measurement of glenoid bone loss. AJR Am J Roentgenol 2012;199(4): 873–8.
35. Dewing CB, McCormick F, Bell SJ, et al. An analysis of capsular area in patients with anterior, posterior, and multidirectional shoulder instability. Am J Sports Med 2008;36(3):515–22.
36. Kim KC, Rhee KJ, Shin HD, et al. Estimating the dimensions of the rotator interval with use of magnetic resonance arthrography. J Bone Joint Surg Am 2007; 89(11):2450–5.
37. Provencher MT, Dewing CB, Bell SJ, et al. An analysis of the rotator interval in patients with anterior, posterior, and multidirectional shoulder instability. Arthroscopy 2008;24(8):921–9.
38. Curtis RJ. Glenohumeral instability in the child. In: DeLee JC, Drez DJ, Miller MD, editors. Delee & Drez's orthopaedic sports medicine, vol. 1. Philadelphia: Saunders/Elsevier; 2010. p. 932–46.
39. Cordischi K, Li X, Busconi B. Intermediate outcomes after primary traumatic anterior shoulder dislocation in skeletally immature patients aged 10 to 13 years. Orthopedics 2009;32(9). http://dx.doi.org/10.3928/01477447-20090728-34. pii: orthopsupersite.com/view/asp?rID:42855.
40. Hovelius L. The natural history of primary anterior dislocation of the shoulder in the young. J Orthop Sci 1999;4(4):307–17.
41. Bottoni CR, Wilckens JH, DeBerardino TM, et al. A prospective, randomized evaluation of arthroscopic stabilization versus nonoperative treatment in patients with acute, traumatic, first-time shoulder dislocations. Am J Sports Med 2002;30(4):576–80.
42. Burkhead WZ Jr, Rockwood CA Jr. Treatment of instability of the shoulder with an exercise program. J Bone Joint Surg Am 1992;74(6):890–6.
43. Takwale VJ, Calvert P, Rattue H. Involuntary positional instability of the shoulder in adolescents and young adults. Is there any benefit from treatment? J Bone Joint Surg Br 2000;82(5):719–23.
44. Kuroda S, Sumiyoshi T, Moriishi J, et al. The natural course of atraumatic shoulder instability. J Shoulder Elbow Surg 2001;10(2):100–4.
45. Misamore GW, Sallay PI, Didelot W. A longitudinal study of patients with multidirectional instability of the shoulder with seven- to ten-year follow-up. J Shoulder Elbow Surg 2005;14(5):466–70.
46. DeBerardino TM, Arciero RA, Taylor DC, et al. Prospective evaluation of arthroscopic stabilization of acute, initial anterior shoulder dislocations in young athletes. Two- to five-year follow-up. Am J Sports Med 2001;29(5):586–92.

47. Owens BD, DeBerardino TM, Nelson BJ, et al. Long-term follow-up of acute arthroscopic Bankart repair for initial anterior shoulder dislocations in young athletes. Am J Sports Med 2009;37(4):669–73.

48. Mazzocca AD, Brown FM Jr, Carreira DS, et al. Arthroscopic anterior shoulder stabilization of collision and contact athletes. Am J Sports Med 2005;33(1): 52–60.

49. Jones KJ, Wiesel B, Ganley TJ, et al. Functional outcomes of early arthroscopic Bankart repair in adolescents aged 11 to 18 years. J Pediatr Orthop 2007;27(2): 209–13.

50. Kraus R, Pavlidis T, Heiss C, et al. Arthroscopic treatment of post-traumatic shoulder instability in children and adolescents. Knee Surg Sports Traumatol Arthrosc 2010;18(12):1738–41.

51. Castagna A, Delle Rose G, Borroni M, et al. Arthroscopic stabilization of the shoulder in adolescent athletes participating in overhead or contact sports. Arthroscopy 2012;28(3):309–15.

52. Jerosch J, Castro WH. Shoulder instability in Ehlers-Danlos syndrome. An indication for surgical treatment? Acta Orthop Belg 1990;56(2):451–3.

53. Altchek DW, Warren RF, Skyhar MJ, et al. T-plasty modification of the Bankart procedure for multidirectional instability of the anterior and inferior types. J Bone Joint Surg Am 1991;73(1):105–12.

54. Cooper RA, Brems JJ. The inferior capsular-shift procedure for multidirectional instability of the shoulder. J Bone Joint Surg Am 1992;74(10):1516–21.

55. Hamada K, Fukuda H, Nakajima T, et al. The inferior capsular shift operation for instability of the shoulder. Long-term results in 34 shoulders. J Bone Joint Surg Br 1999;81(2):218–25.

56. Pollock RG, Owens JM, Flatow EL, et al. Operative results of the inferior capsular shift procedure for multidirectional instability of the shoulder. J Bone Joint Surg Am 2000;82(7):919–28.

57. Choi CH, Ogilvie-Harris DJ. Inferior capsular shift operation for multidirectional instability of the shoulder in players of contact sports. Br J Sports Med 2002; 36(4):290–4.

58. Bak K, Spring BJ, Henderson JP. Inferior capsular shift procedure in athletes with multidirectional instability based on isolated capsular and ligamentous redundancy. Am J Sports Med 2000;28(4):466–71.

59. Wiater JM, Vibert BT. Glenohumeral joint volume reduction with progressive release and shifting of the inferior shoulder capsule. J Shoulder Elbow Surg 2007;16(6):810–4.

60. Kim SH, Noh KC, Park JS, et al. Loss of chondrolabral containment of the glenohumeral joint in atraumatic posteroinferior multidirectional instability. J Bone Joint Surg Am 2005;87(1):92–8.

61. Kim SH, Kim HK, Sun JI, et al. Arthroscopic capsulolabroplasty for posteroinferior multidirectional instability of the shoulder. Am J Sports Med 2004;32(3): 594–607.

62. Lyons TR, Griffith PL, Savoie FH 3rd, et al. Laser-assisted capsulorrhaphy for multidirectional instability of the shoulder. Arthroscopy 2001;17(1): 25–30.

63. Favorito PJ, Langenderfer MA, Colosimo AJ, et al. Arthroscopic laser-assisted capsular shift in the treatment of patients with multidirectional shoulder instability. Am J Sports Med 2002;30(3):322–8.

64. Anderson K, Warren RF, Altchek DW, et al. Risk factors for early failure after thermal capsulorrhaphy. Am J Sports Med 2002;30(1):103–7.

65. Levine WN, Clark AM Jr, D'Alessandro DF, et al. Chondrolysis following arthroscopic thermal capsulorrhaphy to treat shoulder instability. A report of two cases. J Bone Joint Surg Am 2005;87(3):616–21.
66. Wong KL, Williams GR. Complications of thermal capsulorrhaphy of the shoulder. J Bone Joint Surg Am 2001;83(Suppl 2 Pt 2):151–5.
67. McIntyre LF, Caspari RB, Savoie FH 3rd. The arthroscopic treatment of multidirectional shoulder instability: two-year results of a multiple suture technique. Arthroscopy 1997;13(4):418–25.
68. Treacy SH, Savoie FH 3rd, Field LD. Arthroscopic treatment of multidirectional instability. J Shoulder Elbow Surg 1999;8(4):345–50.
69. Gartsman GM, Roddey TS, Hammerman SM. Arthroscopic treatment of multidirectional glenohumeral instability: 2- to 5-year follow-up. Arthroscopy 2001; 17(3):236–43.
70. Baker CL 3rd, Mascarenhas R, Kline AJ, et al. Arthroscopic treatment of multidirectional shoulder instability in athletes: a retrospective analysis of 2- to 5-year clinical outcomes. Am J Sports Med 2009;37(9):1712–20.
71. Harryman DT 2nd, Sidles JA, Harris SL, et al. The role of the rotator interval capsule in passive motion and stability of the shoulder. J Bone Joint Surg Am 1992;74(1):53–66.
72. Provencher MT, Mologne TS, Hongo M, et al. Arthroscopic versus open rotator interval closure: biomechanical evaluation of stability and motion. Arthroscopy 2007;23(6):583–92.
73. Mologne TS, Zhao K, Hongo M, et al. The addition of rotator interval closure after arthroscopic repair of either anterior or posterior shoulder instability: effect on glenohumeral translation and range of motion. Am J Sports Med 2008;36(6): 1123–31.
74. Jost B, Koch PP, Gerber C. Anatomy and functional aspects of the rotator interval. J Shoulder Elbow Surg 2000;9(4):336–41.
75. Gerber C, Werner CM, Macy JC, et al. Effect of selective capsulorrhaphy on the passive range of motion of the glenohumeral joint. J Bone Joint Surg Am 2003; 85(1):48–55.
76. Plausinis D, Bravman JT, Heywood C, et al. Arthroscopic rotator interval closure: effect of sutures on glenohumeral motion and anterior-posterior translation. Am J Sports Med 2006;34(10):1656–61.

Posterior Shoulder Instability in the Contact Athlete

Eric P. Tannenbaum, MD[a], Jon K. Sekiya, MD[b],*

KEYWORDS

- Posterior shoulder instability • Contact athlete • Reverse Bankart
- Reverse Hill-Sachs

KEY POINTS

- The shoulder joint is the most mobile joint in the body; however, it is also the most unstable.
- Athletes may develop posterior shoulder instability through either repetitive microtrauma to the shoulder over time or a single traumatic episode.
- The contact sports most commonly associated with posterior shoulder instability include football, wrestling, hockey, rugby, and lacrosse.
- An initial conservative course of at least 6 months of activity modification and physical therapy to strengthen the dynamic muscular stabilizers is recommended before pursuing surgical options.
- Surgery focuses on correcting either bony and/or soft tissue anatomy to increase the stability of the joint.

INTRODUCTION

Posterior shoulder instability is much less common than anterior instability, affecting between 2% and 10% of all reported cases of instability.[1–3] Consequently, it is commonly missed or underdiagnosed by many orthopedic surgeons. Competitive athletes involved in contact sports, such as wrestling, hockey, rugby, lacrosse, or football, are at a higher risk for developing posterior instability because of their shoulders being commonly subjected to blunt force. In addition, athletes who compete in sports requiring repetitive overhand throwing and/or motion, such as volleyball, baseball,

Disclosures: Jon K. Sekiya: receives royalties and stock options from Arthrex, Inc, OrthoDynamix, LLC (royalties), OrthoDynamix, LLC (stock), and Elsevier (book royalties) and is a consultant for Arthrex, Inc (paid) and OrthoDynamix, LLC (unpaid). Eric P. Tannenbaum: no disclosures.
a Department of Orthopaedic Surgery, University of Michigan, 1500 East Medical Center Drive, Ann Arbor, MI 48109, USA; b MedSport, University of Michigan, 24 Frank Lloyd Wright Drive, PO Box 0391, Ann Arbor, MI 48106-0391, USA
* Corresponding author.
E-mail address: sekiya@med.umich.edu

Clin Sports Med 32 (2013) 781–796
http://dx.doi.org/10.1016/j.csm.2013.07.011
0278-5919/13/$ – see front matter © 2013 Elsevier Inc. All rights reserved.

tennis, and swimming, are also at higher risk for developing posterior shoulder instability secondary to overuse or microtrauma.

Orthopedic surgeons must have a high index of suspicion for athletes participating in contact sports presenting with complaints of shoulder pain and/or instability. A solid understanding of the complex pathoanatomy of the shoulder and the use of appropriate clinical and diagnostic tools is necessary to make the correct diagnosis. In addition, a comprehensive understanding of the surgical and nonsurgical options and indications is necessary to appropriately treat this patient population and get them back to their prior level of competition.

ANATOMY

The shoulder is often described as resembling a golf ball in a tee, with the golf ball representing the humeral head and the tee representing the glenoid. As suggested by this model, the joint is the least stable in the body, with less than one-third of the humeral head articulating with the glenoid fossa at any given time. However, it is also the most mobile joint in the body, providing a tremendous range of motion in adduction, abduction, flexion, extension, internal rotation, external rotation, and 360° circumduction.

The relative instability of the shoulder joint is compensated for by static and dynamic stabilization. The geometric conformity of articular cartilage surfaces, glenoid labrum, and capsular ligaments, and negative intra-articular pressure all function as static stabilizers. Furthermore, the bony morphology of the joint, including the glenoid and humeral versions, glenoid inclination, glenoid size, and joint congruency, help contributes to static stability. Any loss in bone stock or structural irregularities, such as posterior glenoid erosion, glenoid hypoplasia, excessive glenoid retroversion, or excessive humeral retroversion, may predispose patients to posterior instability. Kim and colleagues[4] compared magnetic resonance imaging (MRI) results of 33 posteroinferiorly unstable shoulders with age-matched controls and reported that the shoulders with posteroinferior instability were more retroverted than the controls.

The depth, concavity, and surface area of the shoulder is increased by the labrum, which is a ring of densely packed fibrocartilage that attaches along the perimeter of the glenoid fossa. The labrum also serves as a stable fibrocartilaginous anchor for the capsular ligaments (superior, middle, and inferior) that act to stabilize the glenohumeral joint at the extremes of motion through resisting joint translation. O'Brien and colleagues[5] demonstrated that the inferior glenohumeral ligament and the posteroinferior capsule were the primary stabilizers of the posterior shoulder in 90° of abduction. The posterior capsule, which is the thinnest portion of the entire shoulder capsule, is defined as the area between the intra-articular portion of the biceps tendon and the posterior band of the inferior glenohumeral ligament, and is recognized as an area of potential capsular weakness.[6]

In addition, the capsuloligamentous rotator interval located between the subscapularis and the supraspinatus tendons, and consisting of the coracohumeral and superior glenohumeral ligaments, has been shown to play a role in preventing excessive posterior translation.[6-10] Therefore, any loss of integrity of the rotator interval may contribute to posterior instability. Harryman and colleagues[9] showed this through sectioning the rotator interval capsule in cadaveric specimens and causing increased posterior and inferior translation, resulting in dislocation. However, Mologne and colleagues[11] did not report any improvement in posterior shoulder instability with arthroscopic rotator interval closure. Furthermore, conflicting evidence exists as to whether the rotator interval size affects stability. In a recent study, Lee and colleagues[12] found that patients with instability have a larger rotator interval. Conversely, Provencher and colleagues[13] found that the overall size of the rotator interval was well preserved in all instability patterns.

The dynamic stabilizers of the shoulder include the rotator cuff muscles, the long head of the biceps, the anterior and middle deltoids, and the pectoralis major. Blasier and colleagues[14] found that the subscapularis was the most significant rotator cuff muscle in preventing posterior subluxation. The shoulder girdle muscles help stabilize the joint through contracting and thus forcing the convex humeral head into the concave glenoid socket in a phenomenon known as the concavity-compression effect.[15,16] Sekiya and colleagues[17] demonstrated how humeral head impression fractures (ie, Hill-Sachs defects) lead to loss of humeral head convexity and can cause loss of the concavity-compression effect, resulting in decreased stability. The dynamic stabilizers work together with the static stabilizers to maintain joint stability within the wide ranges of motion of the shoulder.

PATHOGENESIS

Contact athletes who experience a frank posterior dislocation from a single traumatic episode may develop a fixed, or locked, posteriorly dislocated shoulder that often requires reduction. Conversely, athletes with instability resulting from repetitive overhand motion or microtrauma to the posterior capsule more commonly experience recurrent posterior shoulder subluxation wherein the humeral head does not dislocate completely out of the glenoid joint. Continuous cycling of the shoulder joint results in posterior capsule weakening and sometimes even tearing, which ultimately leads to posterior instability. McLaughlin[3] first recognized the aforementioned distinction between fixed dislocation and recurrent subluxation in 1952.

Recurrent posterior subluxation is a much more common entity than frank posterior dislocation,[18] which is generally only seen in traumas, seizures, electrocutions, and contact sports. Some contact athletes, such as football players, may experience repetitive microtrauma from blocking with an outstretched arm, while also being vulnerable to acute traumatic dislocation from a particularly forceful block.

The mechanism of injury commonly causing posterior dislocation in contact sports is a direct force applied to the anterior shoulder (ie, a wrestler thrown onto his shoulder) or an indirect posterior force applied through the arm up to the shoulder (ie, a defensive lineman locking out his elbows to block).[19] In his article on posterior shoulder dislocations, McLaughlin[3] gave examples of some of the patients he treated, including "a wrestler who fell while held by a 'hammer lock', a boxer in the act of punching with an internal rotation twist of the arm, a gymnast 'doing a dip' on parallel bars and a football player who fell on his elbow with the forearm caught behind his back." Athletes' shoulders tend to become unstable during competition as their dynamic stabilizers begin to fatigue, and thus do not function as well. Thus, athletes with already unstable shoulders are at greater risk for subluxation or dislocation the longer they are in the competition, because they are relying more on their static stabilizers while still ranging their shoulders.

Athletes who have had at least one traumatic posterior subluxation/dislocation are at risk for a posterior labral detachment known as a *reverse Bankart lesion*. With the labrum torn off the posterior aspect of the glenoid rim, the labrum cannot provide a sufficient "bumper" and the humeral head is thus more inclined to dislocate.

Abnormalities in bone morphology or lesions can also lead to posterior instability. In addition to the previously mentioned anatomic variations (ie, excessive glenoid retroversion or hypoplasia) that may predispose athletes to instability, specific bony defects can also occur as a result of previous episodes of subluxation/dislocation. For instance, a reverse bony Bankart occurs when a piece of the glenoid rim is avulsed along with the labrum. A reverse Hill-Sachs defect (ie, McLaughlin lesion) is another bony lesion that can occur after an acute posterior dislocation when the humeral head becomes caught on the posterior glenoid rim and forms a notch or impression fracture in the anterior humeral head. This lesion often makes the shoulder more difficult to reduce and increases the risk for instability through lessening the concavity-compression effect.[17]

CLINICAL EVALUATION
Patient History

Patients often present with subtle findings and nonspecific complaints of pain with certain motion or actions, and thus physicians must maintain a high index of suspicion to not miss the diagnosis. The diagnosis is often further complicated by the fact that these athletes commonly have other abnormalities in the shoulder, such as impingement syndrome secondary to abnormal biomechanics resulting from the instability.

Physicians should also be familiar with the sports that place athletes at a higher risk for developing posterior instability, including football (specifically for linemen), wrestling, hockey, rugby, and lacrosse. Bonza and colleagues[20] evaluated shoulder injuries in high school athletes and found that in the 9 sports examined, football players were at the highest risk for shoulder injuries, followed by wrestlers. Kerr and colleagues[21] confirmed this assertion in a recent study examining dislocation/separation injuries among US high school athletes. Furthermore, they reported the shoulder to be the most commonly injured joint (54.9%), and found the most common mechanisms of injury to be contact with another player (52.4%) and contact with the playing surface (26.4%).

Kaplan and colleagues[22] examined the epidemiology of shoulder injuries reported during the National Football League Combine and found that 50% of players reported a history of shoulder injury, with 4% involving posterior shoulder instability. Recurrent posterior instability has even been reported in competitive rifle shooting.[23] All of these sports either place the shoulder at risk for a direct anterior blow or an indirect force transmitted through the arm.

When asked about the position of the arm that most commonly reproduces or intensifies their symptoms, patients will often demonstrate the arm in forward flexion, adduction, and internal rotation.[19] Patients may report a specific inciting traumatic event that caused their symptoms or an episode of frank posterior dislocation. Although the specific location of their pain is often difficult for them to pinpoint, they often complain of pain along the posterior joint line, superior aspect of the shoulder (rotator cuff), or the biceps tendon. In addition to pain, athletes often report a feeling of apprehension when putting their arm through certain ranges of motion. Some patients report clicking or crepitation; however, no neurologic or vascular symptoms should be present.

Lastly, it is important to ask about specific connective tissue disorders or other family members with instability problems when reviewing the family history. Connective tissue disorders such as Ehlers-Danlos or Marfan syndrome predispose patients to joint dislocation/subluxation.

PHYSICAL EXAMINATION

When clinically assessing the patient, orthopedists must understand the difference between posterior shoulder joint laxity versus posterior shoulder joint instability. Many athletes develop joint laxity, allowing for excessive range of motion and joint translation; however, they never report a subjective feeling of pain or apprehension. Therefore, these patients are said to have joint laxity, but not instability. For a patient to be diagnosed with shoulder instability, they must have symptoms of pain/discomfort or a feeling that the shoulder is going to "come out" (ie, apprehension) in addition to extreme translation of the shoulder.[24,25] In other words, excessive symptomatic translation of the humeral head.

Bilateral physical examination of the shoulders should always be performed to provide a comparison. The examination should include visual inspection, palpation, active and passive range of motion, and motor and sensory testing. Although the physical examination is generally benign, patients commonly are tender to palpation along the posterior joint line, possibly from synovitis caused by multiple episodes of instability.[26] Furthermore, a skin dimple over seen over the posteromedial deltoid of both shoulders was found to be 92% specific and 62% sensitive for detecting posterior instability.[27]

In addition to the routine shoulder examination, multiple specific provocative tests have been described to assess for posterior shoulder instability. These tests include the posterior drawer (**Fig. 1**), jerk (**Fig. 2**), and Kim (**Fig. 3**) tests. The Kim test was found to be 97% sensitive for detecting a posteroinferior labral lesion when combined with the jerk test.[28]

DIAGNOSTIC IMAGING

Athletes with instability should be sent for a standard 3-view radiographic series that includes an anterior posterior, an axillary (or West Point), and a supraspinatus outlet view (or an apical oblique view). Although these radiographs are often normal, the

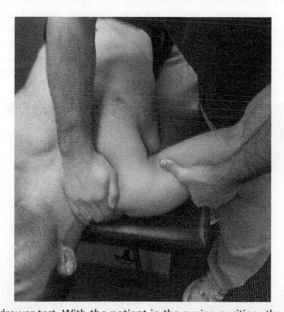

Fig. 1. Posterior drawer test. With the patient in the supine position, the shoulder is stabilized with one hand by placing the palm anteriorly between the clavicle and coracoid, and the fingers posteriorly along the spine of the scapula. The other hand grasps the proximal humerus and presses the humeral head medially into the center of the glenoid to confirm neutral joint position. A posterior stress is then applied with the hand gripping the humerus to evaluate the shoulder for excessive passive posterior translation.

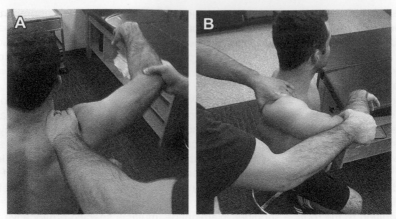

Fig. 2. Jerk test. (*A*) With the patient seated, the shoulder is stabilized with one hand by placing the thumb posteriorly over the scapular spine and the fingers anteriorly over the clavicle. The examiner's other hand grasps the elbow and abducts the arm to 90° while internally rotating and applying an axial load directed to the shoulder. (*B*) The patient's arm is then horizontally adducted while maintaining an axial load. A sudden clunk or jerk occurs when the humeral head slides off the back of the glenoid, and these results are considered positive.

combination of these 3 views will allow the clinician to appropriately assess the patient's shoulder for anterior or posterior translation/dislocation, Hill-Sachs lesions, excessive glenoid retroversion, fracture/erosion of posterior glenoid, reverse bony Bankart lesions, anteroinferior glenoid rim abnormalities, glenoid dysplasia, or even a lesser tuberosity fracture that can indicate a posterior dislocation.

In addition to roentgenography, MRI can be used to achieve a better view of potential soft tissue or cartilaginous abnormalities contributing to the instability, and computed tomography (CT) will provide better imaging of any bony abnormalities.

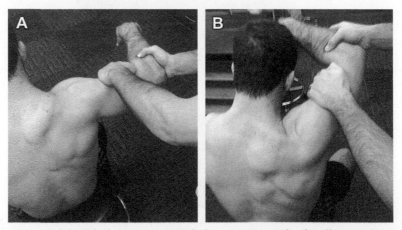

Fig. 3. Kim test. (*A*) With the patient seated, the examiner grabs the elbow with one hand and cups the other over the patient's biceps. (*B*) The arm is then passively elevated an additional 45° while applying a downward and posterior force to the upper arm and an axial load to the elbow. Positive results are indicated by pain and posterior subluxation of the shoulder.

CT is the best imaging modality available for evaluating the size of reverse Hill-Sachs lesions because it permits one to determine what percentage of the humeral articular cartilage the impression fracture involves. Lastly, in the hands of an experienced clinician, dynamic ultrasound can be used as a quick and inexpensive tool to objectively quantify glenohumeral laxity.[29,30]

NONOPERATIVE MANAGEMENT

An initial conservative course of at least 6 months of activity modification and physical therapy to strengthen the dynamic muscular stabilizers is generally recommended and has had positive outcomes in certain patients.[18,19,26,31–34] However, Burkhead and Rockwood[31] showed that only 16% of patients with traumatic instability will improve with an exercise program alone, compared with a success rate of 80% seen in patients with a history of atraumatic instability. If conservative management fails to improve symptoms, surgery should be considered.

OPERATIVE MANAGEMENT

The surgical options can be separated into 2 categories: operations performed to correct osseous defects, and operations performed to correct soft tissue abnormalities. Of course, some operations may require repair of both bony and soft tissue anatomy, such as reverse bony Bankart lesions. In general, procedures involving the correction of osseous defects are performed open, whereas the soft tissue procedures can almost always be performed arthroscopically with comparable results. Unfortunately, no consensus exists in the literature regarding specific indications for each procedure, and because the injury is so rare, many of the current articles reporting on outcomes are case reports. Thus, surgeons must plan procedures on a case-by-case basis, making sure to factor in not only the anatomic abnormality of the patient but also patient expectations, such as how soon they want to return to play.

Management is often further complicated by the fact that patients with posterior instability generally have some component of anterior and/or inferior instability (multidirectional instability) that may also need to be surgically addressed at the same time. Moreover, the patient may have more than one defect contributing to the posterior instability. If other defects or components of instability exist and are not surgically addressed, symptoms of instability may persist after surgery and the patient may potentially require a second operation. Lastly, multiple variations in surgical techniques have been described in the literature, making surgical outcomes difficult to compare objectively.

SOFT TISSUE DEFECTS AND PROCEDURES

The most commonly described soft tissue procedures involve tightening the redundant posterior capsule (ie, vertical posterior capsular shift), reverse Bankart repair (**Fig. 4**), or tendon tenodesis (ie, reverse Putti-Platt). Thermal capsulorrhaphy has shown poor outcomes and is no longer considered an acceptable treatment option.[35,36] If an athlete presents with posterior shoulder instability without any bony abnormalities present on preoperative imaging, the surgeon should focus on fixing the attenuated posterior capsule, the posterior labrum, or often both.

Although open and arthroscopic procedures have shown positive outcomes, arthroscopic techniques are becoming more favorable.[37,38] Arthroscopic surgery is less invasive (less scaring and better preservation of the native shoulder anatomy) and provides better visualization of intra-articular anatomy and other potential lesions (ie, superior labrum anterior-posterior tears) that can be repaired concurrently. In a prospective

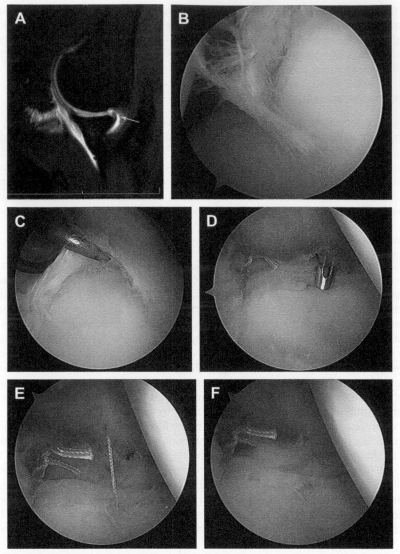

Fig. 4. Reverse Bankart and superior labrum anterior-posterior (SLAP) repair. (*A*) MRI showing reverse Bankart lesion (*white arrow*). (*B*) Reverse Bankart lesion identified arthroscopically. (*C*) Concurrent SLAP tear in the same patient. (*D–F*) Arthroscopic repair of reverse Bankart tear using suture anchors.

study evaluating 100 athletes with unidirectional posterior shoulder instability, Bradley and colleagues[39] reported 91% good to excellent results after arthroscopic capsulolabral reconstruction at a follow-up of 27 months. Of the athletes treated, 51 participated in contact sports and 90% were stable, with either good or excellent results at a mean follow-up of 28 months. Of the 5 contact athletes for whom the procedure was unsuccessful, 4 had undergone capsular plication without suture anchors.

The most commonly used arthroscopic technique involves the use of suture anchor fixation of the posterior labrum with or without capsular plication to tighten the posterior capsule. This technique is generally performed using 2 portals (anterior and posterior). Savoie and colleagues[38] described 3 different arthroscopic techniques for repairing the posterior capsule and labrum. They recommended using a suture anchor technique in the presence of damage to the labrum and/or capsule. A suture capsulorrhaphy was recommended for patients with more extensive damage to the posterior inferior capsulolabral complex, those with an absent posterior capsule from prior surgery, or those with posterior inferior capsule tears near the labrum. Lastly, they described a combined tendon/capsule plication or "mini-open technique" for patients with extensive damage to the posterior capsule and the infraspinatus and teres minor tendons (as seen in competitive weightlifters). They reported a 97% overall success rate of arthroscopic posterior reconstruction based on the Neer-Foster rating at an average follow-up of 28 months.

The last noteworthy soft tissue procedure is the reverse Putti-Platt procedure, first described by Severin[40] in 1953. Although this procedure is not commonly performed compared with the posterior capsulorrhaphy or reverse Bankart repair, it remains an option in patients in whom stabilization attempts failed. The surgery is performed through a posterior approach to the shoulder. The goal is to shorten the infraspinatus tendon (and sometimes the teres minor tendon) through imbrication, therefore creating a firm fibrous buttress at the posterior margin of the glenoid rim. This procedure has been shown to be successful in reducing posterior shoulder instability; however, it is not strongly recommended in athletes because it often causes a significant loss of internal rotation.

OSSEOUS DEFECTS AND PROCEDURES

The osseous procedures involve either correcting humeral head defects (ie, reverse Hill-Sachs lesions) or correcting glenoid rim defects (ie, excessive retroversion, glenoid hypoplasia, or posterior glenoid deficiency). A surgical approach is generally recommended in patients with reverse Hill-Sachs lesions experiencing persistent posterior shoulder instability/dislocations or impression fractures affecting more than 25% to 30% of the humeral articular morphology.[41,42] Many nonanatomic and anatomic techniques for correction of reverse Hill-Sachs lesions have been described with the common goal of restoring stability throughout a functional range of motion.

In 1952, McLaughlin[3] described a nonanatomic technique to limit maximal internal rotation and prevent the edges of reverse Hill-Sachs defects from dropping behind the posterior glenoid rim. This so-called McLaughlin procedure involves transferring the subscapularis into the humeral head defect. Using a deltopectoral approach, McLaughlin released the subscapularis tendon and retracted it medially. He then reduced the posteriorly locked shoulder using a lever and reattached the subscapularis to the humerus in the defect using mattress sutures passed through drill holes in the bone.[3] The Neer modification of the McLaughlin procedure is another technique that involves transferring the subscapularis tendon in continuity with an osteotomized lesser tuberosity.[41,43–48] This procedure is especially useful when an associated fracture of the lesser tuberosity occurs in conjunction with a reverse Hill-Sachs lesion.[45] Another nonanatomic procedure that has been described involves a rotational osteotomy of the proximal part of the humerus, but this is not widely used because it is technically challenging and poses a risk of humeral head devascularization.[49,50]

In addition to the techniques described earlier, anatomic reconstruction using autogenous bone grafting from the iliac crest may also be used to fill smaller defects (<25% of the humeral head articular surface); however, allogenous osteochondral bone grafting is more commonly recommended for larger defects occupying 40% to 50% of the articular surface (**Fig. 5**).[43,45,51–58] Patients in whom the diagnosis has

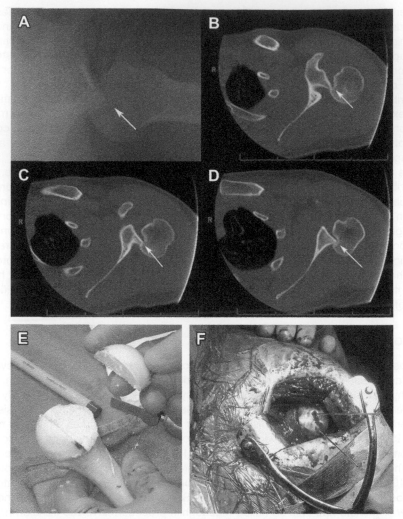

Fig. 5. Reverse Hill-Sachs defect repaired with allograft. (*A*) Cross-table lateral radiograph showing reverse Hill-Sachs lesion (*white arrow*). (*B–D*) CT images showing reverse Hill-Sachs lesion with a posteriorly dislocated shoulder (*white arrows*). (*E*) Humeral head allograft. (*F*) Posterior humeral head defect filled with allograft fixed in place with pins.

been delayed may develop osteoarthritis of the articular surface and may require arthroplasty.[43,51,59–61] Therefore, it is crucial to recognize and treat reverse Hill-Sachs lesions in a timely manner.

Posterior instability caused by posterior glenoid deficiency from an osteochondral fracture, hypoplasia, and/or excessive retroversion can be corrected using either a posterior iliac bone block[62–68] or a posterior glenoid opening wedge osteotomy.[33,69–73] Both of these posterior glenoplasty procedures aim to reinforce posterior glenoid rim deficiency, but they can also be used in patients who have had a previous capsular plication or shift that failed to prevent recurrent instability (**Fig. 6**).

The posterior bone block procedure is most commonly performed through a posterior approach with the patient in the lateral decubitus position. A 6-cm posterior

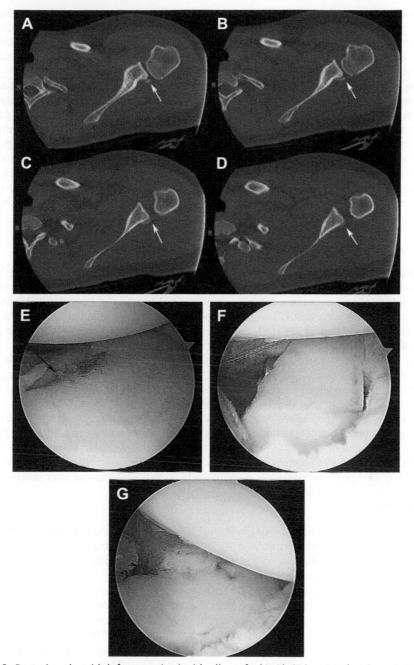

Fig. 6. Posterior glenoid defect repaired with allograft. (*A–D*) CT images showing posterior glenoid bone loss (*white arrows*). (*E*) Posterior glenoid bone loss observed arthroscopically (*black arrow*). (*F*) Posterior glenoid allograft filling glenoid defect. (*G*) Posterior glenoid allograft fixed in place and capsule repaired.

vertical incision is made following the major posterior axillary crease, the deltoid is split, the interval between the infraspinatus and teres minor is split, a capsulotomy is performed, the posterior edge of the glenoid cavity is abraded, and the bone block graft harvested from the iliac crest is secured with two 4.5-mm malleolar compression screws to extend approximately 5 mm from the posterior glenoid rim.[62,63]

The posterior open wedge osteotomy is performed through a similar approach; however, once the shoulder posterior glenoid rim is exposed, a scapular neck osteotomy is made 1 cm medial to the glenoid face and parallel to it.[74] A drill hole is used to guide the osteotome in the correct plane and distance (three-fourths of the depth of the glenoid). The osteotomy is then opened with successive levering steps to bend the glenoid open without fracturing it. An osteochondral allograft can then be harvested from a fresh or fresh/frozen glenoid.[73,75–78] Other allografts include distal tibia or femoral head allograft.[79] The bone is then fixed into place using 3.5- versus 4.0-mm screws. Alternatively, Thompson and colleagues[80] described a technique involving the use of a small T plate to secure the graft in place.

POSTOPERATIVE REHABILITATION

Immediately after surgery, cryotherapy is used to control postoperative swelling. The patient is kept in a sling for the first month to maintain abduction and relative external or neutral rotation to release tension in the posterior capsule. Between 1 and 2 months after surgery, the sling should be discontinued and passive and active assisted range of motion therapy can be initiated, while carefully limiting end ranges of motion in positions that maximally stress the posterior capsule (ie, internal rotation).

The authors recommend starting isometric rotator cuff and periscapular muscle strengthening exercises 2 to 5 months postoperatively, with the goal of returning to full range of motion within 2 to 3 months. The patient should be pain-free by 4 months after the surgery, and between 5 and 8 months athletes may begin returning to their previous level of play gradually and under controlled conditions. Of course, return to full play for contact athletes should be determined on a case-by-case basis, and depends on the patient's ability to achieve full range of motion without symptoms of pain or tenderness and with suitable strength (at least 80% compared with the contralateral shoulder). This goal can generally be achieved within 6 to 9 months after surgery.

SUMMARY

Historically, posterior shoulder instability has been a challenging problem for contact athletes and orthopedic surgeons alike. A complete understanding of the normal shoulder anatomy and biomechanics and the pathoanatomy responsible for the instability is necessary for a successful clinical outcome. In addition, the surgeon must be familiar with the diagnostic imaging and physical examination maneuvers required for the correct diagnosis without missing any other concurrent abnormalities. This understanding will allow orthopedists to plan and execute the appropriate management, whether this may involve conservative or surgical intervention. The goal should always be to correct the abnormality and have the patient return to play with full strength and no recurrent instability.

REFERENCES

1. Antoniou J, Duckworth DT, Harryman DT 2nd. Capsulolabral augmentation for the management of posteroinferior instability of the shoulder. J Bone Joint Surg Am 2000;82(9):1220.

2. Boyd HB, Sisk TD. Recurrent posterior dislocation of the shoulder. J Bone Joint Surg Am 1972;54(4):779.
3. McLaughlin H. Posterior dislocation of the shoulder. J Bone Joint Surg Am 1952; 24:584–90.
4. Kim SH, Noh KC, Park JS, et al. Loss of chondrolabral containment of the glenohumeral joint in atraumatic posteroinferior multidirectional instability. J Bone Joint Surg Am 2005;87(1):92.
5. O'Brien SJ, Schwartz RS, Warren RF, et al. Capsular restraints to anterior-posterior motion of the abducted shoulder: a biomechanical study. J Shoulder Elbow Surg 1995;4(4):298.
6. Pagnani MJ, Warren RF. Stabilizers of the glenohumeral joint. J Shoulder Elbow Surg 1994;3(3):173.
7. Neer CS 2nd, Foster CR. Inferior capsular shift for involuntary inferior and multidirectional instability of the shoulder: a preliminary report. 1980. J Bone Joint Surg Am 2001;83(10):1586.
8. Cole BJ, Rodeo SA, O'Brien SJ, et al. The anatomy and histology of the rotator interval capsule of the shoulder. Clin Orthop Relat Res 2001;(390):129–37.
9. Harryman DT 2nd, Sidles JA, Harris SL, et al. The role of the rotator interval capsule in passive motion and stability of the shoulder. J Bone Joint Surg Am 1992;74(1):53.
10. Gaskill TR, Braun S, Millett PJ. Multimedia article. The rotator interval: pathology and management. Arthroscopy 2011;27(4):556.
11. Mologne TS, Zhao K, Hongo M, et al. The addition of rotator interval closure after arthroscopic repair of either anterior or posterior shoulder instability: effect on glenohumeral translation and range of motion. Am J Sports Med 2008;36(6):1123.
12. Lee HJ, Kim NR, Moon SG, et al. Multidirectional instability of the shoulder: rotator interval dimension and capsular laxity evaluation using MR arthrography. Skeletal Radiol 2013;42(2):231–8.
13. Provencher MT, Dewing CB, Bell SJ, et al. An analysis of the rotator interval in patients with anterior, posterior, and multidirectional shoulder instability. Arthroscopy 2008;24(8):921.
14. Blasier RB, Soslowsky LJ, Malicky DM, et al. Posterior glenohumeral subluxation: active and passive stabilization in a biomechanical model. J Bone Joint Surg Am 1997;79(3):433.
15. Lippitt S, Matsen F. Mechanisms of glenohumeral joint stability. Clin Orthop Relat Res 1993;(291):20.
16. Lippitt SB, Vanderhooft JE, Harris SL, et al. Glenohumeral stability from concavity-compression: a quantitative analysis. J Shoulder Elbow Surg 1993;2(1):27.
17. Sekiya JK, Wickwire AC, Stehle JH, et al. Hill-Sachs defects and repair using osteoarticular allograft transplantation: biomechanical analysis using a joint compression model. Am J Sports Med 2009;37(12):2459.
18. Hawkins RJ, Koppert G, Johnston G. Recurrent posterior instability (subluxation) of the shoulder. J Bone Joint Surg Am 1984;66(2):169.
19. Tibone JE, Bradley JP. The treatment of posterior subluxation in athletes. Clin Orthop Relat Res 1993;(291):124.
20. Bonza JE, Fields SK, Yard EE, et al. Shoulder injuries among United States high school athletes during the 2005–2006 and 2006–2007 school years. J Athl Train 2009;44(1):76.
21. Kerr ZY, Collins CL, Pommering TL, et al. Dislocation/separation injuries among US high school athletes in 9 selected sports: 2005–2009. Clin J Sport Med 2011; 21(2):101.

22. Kaplan LD, Flanigan DC, Norwig J, et al. Prevalence and variance of shoulder injuries in elite collegiate football players. Am J Sports Med 2005;33(8):1142.
23. Cho JH, Chung NS, Song HK, et al. Recurrent posterior shoulder instability after rifle shooting. Orthopedics 2012;35(11):e1677.
24. Kuhn JE. A new classification system for shoulder instability. Br J Sports Med 2010;44(5):341.
25. Silliman JF, Hawkins RJ. Classification and physical diagnosis of instability of the shoulder. Clin Orthop Relat Res 1993;(291):7.
26. Pollock RG, Bigliani LU. Recurrent posterior shoulder instability. Diagnosis and treatment. Clin Orthop Relat Res 1993;(291):85.
27. Von Raebrox A, Campbell B, Ramesh R, et al. The association of subacromial dimples with recurrent posterior dislocation of the shoulder. J Shoulder Elbow Surg 2006;15(5):591.
28. Kim SH, Park JS, Jeong WK, et al. The Kim test: a novel test for posteroinferior labral lesion of the shoulder–a comparison to the jerk test. Am J Sports Med 2005;33(8):1188.
29. Borsa PA, Jacobson JA, Scibek JS, et al. Comparison of dynamic sonography to stress radiography for assessing glenohumeral laxity in asymptomatic shoulders. Am J Sports Med 2005;33(5):734.
30. Borsa PA, Scibek JS, Jacobson JA, et al. Sonographic stress measurement of glenohumeral joint laxity in collegiate swimmers and age-matched controls. Am J Sports Med 2005;33(7):1077.
31. Burkhead WZ Jr, Rockwood CA Jr. Treatment of instability of the shoulder with an exercise program. J Bone Joint Surg Am 1992;74(6):890.
32. Fronek J, Warren RF, Bowen M. Posterior subluxation of the glenohumeral joint. J Bone Joint Surg Am 1989;71(2):205.
33. Norwood LA, Terry GC. Shoulder posterior subluxation. Am J Sports Med 1984; 12(1):25.
34. Wilk KE, Macrina LC, Reinold MM. Non-operative rehabilitation for traumatic and atraumatic glenohumeral instability. N Am J Sports Phys Ther 2006;1(1):16.
35. Toth AP, Warren RF, Petrigliano FA, et al. Thermal shrinkage for shoulder instability. HSS J 2011;7(2):108.
36. Lubowitz JH, Poehling GG. Glenohumeral thermal capsulorrhaphy is not recommended–shoulder chondrolysis requires additional research. Arthroscopy 2007; 23(7):687.
37. Bottoni CR, Franks BR, Moore JH, et al. Operative stabilization of posterior shoulder instability. Am J Sports Med 2005;33(7):996.
38. Savoie FH 3rd, Holt MS, Field LD, et al. Arthroscopic management of posterior instability: evolution of technique and results. Arthroscopy 2008;24(4):389.
39. Bradley JP, Baker CL 3rd, Kline AJ, et al. Arthroscopic capsulolabral reconstruction for posterior instability of the shoulder: a prospective study of 100 shoulders. Am J Sports Med 2006;34(7):1061.
40. Severin E. Anterior and posterior recurrent dislocation of the shoulder: the Putti-Platt operation. Acta Orthop Scand 1953;23(1):14.
41. Cicak N. Posterior dislocation of the shoulder. J Bone Joint Surg Br 2004;86(3): 324.
42. Robinson CM, Aderinto J. Posterior shoulder dislocations and fracture-dislocations. J Bone Joint Surg Am 2005;87(3):639.
43. Hawkins RJ, Neer CS 2nd, Pianta RM, et al. Locked posterior dislocation of the shoulder. J Bone Joint Surg Am 1987;69(1):9.

44. Hughes M, Neer CS 2nd. Glenohumeral joint replacement and postoperative rehabilitation. Phys Ther 1975;55(8):850.
45. Finkelstein JA, Waddell JP, O'Driscoll SW, et al. Acute posterior fracture dislocations of the shoulder treated with the Neer modification of the McLaughlin procedure. J Orthop Trauma 1995;9(3):190.
46. Aparicio G, Calvo E, Bonilla L, et al. Neglected traumatic posterior dislocations of the shoulder: controversies on indications for treatment and new CT scan findings. J Orthop Sci 2000;5(1):37.
47. Kokkalis ZT, Mavrogenis AF, Ballas EG, et al. Bilateral neglected posterior fracture-dislocation of the shoulders. Orthopedics 2012;35(10):e1537.
48. Hart R, Pasa L, Kocis J, et al. Inveterated posterior glenohumeral dislocation treated surgically from the anterior approach. Acta Chir Orthop Traumatol Cech 2011;78(1):34 [in Czech].
49. Walch G, Boileau P, Martin B, et al. Unreduced posterior luxations and fractures-luxations of the shoulder. Apropos of 30 cases. Rev Chir Orthop Reparatrice Appar Mot 1990;76(8):546 [in French].
50. Keppler P, Holz U, Thielemann FW, et al. Locked posterior dislocation of the shoulder: treatment using rotational osteotomy of the humerus. J Orthop Trauma 1994;8(4):286.
51. Checchia SL, Santos PD, Miyazaki AN. Surgical treatment of acute and chronic posterior fracture-dislocation of the shoulder. J Shoulder Elbow Surg 1998;7(1): 53.
52. Mestdagh H, Maynou C, Delobelle JM, et al. Traumatic posterior dislocation of the shoulder in adults. Apropos of 25 cases. Ann Chir 1994;48(4):355 [in French].
53. Khayal T, Wild M, Windolf J. Reconstruction of the articular surface of the humeral head after locked posterior shoulder dislocation: a case report. Arch Orthop Trauma Surg 2009;129(4):515.
54. Shenoy R, Kamineni S. Lateral clavicular autograft for repair of reverse Hill-Sachs defect. Open Orthop J 2011;5:49.
55. Rodia F, Ventura A, Touloupakis G, et al. Missed posterior shoulder dislocation and McLaughlin lesion after an electrocution accident. Chin J Traumatol 2012; 15(6):376.
56. Patrizio L, Sabetta E. Acute posterior shoulder dislocation with reverse hill-sachs lesion of the epiphyseal humeral head. ISRN Surg 2011;2011:851051.
57. Gerber C, Lambert SM. Allograft reconstruction of segmental defects of the humeral head for the treatment of chronic locked posterior dislocation of the shoulder. J Bone Joint Surg Am 1996;78(3):376.
58. Connor PM, Boatright JR, D'Alessandro DF. Posterior fracture-dislocation of the shoulder: treatment with acute osteochondral grafting. J Shoulder Elbow Surg 1997;6(5):480.
59. Rowe CR, Zarins B. Chronic unreduced dislocations of the shoulder. J Bone Joint Surg Am 1982;64(4):494.
60. Cheng SL, Mackay MB, Richards RR. Treatment of locked posterior fracture-dislocations of the shoulder by total shoulder arthroplasty. J Shoulder Elbow Surg 1997;6(1):11.
61. Pritchett JW, Clark JM. Prosthetic replacement for chronic unreduced dislocations of the shoulder. Clin Orthop Relat Res 1987;(216):89.
62. Servien E, Walch G, Cortes ZE, et al. Posterior bone block procedure for posterior shoulder instability. Knee Surg Sports Traumatol Arthrosc 2007;15(9):1130.

63. Barbier O, Ollat D, Marchaland JP, et al. Iliac bone-block autograft for posterior shoulder instability. Orthop Traumatol Surg Res 2009;95(2):100.

64. Sirveaux F, Leroux J, Roche O, et al. Surgical treatment of posterior instability of the shoulder joint using an iliac bone block or an acromial pediculated bone block: outcome in eighteen patients. Rev Chir Orthop Reparatrice Appar Mot 2004;90(5):411 [in French].

65. Meuffels DE, Schuit H, van Biezen FC, et al. The posterior bone block procedure in posterior shoulder instability: a long-term follow-up study. J Bone Joint Surg Br 2010;92(5):651.

66. Gosens T, van Biezen FC, Verhaar JA. The bone block procedure in recurrent posterior shoulder instability. Acta Orthop Belg 2001;67(2):116.

67. Essadki B, Dumontier C, Sautet A, et al. Posterior shoulder instability in athletes: surgical treatment with iliac bone block. Apropos of 6 case reports. Rev Chir Orthop Reparatrice Appar Mot 2000;86(8):765 [in French].

68. Levigne C, Garret J, Grosclaude S, et al. Surgical technique arthroscopic posterior glenoidplasty for posterosuperior glenoid impingement in throwing athletes. Clin Orthop Relat Res 2012;470(6):1571.

69. Bessems JH, Vegter J. Glenoplasty for recurrent posterior shoulder instability. Good results in 13 cases followed for 1-16 years. Acta Orthop Scand 1995; 66(6):535.

70. Brewer BJ, Wubben RC, Carrera GF. Excessive retroversion of the glenoid cavity. A cause of non-traumatic posterior instability of the shoulder. J Bone Joint Surg Am 1986;68(5):724.

71. Wirth MA, Seltzer DG, Rockwood CA Jr. Recurrent posterior glenohumeral dislocation associated with increased retroversion of the glenoid. A case report. Clin Orthop Relat Res 1994;(308):98.

72. Millett PJ, Clavert P, Hatch GF 3rd, et al. Recurrent posterior shoulder instability. J Am Acad Orthop Surg 2006;14(8):464.

73. Kropf EJ, Sekiya JK. Management of bony defects in shoulder instability. In: Cole BJ, Sekiya JK, editors. Surgical techniques of the shoulder, elbow, and knee in sports medicine. Philadelphia: Elsevier; 2008. p. 131.

74. Scott DJ Jr. Treatment of recurrent posterior dislocations of the shoulder by glenoplasty. Report of three cases. J Bone Joint Surg Am 1967;49(3):471.

75. Skendzel JG, Sekiya JK. Arthroscopic glenoid osteochondral allograft reconstruction without subscapularis takedown: technique and literature review. Arthroscopy 2011;27(1):129.

76. Skendzel JG, Sekiya JK. Treatment of combined bone defects of humeral head and glenoid: arthroscopic and open techniques. In: Cole BJ, Sekiya JK, editors. Surgical techniques of the shoulder, elbow, and knee in sports medicine. Philadelphia: Elsevier; 2013. p. 161–74.

77. Tjoumakaris FP, Kropf EJ, Sekiya JK. Osteoarticular allograft reconstruction of a large glenoid and humeral head defect in recurrent shoulder instability. Tech Shoulder Elbow Surg 2007;8(1):98.

78. Tjoumakaris FP, Sekiya JK. Combined glenoid and humeral head allograft reconstruction for recurrent anterior glenohumeral instability. Orthopedics 2008;31(5):497.

79. Provencher MT, Ghodadra N, LeClere L, et al. Anatomic osteochondral glenoid reconstruction for recurrent glenohumeral instability with glenoid deficiency using a distal tibia allograft. Arthroscopy 2009;25(4):446.

80. Thompson SR, Cabot J, Litchfield RB. A modified technique of glenoid osteotomy for posterior shoulder instability. Tech Should Surg 2012;13(3):128.

Posterior Instability Caused by Batter's Shoulder

Richard W. Kang, MS, MD[a],*, Gregory T. Mahony, BA[b],
Thomas C. Harris, MS[c], Joshua S. Dines, MD[d]

KEYWORDS

• Posterior instability • Posterior labral repair • Batter's shoulder • Shoulder injury

KEY POINTS

• Batter's shoulder is posterior instability of the lead shoulder due to repetitive batting swings, especially with missed balls.
• Posterior labral repair can be performed after 12 weeks of failed nonoperative management.
• Initial results promising with greater than 90% good to excellent results in a recent case series by Wanich and colleagues.
• Return to play is possible in approximately 6 to 7 months.

INTRODUCTION

Baseball players and fans alike appreciate the towering homeruns hit by the game's power hitters. However, little attention is paid toward the potential deleterious effects of the forces imparted on the shoulder during the swing. The lead shoulder of a swing can undergo tremendous forces, especially when a pitch is missed. Repetitive loads on the shoulder can lead to posterior instability, sometimes called batter's shoulder.

This article reviews the pathomechanics, clinical presentation, imaging, treatment options, and initial clinical results of batter's shoulder.

MECHANICS OF BATTING

Shaffer and colleagues[1] have divided the batting swing into four distinct phases: (1) wind up, (2) preswing, (3) swing, and (4) follow-through. The swing phase can also be subdivided into early, middle, and late phases. The same investigators also

[a] Department of Sports Medicine and Shoulder Surgery, Sports Medicine and Shoulder Surgery, Hospital for Special Surgery, 535 East 70th Street, New York, NY 10021, USA; [b] Department of Sports Medicine and Shoulder Surgery, Hospital for Special Surgery, 535 East 70th Street, New York, NY 10021, USA; [c] Department of Radiation Oncology, Massachusetts General Hospital, 55 Fruit Street, Boston, MA 02114, USA; [d] Department of Sports Medicine and Shoulder Surgery, Hospital for Special Surgery, 519 East 72nd Street, Suite 203A, New York, NY 10021, USA
* Corresponding author.
E-mail address: rwkang.md@gmail.com

Clin Sports Med 32 (2013) 797–802
http://dx.doi.org/10.1016/j.csm.2013.07.012
0278-5919/13/$ – see front matter © 2013 Elsevier Inc. All rights reserved.

evaluated the degree of muscle activation in each phase of batting. Most of the force is generated in the core and lower extremity and translated into rotational velocities of 937° per second at the shoulder and 1160° per second at the arm. These forces allow the bat to rotate at 1588° per second with a resulting linear bat velocity of 31 m per second.[2]

PATHOPHYSIOLOGY

The high rotational velocities coupled with the weight of the bat leads to a tremendous amount of force at the shoulders. Repetitive exposure to these forces can result in batter's shoulder, which is defined as posterior instability leading to episodic subluxation of the lead shoulder during the baseball swing.[3] The lead shoulder of the batter is subject to this condition.

A missed outside pitch is considered the predominant proposed mechanism of injury that leads to batter's shoulder.[4] When the bat fails to make contact with the pitched ball, there is no counterforce to offset the dynamic posterior pulling force of 500 N during a swing.

In addition, reaching for an outside pitch increases the abduction angle of the shoulder during the swing. This increase in abduction angle can also result in increased glenohumeral shear forces. In a preliminary study, Philips and colleagues[4] found an average shoulder-abduction angle of 105° for outside pitches versus 90° for inside pitches. The American Sports Medicine Institute group hypothesized that the increased shoulder abduction angle may increase shear forces across the joint. Given these angles, the torque generated for an outside pitch can be approximately 13.5% greater than that of an inside pitch. The hypothesis is that during a missed pitch there is no counterforce to the momentum from the baseball swing, which leads to greater dynamics in the shoulder and an excessive pulling force.

Additionally, the stabilizing muscles around the shoulder are recruited when the bat makes contact with the ball. A missed ball can lead to failed recruitment of these surrounding muscles, which are important for conferring shoulder stability.

CLINICAL PRESENTATION

Patients typically recall a specific event in which they felt a sensation of instability after reaching for an outside pitch or missing a pitch. Thereafter, patients may have felt discomfort or pain with certain provocative positions, especially with forward flexion, adduction, and internal rotation.[5]

The physical examination may be positive for a positive load and shift test, jerk test, or Kim test. The combination of the jerk and Kim tests has been shown to be about 97% sensitive for a posteroinferior labral lesion.[6]

IMAGING

Plain radiographs should include an axillary view in addition to the standard views of the shoulder. The radiographs should rule out any fractures or dislocations. Additionally, the radiographs should be evaluated for reverse Hill-Sachs lesions, glenoid hypoplasia, or retroversion, as well as any bony avulsions of the glenohumeral ligaments.

MRI is used to evaluate the labrum and capsule, and any associated chondral lesions. The presence of a Kim lesion should also be ruled out on the MRI.[7]

A CT scan, although used less frequently in the setting of batter's shoulder, can be used to evaluate for glenoid version, humeral version, and reverse Hill-Sachs lesions.

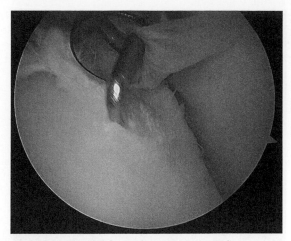

Fig. 1. Torn posterior labrum viewed from the anterior portal.

TREATMENT

The authors' initiate the patient on a course of conservative therapy. This entails physical therapy directed toward rotator cuff strengthening, scapular stabilizing exercises, and improving range of motion. Surgical management is indicated if the patient fails at least 12 weeks of concerted nonoperative management.

Surgical treatment will likely involve an arthroscopic posterior labral repair. Although the operation can be performed in a beach chair position, our preference is the lateral decubitus position. Before prepping and draping, an examination under anesthesia is performed to determine the degree of instability. The posterior portal is made slightly more lateral than usual to facilitate anchor placement for the posterior labral repair. A complete diagnostic arthroscopy is performed initially. Then, the arthroscope is switched to the anterior portal to visualize the torn posterior labrum (**Fig. 1**). The labrum is mobilized using an elevator through the posterior portal. The bony surface is then prepared with the mechanical shaver (**Fig. 2**). Anchors are then placed starting

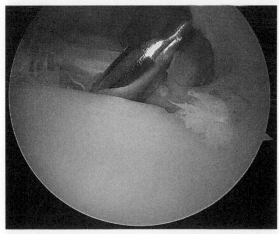

Fig. 2. Preparation of bony glenoid surface and debridement of frayed labral tissue using mechanical shaver.

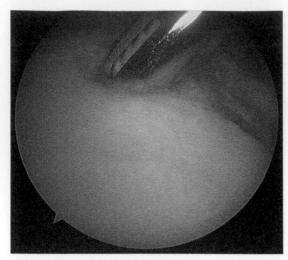

Fig. 3. Implantation of suture anchor onto glenoid rim.

at about the 5:30 position relative to the face of the glenoid in a left shoulder (**Fig. 3**). Using an accessory posterior portal, a tissue-piercing device is used to capture the appropriate amount of capsulolabral tissue to incorporate into the repair (**Fig. 4**). Arthroscopic knots are used to secure the labrum to the glenoid (**Fig. 5**). This sequence is repeated moving superiorly along the face of the glenoid with sequential anchors being placed at 4:30 and 3:30. Occasionally, more anchors are needed if the tear extends into the biceps anchor.

The postoperative rehabilitation protocol involves a sling for 2 weeks. This is followed by physical therapy with a focus on passive range of motion for 6 weeks. After 6 weeks, active range of motion can begin. Then, after the 12-week mark, strength training and hitting off a tee can be started. The patient can progress to taking live pitches at 6 months after the operation.

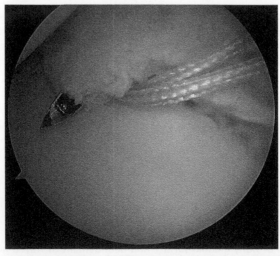

Fig. 4. Tissue-piercing device used to shuttle suture through the capsulolabral complex.

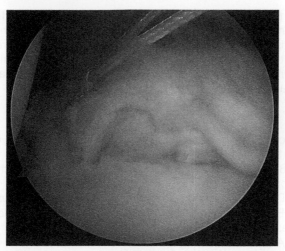

Fig. 5. Arthroscopic knot to bring the capsulolabral complex to the glenoid rim.

CLINICAL RESULTS

Wanich and colleagues[8] conducted the only published study on batter's shoulder. Their retrospective review had 14 participants with an average age of 20 years old (range 17–33 years old). The study consisted of four professional, six college, and four high school athletes. The inclusion criteria consisted of a history of batting-induced shoulder instability. Participants were excluded if they had a history of traumatic injury to the shoulder or a prior shoulder condition. The average follow-up was 1.2 years (range 7–35 months). Posterior laxity was demonstrated on all 14 participants and 12 of 14 had a positive O'Brien sign, 12 out of 14 participants also demonstrated evidence of posterior labral tearing on MRI, 12 out of 14 failed conservative management and went on to surgical treatment, 10 underwent arthroscopic posterior labral repair, and 2 underwent labral debridement without repair. The average return to sport was 6.5 months. Both conservatively managed players had excellent outcomes. Of the surgically treated players, 11 out of 12 (92%) had excellent outcomes. The single player with a poor outcome also had a concomitant glenoid osteochondral lesion that may have contributed to the lack of improvement despite operative intervention. The investigators admitted to several limitations to their study, including the retrospective study design, limited numbers of participants, and lack of long-term follow-up.

SUMMARY

In summary, batter's shoulder is a rare and only recently recognized entity. This condition is posterior shoulder instability caused by a missed attempt at hitting a pitch, especially with an outside pitch. The lack of counterforce from hitting a ball produces increased forces imparted on the posterior capsulolabral complex of the lead shoulder during batting.

If the player fails conservative management, she or he can undergo an arthroscopic posterior labral repair instead of debridement. After treatment, the player can expect to return to play after approximately 6 to 7 months. Initial results from a small, retrospective series demonstrate greater than 90% excellent results.[8] These findings are similar to current literature for arthroscopic treatment of posterior instability, which reports success rates that range from 75% to 91%.[9–13] Longer-term follow-up will be needed to determine the natural history and prognosis for batter's shoulder.

Based on initial results, the authors predict good to excellent results for most players with batter's shoulder who undergo proper treatment. Additionally, with the exception of switch hitters, the nonthrowing arm is affected. This can also improve the athlete's return to play.

REFERENCES

1. Shaffer B, Jobe FW, Pink M, et al. Baseball batting. An electromyographic study. Clin Orthop Relat Res 1993;(292):285–93.
2. Welch CM, Banks SA, Cook FF, et al. Hitting a baseball: a biomechanical description. J Orthop Sports Phys Ther 1995;22(5):193–201.
3. Fleisig GS, Dun S, Kingsley D. Biomechanics of the shoulder during sports. vol. In: Wilk KE, Reinold MM, Andrews JR, editors. The athlete's shoulder. 2nd edition. Philadelphia: Churchill Livingstone; 2009. p. 380.
4. Philips BB, Andrews JR, Fleisig GS. Batter's shoulder: posterior instability of the lead shoulder, A Biomechanical Evaluation. Paper presented at: Alabama Sports Medicine and Orthopaedic Center. Birmingham, 2000.
5. Hawkins RJ, Koppert G, Johnston G. Recurrent posterior instability (subluxation) of the shoulder. J Bone Joint Surg Am 1984;66:169.
6. Kim SH, Park JS, Jeong WK, et al. The Kim test: a novel test for posteroinferior labral lesion of the shoulder–a comparison to the jerk test. Am J Sports Med 2005;33(8):1188–92.
7. Kim SH, Ha KI, Yoo JC, et al. Kim's lesion: an incomplete and concealed avulsion of the posteroinferior labrum in posterior or multidirectional posteroinferior instability of the shoulder. Arthroscopy 2004;20(7):712–20.
8. Wanich T, Dines J, Gambardella RA, et al. Batter's shoulder': can athletes return to play at the same level after operative treatment? Clin Orthop Relat Res 2012; 470(6):1565–70.
9. Bradley JP, Baker CL, Kline AJ, et al. Arthroscopic capsulolabral reconstruction for posterior instability of the shoulder. Am J Sports Med 2006;34(7):1061–71.
10. Kim SH, Ha KI, Park JH, et al. Arthroscopic posterior labral repair and capsular shift for traumatic unidirectional recurrent posterior subluxation of the shoulder. J Bone Joint Surg Am 2003;85(8):1479–87.
11. Provencher MT, Bell SJ, Menzel KA, et al. Arthroscopic treatment of posterior shoulder instability: results in 33 patients. Am J Sports Med 2005;33(10): 1463–71.
12. Williams RJ 3rd, Strickland S, Cohen M, et al. Arthroscopic repair for traumatic posterior shoulder instability. Am J Sports Med 2003;31(2):203–9.
13. Wolf EM, Eakin CL. Arthroscopic capsular plication for posterior shoulder instability. Arthroscopy 1998;14(2):153–63.

Shoulder Instability in Ice Hockey Players
Incidence, Mechanism, and MRI Findings

Tim Dwyer, MBBS, FRACS, FRCSC[a,*], Massimo Petrera, MD[a],
Robert Bleakney, MD, FRCPC[b],
John S. Theodoropoulos, MD, MSc, FRCSC[a,c]

KEYWORDS

- Ice hockey • Traumatic injury • Hill-Sachs lesions • Magnetic resonance imaging

KEY POINTS

- The incidence of injury in ice hockey has been shown to increase with the progression from youth hockey, to college, and professional hockey, likely due to increased player contact and body checking.
- The reported rate of injury to the shoulder in ice hockey ranges between 8.6% and 21.9%, with 1 prospective study identifying that shoulder sprains and dislocations made up 11% of all injuries.
- In this study, 75% of players seen following a traumatic episode of shoulder instability had a Bankart lesion; nearly 80% of these players had a Hill-Sachs lesion.
- The high rate of Hill-Sachs lesions may contribute to failure of shoulder stabilization procedures, and may require additional procedures to address the humeral head defect.

INTRODUCTION

Ice hockey players are a category of athletes at high risk for traumatic injuries because of the aggressive nature of this contact sport. The most common cause of injury is from body checking or player contact.[1] Furthermore

- Reports indicate that players are up to 25 times more likely to be injured in an actual game than during practice.[2–4]

Disclosure: The authors listed have identified no professional or financial affiliations for themselves or their spouse/partner: Tim Dwyer, Massimo Petrera, Robert Bleakney; The authors listed have identified the following professional or financial affiliations for themselves or their spouse/partner: John S. Theodoropoulos is a paid consultant for Smith and Nephew.
[a] Department of Surgery, Women's College Hospital, University of Toronto Orthopaedic Sports Medicine, 76 Grenville Street, Toronto, Ontario M5S 1B2, Canada; [b] Department of Medical Imaging, Mount Sinai Hospital, 600 University Avenue, Toronto, Ontario M5G 1X5, Canada; [c] Department of Surgery, Mount Sinai Hospital, 600 University Avenue, Suite 476C, Toronto, Ontario M5G 1X5, Canada
* Corresponding author.
E-mail address: tim.dwyer@wchospital.ca

Clin Sports Med 32 (2013) 803–813
http://dx.doi.org/10.1016/j.csm.2013.07.013
0278-5919/13/$ – see front matter © 2013 Elsevier Inc. All rights reserved.

- A Swedish study identified that foul play (as defined by an injury associated with a penalty call) was responsible for 50% of all injuries resulting in a player missing practice or a game.[2]

Interestingly, it has been shown that mandatory rules, such as those that restrict body checking in minor hockey leagues, are effective at reducing injury rates.[5] The following factors have been shown to increase the incidence of injury in ice hockey:

- The progression from youth and high school hockey, through to college and professional teams[6]
- The rate of injury increases with the age of hockey players, becoming higher especially in those over 30 years of age[7]
- The rate of injury increases as the level of competition, and subsequently the incidence of player contact increases

Although injuries to the face and concussion are the most commonly reported in ice hockey, up to 32% of all major injuries sustained in ice hockey are to the upper limb.[4,8–10] Although the shoulder is protected by ice hockey equipment, it is thought that the relative flexibility of the shoulder pads in ice hockey (compared with American football) may be problematic.[11] The reported rate of injury to the shoulder in ice hockey ranges between 8.6% and 21.9%[12]:

- In 1 study, reporting on junior hockey players followed for a season, Stuart and colleagues[13] identified that the shoulder and arm were the most common anatomic sites injured (22% each).
- In a prospective study of youth ice hockey teams in Canada, shoulder sprains and dislocations made up to 11% of all injuries.[14]
- Mölsä and colleagues[7] retrospectively analyzed 760 upper limb injuries in Finnish ice hockey players; 70% occurred during games, and most injuries to the shoulder were the result of body checking or player contact.
- Frank shoulder dislocation made up to 2% (20 of 760 injuries) of this cohort, similar to the rate of grade 3 acromioclavicular joint (ACJ) separations. However, another 107 of 760 (12%) injuries were categorized as shoulder sprains, a category that included an unreported number of shoulder subluxations.[7]

Most traumatic shoulder dislocations and subluxations occur in the anterior direction. The Bankart lesion is the most common finding in the setting of recurrent anterior dislocation.[15–17] Other lesions seen include

- Bankart variants such as anterior labral periosteal sleeve avulsion (ALSPA) lesions, Perthes lesions, and glenolabral articular disruption (GLAD) lesions[18]
- A smaller number of patients with glenohumeral instability will have injuries to the superior anterior to posterior labrum (SLAP),[19] and more rarely, humeral avulsion glenohumeral ligament (HAGL) lesions[20]
- Bony lesions of the glenoid and humeral head (Hill-Sachs) defects[21,22]
- Tears or avulsions of the supraspinatus tendon, avulsion of the subscapularis tendon, and fractures of the greater tuberosity may be seen in first-time shoulder dislocation, especially in patients older than 35 years[23]

The aim of this study is to describe the injury patterns on MRI/MRA in ice hockey players presenting after an episode of traumatic shoulder instability. The authors hypothesized that because of the aggressive nature of ice hockey as a contact sport, players presenting after shoulder injury would demonstrate more complex and severe injury patterns than those described in the general population, and in noncontact athletes.

METHODS

The authors reviewed a consecutive series of professional ice hockey players presenting to the senior author (JT) between 2010 and 2013. Each player had sustained a significant trauma to the shoulder, and described a history of acute subluxation or dislocation. Each athlete underwent a 1.5T MRI or MRA, which was independently reviewed by a musculoskeletal radiologist (RB). Patients with isolated injury to the acromioclavicular (AC) joint were excluded.

Each MRI was assessed for pathology, including soft tissue or bony Bankart lesions, posterior labral lesions, SLAP lesions, Hill-Sachs lesions, chondral defects, rotator cuff tears, and any associated pathology. Any concomitant pathology was also noted. All Hill-Sachs lesions were quantified in 3 dimensions, and classified using the system described by Rowe (mild defect: 2 cm wide and 0.3 cm deep, moderate defect: 4 cm wide and 0.5 cm deep, severe defect: 4 cm wide and 1 cm deep).[24] Bony Bankart lesions were classified as none, less than 25%, or greater than 25%[25–27] using an en face view of the glenoid, and calculating the percentage glenoid area loss based on a best-fit circle.[27–29]

Player information regarding level of play was collected, as well as age and position of play. The number of episodes of dislocation and/or subluxation was recorded, as well as any surgery required.

RESULTS

Twenty-four players (24 shoulders) were included in this study, with an average age of 26.6 years (range, 18–37). MRI was used most, with 5 of 25 (20%) players undergoing MRA. **Tables 1** and **2** detail the player demographics, as well as the pathology identified on MRI. The majority of players played in the National Hockey League (NHL) (18/24, 75%), while 2 of 24 (8.3%) players played in the Ontario Hockey League (OHL), and 3 of 24 (12.5%) plyers played in Junior A. The average number of dislocations was 1.6 (range, 1–3).

An anterior labral lesion/Bankart lesion was seen in 18 of 24 shoulders (75%), with the extent of the labral tear variable; the location and extent of all labral lesions identified is demonstrated in **Fig. 1**. A total of 13 of 24 (54.2%) shoulders had a Hill-Sachs lesion. In 10 of 13 cases (77%), the defect was moderate-to-severe, with an average depth of 0.9 mm. Only 5 of 24 (20.8%) players with Bankart lesions did not have a Hill-Sachs lesion. Five of the patients (20.8%) had a type 2 SLAP tear, with 1 extending to the posterior labrum; 2 of 24 (8.3%) patients had an isolated posterior labral tear. Only 3 shoulders (12.5%) had glenoid bony defects, all of which were less than 25% of the anteroinferior glenoid. The variety of lesions seen is demonstrated in **Figs. 2–5**.

Various concomitant lesions were encountered. Two patients had tears of inferior glenohumeral ligament (IGHL), while cartilage lesions of the humeral head, and osteoarthritis of the glenohumeral joint, were seen in 1 player each. One player had a subscapularis tear and a subluxed biceps tendon in association with a Bankart lesion, while another patient had a retear of a previously repaired rotator cuff lesion in conjunction with their Bankart lesion.

DISCUSSION

This investigation has demonstrated that ice hockey players have complex injury patterns in the setting of shoulder instability. In this consecutive series of players with a traumatic episode of shoulder instability, most athletes had a Bankart lesion in

Table 1
Pathology identified on MRI/MRA in each ice hockey player presenting after traumatic injury, with a history suggestive of glenohumeral joint subluxation or dislocation. Players with isolated injury to the ACJ were excluded. All labral lesions have been described relative to a clockface on a right shoulder for simplicity (anterior labrum between 12 o'clock and 6 o'clock)

Player Age	Level	Number of Dislocations	Bankart	ALPSA/Perthes	SLAP	Posterior Labrum	Glenoid Bone Loss	Hill-Sachs (Length cm × Width cm × Depth cm)	Other Lesion	Surgery
18	OHL	2	3-6	—	—	—	—	2 × 0.7 × 0.6	—	—
19	NHL	1	1-6	Yes	—	—	—	—	Tear IGHL	AB
22	NHL	2	3-6	—	—	—	—	2.2 × 1.6 × 0.4	—	AB
32	NHL	1	2-6	Yes	—	—	<25%	2.5 × 1.4 × 0.8	—	—
30	NHL	1	2-6	Yes	—	—	<25%	3 × 2.5 × 0.7	—	—
27	NHL	2	—	—	12-10	—	—	—	—	—
31	NHL	2	3-6	Yes	—	12-6	<25%	1.5 × 1.3 × 0.3	SSC tear, subluxed biceps	A 360
37	NHL	3	—	—	1-11	—	—	—	—	—
23	NHL	2	12-6	Yes	—	—	—	2.2 × 2.2 × 0.6	—	AB
31	NHL	2	2-6	—	—	—	—	—	Chondral lesion humeral head	AB
23	NHL	1	2-6	—	—	—	—	2.5 × 1.2 × 0.7	—	AB

29	NHL	2	—	—	—	—	—	—	APL
29	NHL	1	1-6	Yes	—	—	2.2 × 2 × 0.9	—	—
28	NHL	1	12-6	—	—	—	2.5 × 1 × 0.8	Tear IGHL	AB
36	NHL	2	—	—	1-7	11-7	—	—	—
26	OHL	1	2-6	—	12-10	1 - 7	1.6 × 1.2 × 0.4	Retear SS	AB
27	OJHL	2	—	—	—	—	—	—	—
27	NHL	2	3-6	—	—	—	—	—	—
21	OJHL	1	12-6	—	—	—	2.2 × 2 × 1.3	—	AB
21	OJHL	2	—	—	12-10	—	—	Moderate GHJ OA	SLAP
36	NHL	1	2-6	—	—	—	2.5 × 2.3 × 0.6	—	AB
26	NHL	1	4-6	—	—	—	—	—	—
22	OHL	2	2-5	—	—	—	—	—	AB
23	NHL	1	2-6	—	—	—	2.6 × 2.5 × 1	—	—

Abbreviations: A 360, arthroscopic 360 degree labral repair; AB, arthroscopic Bankart repair; APL, arthroscopic posterior labral repair; GHJ, glenohumeral joint; OJHL, Ontario Junior Hockey League; SS, supraspinatus.

Table 2
Pathology based on player position

Position	Number	Bankart	Hill-Sachs	SLAP	Posterior Labrum
Center	7	7 (100%)	7 (100%)	—	—
Right wing	5	3 (60%)	3 (60%)	1 (20%)	1 (20%)
Left wing	5	5 (100%)	4 (80%)	—	—
Defenseman	7	4 (57.1%)	3 (42.9%)	3 (42.9%)	—
Goalie	0	—	—	—	—

association with a significant Hill-Sachs lesion. The incidence of major glenoid defects was low.

An anterior labral lesion was seen in 75% of athletes, with a Hill-Sachs in 54% of shoulders, and an SLAP lesion in 20%. These results are consistent with other imaging studies in the setting of shoulder instability, although these do not focus on professional athletes in contact sports:

- Antonio and colleagues[30] reviewed the MRA images of 66 patients after a first time dislocation. seventy-three percent had an anteroinferior labral lesion; 14% had an SLAP lesion, and 71% had a Hill-Sachs defect.
- In a review of 61 MRI images in patients presenting with traumatic shoulder dislocation, Widjaja and colleagues[31] identified that 73% of patients had a Bankart lesion, while 67% had a Hill-Sachs lesion.

In the authors' study, only 21% of the players with Bankart lesions did not have a Hill-Sachs lesion. The high incidence of concomitant Bankart and Hill-Sachs lesion in the authors' series may be in relation to the high energy of trauma sustained during a player contact or collision. The reported incidence of Hill-Sachs lesions varies, but is estimated to be as high as 93%.[24,32,33] The cause of this variation is unknown, but is thought to be related to

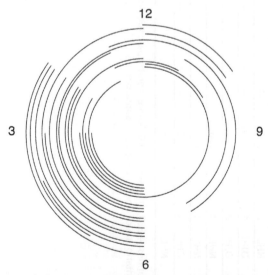

Fig. 1. Representation of the extent of the labral tears identified on MRI/MRA in the 24 shoulders. On this diagram, 12 o'clock represents superior; 3 o'clock represents anterior, and 9 o'clock represents posterior.

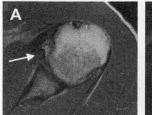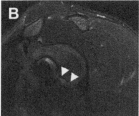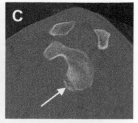

Fig. 2. Conventional MRI demonstrating a bony and fibrocartilagenous Bankart lesion. (*A*) Axial proton density sequence demonstrating the torn displaced labrum anteriorly (*white arrow*). (*B*) Oblique sagittal T2 fat saturated sequence demonstrating the blunted and truncated anteroinferior glenoid (*white arrow heads*). (*C*) Oblique sagittal CT image demonstrating the small (<25%) bony Bankart (*white arrow*).

- The number of actual shoulder dislocations sustained—a study comparing patients with a single shoulder dislocation to those with more than 2 dislocations, noted that both the size and the incidence of the Hill-Sachs lesions increased (67.2% vs 83.9%)[32]
- The method of detection (radiograph vs computed tomography (CT) vs MRI)[34]
- The degree of trauma

It is recognized that athletes involved in contact or collision sports, such as ice hockey, are at increased risk of recurrence following stabilization, compared with noncontact athletes.[35,36] The high incidence of significant humeral bone loss in the authors' series is concerning, as there are reports of increased failure rates after shoulder stabilization in the setting of large Hill-Sachs lesions.[24,37–39] This is supported by the study by Kurokawa and colleagues,[38] identifying that the incidence of an engaging Hill-Sachs lesion was 7%. Interestingly, the authors did not observe any case of glenoid bone loss greater than 25% of the anteroinferior glenoid. This is in contrast to the report by Burkhart and De Beer, demonstrating that 10% of collision athletes treated for recurrent instability had significant glenoid bony defects.[37]

Twenty-one percent of the hockey players in this study group had a type 2 SLAP tear, with 1 tear extending into the posterior labrum. As reported by Snyder and colleagues,[40] the SLAP lesion describes a complex injury of the superior labrum

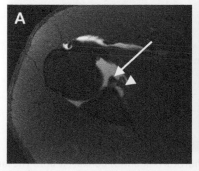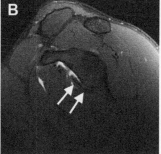

Fig. 3. MRI arthrogram demonstrating an anterior labral periosteal sleeve avulsion (ALSPA). (*A*) Axial T1 fat saturated sequence demonstrating a displaced anterior labrum (*white arrow*) with an intact periosteal sleeve attachment. (*B*) Oblique sagittal T1 fat saturated sequence demonstrating the displaced torn labrum anteroinferiorly (*white arrows*).

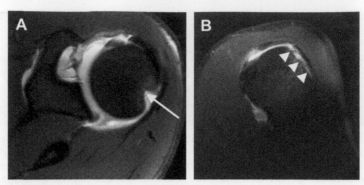

Fig. 4. MRI arthrogram demonstrating a Hill Sachs impaction fracture. (*A*) Axial T1 fat saturated sequence demonstrating the "hatchet"-type defect to the posterior superior aspect of the humeral head (*white arrow*). (*B*) Oblique sagittal T1 fat saturated sequence demonstrating the craniocaudal extent of the Hill-Sachs impaction fracture (*white arrow heads*).

extending from anterior to posterior, thought to be related to a tensile failure of the biceps root secondary to compression loading with the shoulder in flexed and abducted position,[41] or secondary to a peel-back mechanism.[42] Although the latter is common in overhead sports, the authors believe a tensile failure of the biceps root to compression loading may be the mechanism behind SLAP lesions in hockey players. The authors believe that players sustaining an SLAP lesion in this manner may experience a sensation of subluxation or dislocation.

Another 8.3% of players had an isolated posterior labral tear. None of these 3 players sustained a frank posterior dislocation requiring reduction; it may be that these tears are the result of a single trauma, or caused by repetitive forced posterior translation of the shoulder from body contact. None of these patients had a reverse Hill-Sachs lesion; as Saupe and colleagues[43] identified that 86% of patients with a documented first-time posterior dislocation had this lesion, the authors suggest that these posterior labral lesions are not the result of frank posterior dislocation.

Analyzing the data in their study group, the authors also tried to identify if a correlation between shoulder injury and player position exists. In a 3-year prospective study

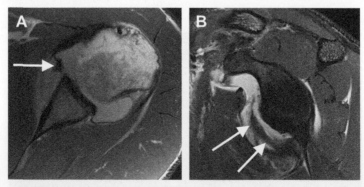

Fig. 5. Conventional MRI demonstrating a fibrocartilagenous Bankart lesion. The large effusion is providing an arthrographic effect. (*A*) Axial proton density sequence demonstrating the torn displaced labrum anteriorly (*white arrow*). (*B*) Oblique sagittal T2 fat saturated sequence demonstrating the displaced labrum (*white arrow heads*) torn off the anteroinferior glenoid.

of a Junior A Hockey League team in the United States, the injury rate was higher (87 injuries per 1000 player game hours) for defenseman than for forwards (134 injuries per 1000 player game hours).[4] Although the authors had only limited numbers for review, there was no evidence that defensemen were more susceptible to traumatic shoulder instability than centers or wingers. Interestingly, a subanalysis by position showed that defenseman had lower prevalence of Bankart lesions, compared with centers and wingers, in this consecutive series. The centers seemed also to be at higher risk for concomitant Bankart and Hill-Sachs lesions.

SUMMARY

Ice hockey is by definition a contact sport, making players at high levels prone to traumatic injuries. The most common cause of injury is from body checking or player contact.[1] A high incidence of concomitant Bankart and significant Hill-Sachs lesions was seen in these professional athletes. These results suggest that a careful assessment and appropriate management of humeral bone loss may be crucial in order to obtain successful outcomes in this challenging group of athletes.

REFERENCES

1. Warsh JM, Constantin SA, Howard A, et al. A systematic review of the association between body checking and injury in youth ice hockey. Clin J Sport Med 2009;19: 134–44.
2. Lorentzon R, Wedren H, Pietila T, et al. Injuries in international ice hockey. A prospective, comparative study of injury incidence and injury types in international and Swedish elite ice hockey. Am J Sports Med 1988;16:389–91.
3. Lorentzon R, Wedren H, Pietila T. Incidence, nature, and causes of ice hockey injuries. A three-year prospective study of a Swedish elite ice hockey team. Am J Sports Med 1988;16:392–6.
4. Stuart MJ, Smith A. Injuries in Junior A ice hockey. A three-year prospective study. Am J Sports Med 1995;23:458–61.
5. Cusimano MD, Nastis S, Zuccaro L. Effectiveness of interventions to reduce aggression and injuries among ice hockey players: a systematic review. CMAJ 2013;185:E57–69.
6. Sutherland GW. Fire on ice. Am J Sports Med 1976;4:264–9.
7. Mölsä J, Kujala U, Myllynen P, et al. Injuries to the upper extremity in ice hockey: analysis of a series of 760 injuries. Am J Sports Med 2003;31:751–7.
8. Molsa J, Airaksinen O, Nasman O, et al. Ice hockey injuries in Finland. A prospective epidemiologic study. Am J Sports Med 1997;25:495–9.
9. Molsa J, Kujala U, Nasman O, et al. Injury profile in ice hockey from the 1970s through the 1990s in Finland. Am J Sports Med 2000;28:322–7.
10. Flik K, Lyman S, Marx RG. American collegiate men's ice hockey: an analysis of injuries. Am J Sports Med 2005;33:183–7.
11. Sim FH, Simonet WT, Scott SG. Ice hockey injuries: Causes, treatment and prevention. J Musculoskelet Med 1989;6:15–44.
12. Sim FH, Simonet WT, Melton LJ 3rd, et al. Ice hockey injuries. Am J Sports Med 1987;15:30–40.
13. Stuart MJ, Smith AM, Nieva JJ, et al. Injuries in youth ice hockey: a pilot surveillance strategy. Mayo Clin Proc 1995;70:350–6.
14. Emery CA, Meeuwisse WH. Injury rates, risk factors, and mechanisms of injury in minor hockey. Am J Sports Med 2006;34:1960–9.

15. Jana M, Srivastava DN, Sharma R, et al. Magnetic resonance arthrography for as-sessing severity of glenohumeral labroligamentous lesions. J Orthop Surg (Hong Kong) 2012;20:230–5.
16. Chandnani VP, Yeager TD, DeBerardino T, et al. Glenoid labral tears: prospective evaluation with MRI imaging, MR arthrography, and CT arthrography. AJR Am J Roentgenol 1993;161:1229–35.
17. Gutierrez V, Monckeberg JE, Pinedo M, et al. Arthroscopically determined degree of injury after shoulder dislocation relates to recurrence rate. Clin Orthop Relat Res 2012;470:961–4.
18. Waldt S, Burkart A, Imhoff AB, et al. Anterior shoulder instability: accuracy of MR arthrography in the classification of anteroinferior labroligamentous injuries. Radi-ology 2005;237:578–83.
19. Volpi D, Olivetti L, Budassi P, et al. Capsulo-labro-ligamentous lesions of the shoulder: evaluation with MR arthrography. Radiol Med 2003;105:162–70.
20. Yiannakopoulos CK, Mataragas E, Antonogiannakis E. A comparison of the spec-trum of intra-articular lesions in acute and chronic anterior shoulder instability. Arthroscopy 2007;23:985–90.
21. Sanders TG, Zlatkin M, Montgomery J. Imaging of glenohumeral instability. Semin Roentgenol 2010;45:160–79.
22. Steinbach LS. MRI of shoulder instability. Eur J Radiol 2008;68:57–71.
23. Neviaser RJ, Neviaser TJ, Neviaser JS. Concurrent rupture of the rotator cuff and anterior dislocation of the shoulder in the older patient. J Bone Joint Surg Am 1988;70:1308–11.
24. Rowe CR, Zarins B, Ciullo JV. Recurrent anterior dislocation of the shoulder after surgical repair. Apparent causes of failure and treatment. J Bone Joint Surg Am 1984;66:159–68.
25. Sugaya H, Moriishi J, Dohi M, et al. Glenoid rim morphology in recurrent anterior glenohumeral instability. J Bone Joint Surg Am 2003;85-A:878–84.
26. Griffith JF, Antonio GE, Yung PS, et al. Prevalence, pattern, and spectrum of gle-noid bone loss in anterior shoulder dislocation: CT analysis of 218 patients. AJR Am J Roentgenol 2008;190:1247–54.
27. Burkhart SS, Debeer JF, Tehrany AM, et al. Quantifying glenoid bone loss arthro-scopically in shoulder instability. Arthroscopy 2002;18:488–91.
28. Lee RK, Griffith JF, Tong MM, et al. Glenoid bone loss: assessment with MR Im-aging. Radiology 2013;267(2):496–502.
29. Huijsmans PE, Haen PS, Kidd M, et al. Quantification of a glenoid defect with three-dimensional computed tomography and magnetic resonance imaging: a cadaveric study. J Shoulder Elbow Surg 2007;16:803–9.
30. Antonio GE, Griffith JF, Yu AB, et al. First-time shoulder dislocation: High preva-lence of labral injury and age-related differences revealed by MR arthrography. J Magn Reson Imaging 2007;26:983–91.
31. Widjaja AB, Tran A, Bailey M, et al. Correlation between Bankart and Hill-Sachs lesions in anterior shoulder dislocation. ANZ J Surg 2006;76:436–8.
32. Spatschil A, Landsiedl F, Anderl W, et al. Posttraumatic anterior-inferior instability of the shoulder: arthroscopic findings and clinical correlations. Arch Orthop Trauma Surg 2006;126:217–22.
33. Cetik O, Uslu M, Ozsar BK. The relationship between Hill-Sachs lesion and recur-rent anterior shoulder dislocation. Acta Orthop Belg 2007;73:175–8.
34. Wilson AJ, Totty WG, Murphy WA, et al. Shoulder joint: arthrographic CT and long-term follow-up, with surgical correlation. Radiology 1989;173:329–33.

35. Mazzocca AD, Brown FM Jr, Carreira DS, et al. Arthroscopic anterior shoulder stabilization of collision and contact athletes. Am J Sports Med 2005;33:52–60.
36. Cho NS, Hwang JC, Rhee YG. Arthroscopic stabilization in anterior shoulder instability: collision athletes versus noncollision athletes. Arthroscopy 2006;22:947–53.
37. Burkhart SS, De Beer JF. Traumatic glenohumeral bone defects and their relationship to failure of arthroscopic Bankart repairs: significance of the inverted-pear glenoid and the humeral engaging Hill-Sachs lesion. Arthroscopy 2000;16: 677–94.
38. Kurokawa D, Yamamoto N, Nagamoto H, et al. The prevalence of a large Hill-Sachs lesion that needs to be treated. J Shoulder Elbow Surg 2013 Mar 1. pii: S1058-2746(13)00009-8.   http://dx.doi.org/10.1016/j.jse.2012.12.033.   [Epub ahead of print].
39. Boileau P, Villalba M, Hery JY, et al. Risk factors for recurrence of shoulder instability after arthroscopic Bankart repair. J Bone Joint Surg Am 2006;88:1755–63.
40. Snyder SJ, Karzel RP, Del Pizzo W, et al. SLAP lesions of the shoulder. Arthroscopy 1990;6:274–9.
41. Andrews JR, Carson WG Jr, McLeod WD. Glenoid labrum tears related to the long head of the biceps. Am J Sports Med 1985;13:337–41.
42. Burkhart SS, Morgan CD. The peel-back mechanism: its role in producing and extending posterior type II SLAP lesions and its effect on SLAP repair rehabilitation. Arthroscopy 1998;14:637–40.
43. Saupe N, White LM, Bleakney R, et al. Acute traumatic posterior shoulder dislocation: MR findings. Radiology 2008;248:185–93.

From the Unstable Painful Shoulder to Multidirectional Instability in the Young Athlete

Haifeng Ren, MD, FRCS(C), Ryan T. Bicknell, MD, MSc, FRCS(C)*

KEYWORDS

- Shoulder • Instability • Pain • Laxity • Athlete • Overhead

KEY POINTS

- Instability as a cause of shoulder pain in the young athlete is a difficult and often missed diagnosis.
- In unstable painful shoulder (UPS), patients are young hyperlax athletes with a history of trauma and have shoulder pain described as deep anterior, reproduced with an anterior apprehension test and relieved with a relocation test.
- In UPS, soft tissue and/or bony lesions consistent with traumatic instability are common and confirm the diagnosis.
- In MDI, patients are young hyperlax athletes with no history of trauma and have shoulder pain described as vague in location and is reproduced with a sulcus and/or hyperabduction test.
- In multidirectional instability (MDI), soft tissue and/or bony lesions consistent with traumatic instability are uncommon, with the exception of capsular laxity.
- Treatment usually consists of arthroscopic surgical reconstruction for UPS and physiotherapy rehabilitation for MDI.

INTRODUCTION

Shoulder pain is one of the leading complaints among athletes. Athletic activities that involve excessive, repetitive, and overhead motion, such as swimming, tennis, pitching, and weightlifting, subject the shoulder to a wide variety of pathological conditions, predominantly associated with pain. The diagnosis of shoulder pain in the young athlete can be difficult and confusing. It is often difficult to diagnose and it is frequently attributed to superior labrum anterior and posterior (SLAP) lesions, internal impingement, partial rotator cuff tears, or biceps tendinitis.[1–7] However, the link between pain and shoulder instability is not well established. In some instances, this pain is related to

Division of Orthopaedic Surgery, Department of Surgery, Kingston General Hospital—Nickle 3, Queen's University, 76 Stuart Street, Kingston, Ontario K7L 2V7, Canada
* Corresponding author.
E-mail address: rtbickne@yahoo.ca

Clin Sports Med 32 (2013) 815–823
http://dx.doi.org/10.1016/j.csm.2013.07.014
0278-5919/13/$ – see front matter © 2013 Elsevier Inc. All rights reserved.

unrecognized instability. This can occur in two forms: the unstable painful shoulder (UPS), which refers to anteroinferior instability of the shoulder without any apparent history of dislocations or subluxations, or increased shoulder laxity, most commonly multidirectional instability (MDI). Misdiagnosis often leads to delayed treatment, progression of the condition, and delayed return to sports. This article discusses the unique points regarding diagnosis, treatment, and outcomes for these two conditions.

UPS

The first description of a UPS, without a history of dislocation or subluxation, came in 1980 from the French surgeon Didier Patte and colleagues.[8] The most recent detailed explanation is by Boileau and colleagues.[9] Although Rowe,[10] Rowe and Zarins,[11] and Blazina and Satzman[12] reported on a recurrent transient anterior subluxation of the shoulder (ie, dead arm syndrome), their patients differed from patients with UPS in that they report awareness of shoulder subluxation with subsequent paralyzing pain, weakness, and a positive apprehension test. Other investigators offer different theories for overstressed anatomic structures, mainly of the anterosuperior part of the shoulder, including the middle glenohumeral ligament (MGHL) and the biceps anchor.[1,5,6] Burkhart and colleagues[2] reported that type II SLAP lesions may be responsible for the dead arm syndrome in overhead-throwing athletes in the late cocking phase. They proposed that abduction and external rotation might stress the bicipital anchor at the posterior glenoid labrum. Furthermore, Castagna and colleagues[3,4] described an acquired instability of the overstressed shoulder and an atraumatic minor shoulder instability.

Diagnosis

The most important factor in diagnosing a UPS is to be aware of this uncommon diagnosis and to consider it a possible cause in the young athlete. The diagnosis of UPS is often missed because the patients do not recall any episode of subluxation or dislocation and, in addition, they do not feel that their shoulders are lax or unstable. Their only complaints are of chronic deep shoulder pain that prohibits overhead activities. They often report persistent symptoms that do not respond to rehabilitation and injections. The pain is not specific and the clinical examination often confounding. This unusual presentation may account for the reported long delay between symptom onset and the final diagnosis (25 ± 23 months) found by Boileau and colleagues.[9] The diagnosis of UPS should be suspected in a young (<30 years old) overhead athlete with deep shoulder pain that is resistant to conservative treatment. Interview of the patient should look for a direct or indirect forgotten trauma of the shoulder with the arm either at the side or in abduction and external rotation. The clinical suspicion that shoulder pain may be due to unrecognized instability is then confirmed by physical examination and the discovery of rollover lesions with imaging or arthroscopy.

History

Features of patients with confirmed UPS was first reported by Boileau and colleagues[9] in 20 subjects with minimum 2-year follow-up. These subjects were often young, with a reported mean age of 22 years at symptom onset; 85% were athletes; 45% engaged in competitive sports; and 80% engaged in contact, overhead, or resisted overhead sports. The dominant arm was affected in 80% and there was a preceding traumatic event in 80% of the cases.

All subjects presented with a complaint of a painful shoulder, without any history of recognized glenohumeral (GH) instability. In 80%, the pain was described as a deep anterior pain. The pain occurred during activity in all subjects, with occasional pain present at rest (15%), and night pain (25%). Only one subject had temporary associ-ated paresthesias in the affected upper extremity. All subjects had to stop sports ac-tivities because of persistent shoulder pain.[9]

Examination

Glenohumeral hyperlaxity was present in 85% of subjects, indicated by external rota-tion with the arm at the side of greater than 85° (anterior hyperlaxity) or greater than 20° difference in hyperabduction compared with the contralateral side (inferior hyperlax-ity). There was anterior GH laxity, indicated by greater than 50% anterior translation on a drawer test in 90%, an asymmetrical inferior drawer (sulcus sign) in 25%, and a posterior drawer in 10% of cases.[9]

Pain was reproduced with the arm in an anterior apprehension position (ie, abduc-tion and external rotation) in all (100%) and was relieved with the Jobe relocation test in 95% of cases.[13,14] It is important to note that the symptom was pain and not appre-hension. Pain was also reproduced with the Gagey hyperabduction test in 85%.[15]

Further tests that reproduce the pain and aid in the diagnosis of UPS have been described by Boileau and colleagues.[9] These include: (1) the comparative (side to-side) hyperabduction test[15] (**Fig. 1**), (2) the KST (**Fig. 2**), and (3) direct palpation of the anterior-inferior glenoid rim lesion through the axilla (**Fig. 3**). Although these tests are noted to be helpful, none are validated for diagnostic decision-making. The comparative hyperabduction test is described previously (**Fig. 1**).[15] It is considered positive when (1) it reproduces the patient's pain (deep anterior pain recognized by the patient), (2) it is asymmetrical when compared with the contralateral side (>20° of difference), and (3) there is a soft end-point (when compared with the firm endpoint of the contralateral side). The knee shoulder test (KST) is positive when the pain is reproduced, the patient can feel his or her shoulder sliding outside the socket, or an anteroinferior drawer is visible (**Fig. 2**).[9] The direct-palpation test of the anteroinferior glenoid rim is positive when it reproduces the patient's pain and discomfort (**Fig. 3**).[9]

Imaging

The diagnosis of a UPS is based on the finding of soft tissue and/or bony lesions commonly associated with anteroinferior instability. This can include any posttrau-matic soft tissue or bony lesion indicating anteroinferior instability, including capsulo-labral detachment (ie, Bankart or humeral avulsion of the glenohumeral ligaments), capsular tears, GH fractures or erosions, or capsular distension allowing excessive GH translation at arthroscopy. The presence of such rollover lesions confirms the

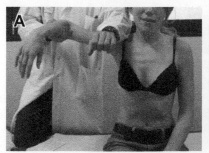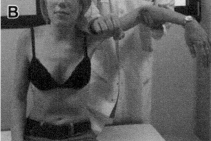

Fig. 1. The comparative hyperabduction test is positive on the left shoulder (*B*) when: (1) it reproduces the patient's pain (deep pain recognized by the patient), (2) it is asymmetrical when compared with the contralateral side (*A*) (>20° of difference) and; (3) there is a soft end-point (when compared with the firm endpoint of the contralateral side).

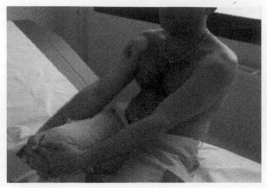

Fig. 2. The KST is considered positive when the pain is reproduced, when the patient can feel his or her shoulder sliding outside the socket, or when an anteroinferior drawer is visible.

history of an unrecognized shoulder subluxation or dislocation. Bony lesions (glenoid fracture or erosion or Hill-Sachs lesion) are rare, presumably because the patients generally have hyperlaxity.

Treatment

The first step of treatment is to perform a diagnostic arthroscopy to confirm the diagnosis. At arthroscopy, detachment of the capsulolabral complex from the anteroinferior glenoid rim was observed in 70% of cases by Boileau and colleagues.[9] However, a capsulolabral detachment can often be quite subtle in this patient population (**Fig. 4**). The Bankart lesion can be limited to a small slot between the labrum and glenoid surface into which the probe can be introduced. The remaining 30% in that series had a distension of the anterior band of the inferior glenohumeral ligament (IGHL) and the capsular pouch, allowing excessive GH translation. Similar to recognized instability, after the diagnosis of a UPS is made, treatment is undertaken according to the specific lesion.

Outcomes

Boileau and colleagues[9] demonstrated that arthroscopic stabilization is effective to relieve pain and improve function in subjects with UPS. Subjectively, 95% of subjects

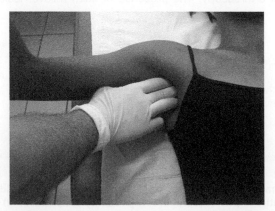

Fig. 3. Direct-palpation test of the anteroinferior glenoid rim that reproduces the patient's pain and discomfort.

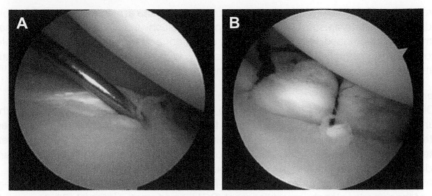

Fig. 4. (A) The anteroinferior capsulolabral detachment is often limited to a small slot between the labrum and glenoid surface into which the probe can be introduced. (B) Subsequent repair.

were very satisfied or satisfied. Subjects had improvement in functional outcomes, with a significant improvement in UCLA, Rowe, and Walch-Duplay scores (P<.05). All subjects returned to work at a mean duration of 5 months (range, 0–18 months). The subjects were able to return to their previous sport at the same level in 75% of cases, at a mean time of 7 months (range, 2–18 months).

MDI

MDI is another form of shoulder instability that often presents predominantly with pain. MDI is defined as symptomatic instability in two or more directions. Repetitive episodes of instability lead to proprioceptive loss from the capsule with repetitive stretching that disrupts the afferent feedback from receptors in the capsule. This may cause muscle patterning and/or recruiting deficits, which in turn disrupt the muscle balance and recruitment pattern. The resultant muscle imbalance is considered one of the major reasons for instability in the lax shoulder. The humeral head fails to center itself on the glenoid with loss of force couples. This leads to pain that may be from a variety of sources, including painful impingement (eg, against the coracoacromial arch), rotator cuff tendinosis, or rotator cuff and periscapular fatigue, thereby converting an asymptomatic laxity to symptomatic instability and creating a vicious cycle further stretching the capsule.[16]

Diagnosis

Clinical suspicion is critical for accurate and prompt identification of MDI, particularly with pain as the chief complaint. Most MDI patients present with insidious onset and nonspecific, activity-related pain. A history of instability is usually vague because instability events are predominantly spontaneously reduced subluxations.

History

The pattern of pain often depends on the direction, or combination of directions, of instability. Anterior instability is often associated with pain with an overhead abducted and externally rotated position, whereas inferior instability leads to symptoms when carrying objects at the side. Posterior instability occurs with the arm in an adducted reaching position. As a result, anterior shoulder pain is common in chronic anterior or MDI, typically aggravated by activities in an abducted-externally rotated position (eg, throwing or overhead activities). Posterior shoulder pain is common in chronic posterior or MDI, typically aggravated by activities with the arm in a position of flexion, adduction, and internal rotation (eg, bench press or push-ups). Overhead athletes may complain of decreased velocity, precision, or distance of throwing. Phases of painful throwing usually signify the direction of instability, with anterior instability causing pain in the cocking phase versus posterior instability causing pain in follow-through.[17,18]

Examination

MDI patients often present with generalized ligamentous laxity. This is assessed by the four Beighton criteria: (1) hyperflexibility of the thumb to touch the forearm, (2) hyperextensibility of the metacarpophalangeal joint of the little finger beyond 90°, (3) hyperextension of the elbows and (4) knees beyond 10°, and (5) the ability to bend forward and place the hands flat on the floor without bending the knees.[19]

A sulcus sign is pathognomonic of MDI. This measures inferior GH laxity and integrity of the superior glenohumeral ligament (SGHL) and rotator interval (RI). The visible dimpling or palpable step-off (1 cm) between the acromion and humeral head, grades the severity of laxity (1+). The test is then repeated in 30° external rotation. If the amount of inferior translation does not decrease with external rotation, it suggests incompetence of the SGHL and RI. A persistent sulcus sign with the arm in external rotation suggests RI laxity.[18]

The Gagey hyperabduction test assesses laxity of the IGHL, with passive abduction (scapular stabilized) of more than 105°. Gagey and Gagey[15] showed that passive abduction from the isolated GH joint has a constant value in 95% in normal subjects. Passive abduction of over 105° versus 90° in the contralateral shoulder was shown in 85% of shoulders with instability (see **Fig. 1**).

Imaging

Radiographs are usually normal in MDI because bony injury is uncommon owing to the protective effect of hyperlaxity. CT or MR arthrogram is often not contributory because MDI is generally a result of generalized ligamentous laxity with an absence of capsulolabral detachment.

Treatment

The mainstay of initial treatment of MDI is physiotherapy rehabilitation, which focuses on scapulothoracic dyskinesia to aid scapular positioning, rotator cuff strengthening to improve concavity-compression, and proprioceptive exercises. Surgery should not be considered until after at least 6 months of appropriate rehabilitation.[20]

Complicated cases may require examination under anesthesia or diagnostic arthroscopy as the gold standard. Typical arthroscopic findings of MDI include patulous capsule, an obvious drive-through sign, and widened RI. Open inferior capsular shift, arthroscopic capsular plication, and RI interval closure have been useful in MDI.[20,21]

In 1980, Neer and Foster[22] pioneered the technique of open inferior capsular shift, which is considered the gold standard to eliminate redundancy and reduce capsular volume in MDI. The subscapularis muscle is tenotomized and superior and inferior capsular flaps are elevated from the humeral neck by a T-shaped incision made between the middle and inferior GH ligaments. The superior leaflet is shifted inferiorly and the inferior leaflet is shifted superiorly, in a pants-over-vest configuration. This technique is performed with the arm in 30° of abduction, external rotation, and forward flexion to minimize loss of motion.

Arthroscopic capsular plication effectively reduces the capsular volume by passing multiple sutures through the capsular tissue and imbricating the capsule into pleats that are anchored to the labrum with or without suture anchors. Anchor fixation was shown in vitro to be mechanically more robust than direct suture repair.[23] Overly aggressive plication risks postoperative motion loss, particularly external rotation. However, the optimal magnitude of plication is not defined, although studies consistently show a correlation with the extent of volume reduction in vitro.[24,25] A recent systematic review showed that in MDI with no structural lesions, arthroscopic capsular plication yielded comparable results to open capsular shift with regard to recurrent instability, return to sport, loss of external rotation, and overall complications.[26] It has become increasingly popular due to its advantages of (1) preservation of the subscapularis without tenotomy; (2) visualization of the entire capsulolabral anatomy, including posterior structures; (3) ability to address selectively anteroinferior and/or posteroinferior capsular or IGHL redundancy using a single approach; and (4) decreased morbidity.[21]

RI closure has been shown to exert an additive effect to anterior stabilization. The current debate regarding its effectiveness in MDI originates from Harryman and colleagues[27] who showed decreased posterior and inferior translation after open medial-to-lateral imbrication of the coracohumeral ligament (CHL), which has not been replicated in later studies.[28,29] The discrepancies may relate to differences in various interval closure techniques. In contrast to the CHL imbrication described by Harryman and colleagues,[27] the typical arthroscopic techniques involve SGHL-to-MGHL closure. Using a cadaveric MDI model, Farber and colleagues[30] proposed an arthroscopic medial-lateral RI closure with a suture anchor in the humeral head as a viable option in MDI, especially in cases with a component of posterior instability with acceptable loss of range of motion. Compared with the superior-inferior RI closure, the medial-lateral RI closure restored range of motion closer to the intact state and decreased posterior translation with the shoulder in abduction and external rotation. The decision whether to supplement the stabilization with RI closure should be weighed against its potential to limit external rotation.

Outcomes

Nonoperative treatment has been shown effective in approximately 80% of patients compliant with their exercise program.[31] Open inferior capsular shift was previously established as the gold standard procedure based on a 95% success rate of subjective clinical outcome scores and long-term stability rates.[32,33] However, a recent systemic review comparing open capsular shift and arthroscopic capsular plication showed similar efficacy between the two procedures with regard to reported outcomes of recurrent instability, postoperative range of motion, and complications. It also noted a trend toward increased return to preoperative level of sports participation for patients treated arthroscopically versus those treated with open capsular shift (86% vs 80%).[26]

SUMMARY

In conclusion, instability as a cause of shoulder pain in the young athlete is a difficult and often missed diagnosis. These young patients often seek treatment of shoulder pain but do not recall any episodes of shoulder instability. As a result, these uncommon, poorly described forms of instability are often misdiagnosed. A heightened clinical suspicion and an accurate, prompt diagnosis of instability is of paramount importance in this athletic group. It dictates appropriate treatment of the condition, avoids treatment delays and failure, provides better outcomes, and ensures timely return to play. UPS and MDI are two forms of this diagnosis.

In UPS, patients at risk are young hyperlax athletes with a history of direct trauma or forceful overextension of the shoulder. They have shoulder pain that is described as deep anterior, reproduced with an anterior apprehension test and relieved with a relocation test. Soft tissue and/or bony lesions consistent with instability (observed on imaging or at arthroscopy) are necessary to confirm the diagnosis of UPS. Once the diagnosis is made, standard arthroscopic techniques with labrum reinsertion and/or anteroinferior capsule plication can lead to predictable good results and return to sport.

In MDI, patients at risk are also young hyperlax athletes. However, these patients often do not have a history of trauma. They have shoulder pain that is often somewhat vague in location and is reproduced with a sulcus and/or hyperabduction test. Soft tissue and/or bony lesions consistent with instability are uncommon, with the exception of capsular laxity. The mainstay of treatment is physiotherapy rehabilitation. When surgery is necessary, open capsular shift and arthroscopic capsular plication are effective.

REFERENCES

1. Andrews JR, Carson WG Jr, McLeod WD. Glenoid labrum tears related to the long head of the biceps. Am J Sports Med 1985;13(5):337–41.
2. Burkhart SS, Morgan CD, Kibler WB. Shoulder injuries in overhead athletes. The "dead arm" revisited. Clin Sports Med 2000;19(1):125–58.
3. Castagna A, Grasso A, Vinanti G. Minor shoulder instability. In: Lajtai G, Snyder S, Applegate GR, et al, editors. Shoulder arthroscopy and MRI technique, vol. 1. Berlin: Springer-Verlag; 2003. p. 193–211.
4. Castagna A, Nordenson U, Garofalo R, et al. Minor shoulder instability. Arthroscopy 2007;23(2):211–5.
5. Savoie FH 3rd, Papendik L, Field LD, et al. Straight anterior instability: lesions of the middle glenohumeral ligament. Arthroscopy 2001;17(3):229–35.
6. Townley CO. The capsular mechanism in recurrent dislocation of the shoulder. J Bone Joint Surg Am 1950;32(2):370–80.
7. Walch G, Boileau P, Noel ED. Impingement of the deep surface of the supraspinatus tendon on the posteriosuperior glenoid rim: an arthroscopic study. J Shoulder Elbow Surg 1992;1:238–45.
8. Patte D, Bernageau J, Rodineau J, et al. Unstable painful shoulders (author's transl). Rev Chir Orthop Reparatrice Appar Mot 1980;66(3):157–65 [in French].
9. Boileau P, Zumstein M, Balg F, et al. The unstable painful shoulder (UPS): as a cause of pain from unrecognized antero-inferior instability in the young athlete. J Shoulder Elbow Surg 2011;20:98–106.
10. Rowe CR. Recurrent transient anterior subluxation of the shoulder. The "dead arm" syndrome. Clin Orthop Relat Res 1987;223:11–9.
11. Rowe CR, Zarins B. Recurrent transient subluxation of the shoulder. J Bone Joint Surg Am 1981;63(6):863–72.
12. Blazina ME, Satzman JS. Recurrent anterior subluxation of the shoulder in athletes—A distinct entity. J Bone Joint Surg Am 1969;51:1037.
13. Jobe FW, Giangarra CE, Kvitne RS, et al. Anterior capsulolabral reconstruction of the shoulder in athletes in overhand sports. Am J Sports Med 1991;19(5):428–34.
14. Kvitne RS, Jobe FW. The diagnosis and treatment of anterior instability in the throwing athlete. Clin Orthop Relat Res 1993;291:107–23.
15. Gagey OJ, Gagey N. The hyperabduction test. J Bone Joint Surg Br 2001;83(1):69–74.

16. Gerber C, Nyffeler RW. Classification of glenohumeral joint instability. Clin Orthop Relat Res 2002;400:65–76 [UI: 12072747].
17. Van Tongel A, Karelse A, Berghs B, et al. Posterior shoulder instability: current concepts review. Knee Surg Sports Traumatol Arthrosc 2011;19(9):1547–53 [UI: 20953863].
18. Owens BD, Dickens JF, Kilcoyne KG, et al. Management of mid-season traumatic anterior shoulder instability in athletes. J Am Acad Orthop Surg 2012;20:518–26 [UI: 22855854].
19. Beighton P, Horan F. Orthopaedic aspects of the Ehlers-Danlos syndrome. J Bone Joint Surg Br 1969;51(3):444–53 [UI: 5820785].
20. Gaskill TR, Taylor DC, Millett PJ. Management of multidirectional instability of the shoulder. J Am Acad Orthop Surg 2011;19(12):758–67 [UI: 22134208].
21. Bell JE. Arthroscopic management of multidirectional instability. Orthop Clin North Am 2010;41(3):357–65 [UI: 20497811].
22. Neer CS 2nd, Foster CR. Inferior capsular shift for involuntary inferior and multi-directional instability of the shoulder. A preliminary report. J Bone Joint Surg Am 1980;62(6):897–908 [UI: 7430177].
23. Provencher MT, Verma N, Obopilwe E, et al. A biomechanical analysis of capsular plication versus anchor repair of the shoulder: can the labrum be used as a suture anchor? Arthroscopy 2008;24(2):210–6 [UI: 18237706].
24. Sekiya JK, Willobee JA, Miller MD, et al. Arthroscopic multi-pleated capsular plication compared with open inferior capsular shift for reduction of shoulder volume in a cadaveric model. Arthroscopy 2007;23(11):1145–51 [UI: 17986400].
25. Flanigan DC, Forsythe T, Orwin J, et al. Volume analysis of arthroscopic capsular shift. Arthroscopy 2006;22(5):528–33 [UI: 16651163].
26. Jacobson ME, Riggenbach M, Wooldridge AN, et al. Open capsular shift and arthroscopic capsular plication for treatment of multidirectional instability. Arthroscopy 2012;28(7):1010–7 [UI: 22365265].
27. Harryman DT 2nd, Sidles JA, Harris SL, et al. The role of the rotator interval capsule in passive motion and stability of the shoulder. J Bone Joint Surg Am 1992;74(1):53–66 [UI: 1734014].
28. Mologne TS, Zhao K, Hongo M, et al. The addition of rotator interval closure after arthroscopic repair of either anterior or posterior shoulder instability: effect on glenohumeral translation and range of motion. Am J Sports Med 2008;36(6):1123–31 [UI: 18319350].
29. Provencher MT, Mologne TS, Hongo M, et al. Arthroscopic versus open rotator interval closure: biomechanical evaluation of stability and motion. Arthroscopy 2007;23(6):583–92 [UI: 17560472].
30. Farber AJ, ElAttrache NS, Tibone JE, et al. Biomechanical analysis comparing a traditional superior-inferior arthroscopic rotator interval closure with a novel medial-lateral technique in a cadaveric multidirectional instability model. Am J Sports Med 2009;37(6):1178–85 [UI: 19282507].
31. Burkhead WZ Jr, Rockwood CA Jr. Treatment of instability of the shoulder with an exercise program. J Bone Joint Surg Am 1992;74:890.
32. Altchek DW, Warren RF, Skyhar MJ, et al. T-plasty modification of the Bankart procedure for multidirectional instability of the anterior and inferior types. J Bone Joint Surg Am 1991;73(1):105–12 [UI: 1985978].
33. Pollock RG, Owens JM, Flatow EL, et al. Operative results of the inferior capsular shift procedure for multidirectional instability of the shoulder. J Bone Joint Surg Am 2000;82(7):919–28 [UI: 10901306].

Results of Shoulder Stabilization Surgery in Athletes

Robert H. Brophy, MD

KEYWORDS

- Glenohumeral dislocation • Anterior instability • Posterior instability
- Arthroscopic stabilization • Open stabilization

KEY POINTS

- Athletes are at risk for glenohumeral instability, with anterior instability significantly more common than posterior instability.
- Anterior shoulder instability in athletes can be treated using open or arthroscopic stabilization, with slightly lower recurrence rates using open techniques compared with arthroscopic techniques, especially for contact or collision athletes.
- Posterior instability in athletes can be treated using open or arthroscopic stabilization, with greater rates of return to play using arthroscopic techniques compared with open techniques.
- Throwing athletes have a lower rate of return to play after surgical stabilization for both anterior and posterior shoulder instability.

INTRODUCTION

Glenohumeral instability is a common occurrence in athletes, particularly for contact sports. Instability episodes have been shown to occur at a rate of 0.12 per 1000 sporting exposures in athletes and high-risk individuals.[1] Contact sports, such as American football, ice hockey, and rugby, are associated with the highest risk for shoulder instability.[1–3] Almost 10% of the collegiate American football players invited to the National Football League (NFL) Combine to evaluate prospects for professional football have a history of shoulder instability,[2] which represents the second most common shoulder disorder in this group of elite athletes.[4]

Traumatic shoulder instability is often classified by the direction, degree of instability, and chronology.[5] Although more than 90% of traumatic shoulder instability is anterior,[6] traumatic posterior instability can also be a significant source of morbidity

Disclosures: None.
Department of Orthopaedic Surgery, Washington University School of Medicine, 14532 South Outer Forty Drive, St. Louis, MO 63017, USA
E-mail address: brophyr@wudosis.wustl.edu

Clin Sports Med 32 (2013) 825–832
http://dx.doi.org/10.1016/j.csm.2013.07.015
0278-5919/13/$ – see front matter © 2013 Elsevier Inc. All rights reserved.

in athletes.[7] After an episode of glenohumeral joint dislocation, patients are at risk for recurrent shoulder dislocation, pain, and weakness. In athletes, these symptoms can be particularly debilitating, limiting their ability to train and compete. Management of instability in the athlete starts with conservative interventions but often requires surgical intervention because of recurrent instability and symptoms.[8,9] Traumatic shoulder instability has been shown to have a high recurrence rate in young, active populations.[8,10] In a series of 38 patients with a primary anterior shoulder dislocation treated nonoperatively at the US Military Academy, there was a 92% recurrence rate.[10]

Almost half of the athletes at the NFL combine with a history of shoulder instability have undergone stabilization surgery (4.7% of all athletes at the combine),[2] accounting for 58% of shoulder surgeries in this population.[4] A history of shoulder instability has been shown to decrease the likelihood that an athlete at the combine will play professional football,[11] particularly for linemen, and shorten an athlete's professional career,[12] particularly for defensive linemen and receivers.[13] Professional rugby players lose an average of 81 days from competition after a shoulder dislocation, with a recurrence rate of 62%.[3]

Considering the impact of shoulder instability on athletes and their frequent need for operative treatment, the outcomes of shoulder stabilization surgery in this population are particularly relevant to the shoulder and sports medicine surgeon. The purpose of this article is to review the literature for outcomes of shoulder stabilization surgery in athletes, focusing on open and arthroscopic techniques for anterior and posterior shoulder instability.

SURGICAL TREATMENT OF ANTERIOR INSTABILITY IN THE ATHLETE
Open Stabilization of Anterior Instability

Open stabilization with a Bankart repair and anterior capsulorrhaphy is the historical gold standard for the treatment of anterior shoulder instability for athletes as well as the general population.[14–17] Numerous studies have reported outcomes of open stabilization for anterior instability in athletic populations.[15–19]

Jobe and colleagues[17] looked at the outcomes of open anterior capsulolabral reconstruction in 25 elite throwing athletes with shoulder pain related to anterior instability. There was no recurrent instability, and clinical outcomes were good or excellent in 92% of these athletes. Seventy-two percent returned to their preinjury level of competition as a throwing athlete.

Bigliani and colleagues[15] reported a 2.9% recurrence rate of dislocation in 63 athletes treated with open Bankart repair and anterior capsulorrhaphy for anterior shoulder instability. Ten percent of the patients reported some mechanical symptoms, such as clicking or snapping at the final follow-up. Sixty-eight percent of these patients were involved in overhead sports (most common sport overall was baseball with 16 athletes) and 13% were involved in contact sports (most common contact sport was football with 8 athletes). Although 94% got back to the sport, only 75% achieved their preinjury level of competition. This number decreased to 50% of the throwing athletes.

Uhorchak and colleagues[19] reported the results of open shoulder stabilization in 66 athletes participating in contact or collision sports at the US Military Academy in West Point, New York. At an average follow-up of 47 months, there was an overall recurrence rate of 23%: 12% had noted less than 3 recurrent subluxations; 8% reported 3 or more recurrent subluxations; and 3% reported recurrent dislocations. The average American Shoulder and Elbow Surgeons (ASES) score was 95 and the average Rowe score was 80 in this cohort at the final follow-up. Of note, all of these athletes returned to their sport and military training after surgery.

Pagnani and Dome[18] reported no recurrent dislocations and 2 recurrent subluxations in 58 American football players treated with open stabilization for traumatic anterior shoulder instability. The clinical outcomes were excellent, with an average postoperative ASES score of 97 and a Rowe and Zarins score of 93.6. A total of 52 out of 58 patients returned to football, and only one patient was forced to retire from football because of recurrent instability. Forty-nine patients restored forward flexion and external rotation to within 5° of the contralateral side.

Although open stabilization surgery has been shown to be successful in reducing recurrent shoulder instability among athletes, the surgery may not be completely restorative. In a study of 19 athletes treated with open shoulder stabilization surgery, there was still a significant reduction of quality of life (9%) and sports activity at minimum 2-year follow-up.[20] It was also noted that shoulder muscle activity and strength were diminished. A study from the NFL combine showed that a history of shoulder stabilization during college or high school, most of which were anterior dislocations treated with open stabilization, decreased an athlete's durability in professional football.[12] This finding was particularly true for linebackers and linemen.

In summary, open stabilization with Bankart repair and capsulorrhaphy is an effective treatment option for recurrent anterior shoulder instability in athletes. The recurrence of frank dislocation is less than 5%, although a larger percentage will have recurrent subluxation episodes. Clinical outcomes are very good, and upwards of 90% of athletes will return to their sport after this procedure. More research is needed to better understand the long-term implications of these surgeries in athletes.

Arthroscopic Stabilization of Anterior Instability

Advances in arthroscopic techniques, particularly the development of suture anchors, have led to more common use of arthroscopic procedures for shoulder stabilization. The potential advantages include decreased pain and morbidity, quicker rehabilitation, and less loss of motion postoperatively. Open stabilization may be associated with a greater loss of external rotation, which is particularly important to throwing athletes.[21] Arthroscopic stabilization may be particularly desirable for athletes who want to return to sport as quickly as possible with preservation of motion, for example, the throwing athlete. Although initial rates of recurrent instability were reported to be higher with arthroscopic stabilization, more recent reports have shown results approaching equivalence with open techniques.[22–24]

DeBerardino and colleagues[25] reported a 12% recurrence rate in 48 shoulders with traumatic anterior shoulder instability treated with arthroscopic stabilization using tissue tacks. All patients with stable shoulders were able to return to their preinjury activity level. They reported that a history of bilateral shoulder instability, a 2+ sulcus sign, and poor capsulolabral tissue at the time of repair were associated with a higher risk of failure. The average Rowe score at the final assessment was 92.

Ide and colleagues[26] reported on 55 athletes, younger than 25 years or participating in a contact sport, with recurrent anterior instability and no significant bone loss treated with arthroscopic stabilization using suture anchors. At a mean follow-up of 42 months, there was a recurrence rate of 7% with an average loss of 4° of external rotation and a mean Rowe score of 92. They did not see a significant difference in the recurrence rate between contact athletes (9.5%) and noncontact athletes (6.0%). Overall, 80% of the athletes got back to the same level of competition as before their injury. However, throwing athletes returned to the same level of competition at a significantly lower rate (68%) than nonthrowing athletes (90%).

Mazzocca and colleagues[27] reported the results of arthroscopic anterior stabilization using suture anchors in 13 collision and 5 contact athletes. At an average follow-up of 37 months, all of the athletes had returned to high school or collegiate competition. The mean ASES score was 88.4 and the mean Rowe score was 92. Overall, 11% (2) of the athletes suffered a recurrent dislocation, both in collision sports. However, no athletes required recurrent stabilization surgery.

Larrain and colleagues[28] reported on the results of arthroscopic stabilization of anterior shoulder instability using suture anchors in rugby players. They treated 39 of 40 (98%) acute patients and 121 of 158 (77%) patients with recurrent instability with an arthroscopic technique. All patients in the acute group and 84% of the recurrent instability group returned to the same level of rugby competition. The mean time to return to play was 5 months in the acute group and 7.5 months in those with recurrent instability. There was a 5.1% recurrence rate in the acute group and an 8.3% recurrence rate in the recurrent group. Good or excellent results using the Rowe scale were reported in 95% of the acute group and 92% of the recurrent instability group. The investigators emphasized the importance of patient selection based on the type of lesion to guide surgical technique, excluding patients with bony defects, poor tissue quality, or humeral avulsion of the glenohumeral ligament lesions from arthroscopic stabilizations.

One study compared arthroscopic stabilization with open stabilization for anterior shoulder instability in an athletic patient population. Rhee and colleagues[29] looked at 48 shoulders in 46 collision athletes, 32 of which were treated with open stabilization and 16 of which were treated with arthroscopic stabilization. Twelve of the shoulders treated arthroscopically were fixed with suture anchors, whereas 4 were treated with Suretacs (Acufex, Mansfield, MA). The mean Rowe score increased from 43 to 88, whereas the mean Constant score increased from 65 to 87, with no significant differences between surgical techniques. Overall, the return to sport (at least 90% of preinjury activity) was 83%, with more of the open patients returning to this level (90% vs 63%, $P = .02$). Overall, there was a 16.5% recurrence rate with 2 postoperative subluxations (4.0%) and 6 recurrent dislocations (12.5%). There was a significantly higher recurrence rate in the arthroscopic group (25.0%) than the open group (12.5%) ($P = .04$). The highest recurrence rate was in wrestling athletes (57%). There were no significant differences between the groups in terms of postoperative shoulder range of motion. The investigators concluded that open stabilization was more reliable in collision athletes.

Overall, the data suggest that arthroscopic stabilization can be successful in athletes, with the potential benefit of better range of motion. Suture anchors are likely better than tissue tacks. Although the evidence suggests the outcomes following arthroscopic surgery are improving, more studies are needed to better characterize the indications for and outcomes of this technique in athletes, especially for collision and contact sports whereby open techniques may result in lower rates of recurrence.

Bony Block Procedures for Anterior Instability

There is growing interest in bony block procedures to address anterior shoulder instability. A recent study reported the long-term results of the Latarjet procedure in athletes.[30] In this study, 37 shoulders in 34 rugby union players with anterior shoulder instability were treated with the Latarjet procedure. At a mean follow-up of 12 years (minimum 5 years), there were no recurrent dislocations or subluxations. On physical examination, 5 patients (14%) were noted to have a persistent apprehension. The mean Rowe score was 93%, and 65% of the athletes returned to rugby union. Only one athlete did not return to sport as a direct result of the shoulder. Radiographic healing of the bone block was noted in 89% of the patients; 30% had minor shoulder arthritis, with no cases of moderate or severe glenohumeral arthritis. The investigators concluded that this technique is a reliable treatment method for athletes in contact sports such as rugby union without a significant increased risk of degenerative change. They emphasized the importance of avoiding lateral overhang of the coracoid graft, which has been shown to be associated with a higher risk of developing osteo-arthritis.[31] Although there is still limited evidence, particularly for athletes, bony block procedures are likely to become an increasingly used treatment option for anterior shoulder instability in an active population.

SURGICAL TREATMENT OF POSTERIOR INSTABILITY IN THE ATHLETE
Open Stabilization of Posterior Instability

Although posterior shoulder instability is less common than anterior shoulder insta-bility,[32] athletes are at risk for this clinical problem.[7] Posterior shoulder instability may be more amenable to conservative treatment than anterior instability,[33–36] but surgical intervention is more likely to be necessary for posterior shoulder instability with a traumatic cause,[33] which is often the case with athletes. A few early studies looked at open treatment of posterior shoulder instability in athletes with staples[37,38] before Tibone and Bradley[39] reported on 40 athletes treated with suture anchors. In their series, a 40% failure rate was attributed to unrecognized ligamentous laxity and multidirectional instability. Only 29% of elite throwing athletes in this cohort returned to competition. Misamore and Facibene[40] reported on the treatment of pos-terior instability in 14 athletes with open posterior capsulorrhaphy. In this series, 13 (93%) reported good to excellent results, with a return to sporting activity at a mean follow-up of 45 months. One shoulder in a college football player had recurrent insta-bility and required revision surgery. Although there are relatively few studies, open sta-bilization is a viable option for the treatment of posterior instability in athletes.

Arthroscopic Stabilization of Posterior Instability

Considering the relative morbidity of an open approach to the posterior shoulder compared with the anterior shoulder, arthroscopic techniques may be particularly attractive for treating posterior shoulder instability. In a series of 9 athletes (8 American football players, 1 lacrosse player) treated with arthroscopic stabilization using tacks, all of them returned to at least one season of sport at an average follow-up of 30 months.[34] Williams and colleagues[41] reported a 92% success rate for arthroscopic posterior shoulder stabilization using tack fixation at a mean follow-up of 5 years in 27 patients. Twenty of the 27 patients were athletes, most commonly injured in American football (11) or weightlifting (4). Kim and colleagues[42] reported that 26 of 27 athletes treated for traumatic unidirectional recurrent posterior subluxation with arthroscopic posterior labral repair and capsular shift using suture anchors returned to sport without limitation at a mean follow-up of 39 months. The mean ASES scores increased from 51 to 97, and the mean Rowe scores increased from 36 to 95. This series included athletes from a variety of sports, with rugby (5) and soccer (4) being the most common. The only athlete who failed was a rugby player who initially returned to sport and suffered a traumatic reinjury.

Bradley and colleagues[43] reported good results for arthroscopic posterior capsulo-labral reconstructions using plication sutures, suture anchors, or some combination in 100 shoulders from 91 athletes. The most common sport played by these athletes was American football (34), followed by baseball/softball (16), wrestling (7) and swimming (7). At a mean follow-up of 27 months, 89% of the athletes got back to their sport, with 67% back to their original level of competition. The mean ASES score improved from

50 preoperatively to 86 at the final follow-up. There were 11 failures (11%), of which 8 (8%) elected to undergo revision surgery. The investigators noted that all failures occurred early, within 7 months of surgery, and attributed the most likely cause of failure to be misdiagnosis with additional inferior and/or multidirectional instability.

In a subsequent study, the same group compared results of arthroscopic capsulolabral repair for unidirectional posterior shoulder instability between throwing and nonthrowing athletes.[44] They compared the results of 27 dominant shoulders in throwing athletes with those for 80 shoulders in nonthrowing athletes. Although there was no difference between the groups in terms of clinical outcomes as measured by the ASES score or failure rate in terms of instability, throwing athletes were less likely to return to their preinjury level of competition (55%) than nonthrowing athletes (71%). The investigators concluded that throwing athletes should be counseled about the difficulty of returning to sport after this surgery.

Pennington and colleagues[45] reported a 93% return to sport with 82% returning to their previous level of competition after arthroscopic repair of posterior labral tears in 28 patients using suture anchors with a minimum 2-year follow-up. The mean ASES scores improved from 48 to 93, and the mean Rowe score improved from 48 to 90. Again, American football was the most common sport (10 of 28). Of note, the investigators reported that only 29% of their patients had posterior shoulder instability on examination under anesthesia in the operating room.

One series of arthroscopic posterior labral repairs has been reported in 11 rugby players.[46] At an average follow-up of 32 months, the mean Constant score increased from 66 to 99. All of the athletes returned to rugby at 3 to 6 months (mean 4.3 months). One player had a loose suture anchor removed at 3 months and returned to play a month after the anchor was removed. Another player suffered an anterior dislocation the next season that was treated surgically, at which time the posterior labrum was noted to have healed.

An arthroscopic approach to posterior instability does seem to have advantages for athletes, particularly in terms of return to sport. However, throwing athletes may still have a difficult time getting back to competition. There are no long-term follow-up studies of this procedure in athletes, and more study is needed to guide indications and technique.

REFERENCES

1. Owens BD, Agel J, Mountcastle SB, et al. Incidence of glenohumeral instability in collegiate athletics. Am J Sports Med 2009;37(9):1750–4.
2. Brophy RH, Barnes R, Rodeo SA, et al. Prevalence of musculoskeletal disorders at the NFL Combine–trends from 1987 to 2000. Med Sci Sports Exerc 2007;39(1): 22–7.
3. Headey J, Brooks JH, Kemp SP. The epidemiology of shoulder injuries in English professional rugby union. Am J Sports Med 2007;35(9):1537–43.
4. Kaplan LD, Flanigan DC, Norwig J, et al. Prevalence and variance of shoulder injuries in elite collegiate football players. Am J Sports Med 2005;33(8):1142–6.
5. Stein DA, Jazrawi L, Bartolozzi AR. Arthroscopic stabilization of anterior shoulder instability: a review of the literature. Arthroscopy 2002;18(8):912–24.
6. Goss TP. Anterior glenohumeral instability. Orthopedics 1988;11(1):87–95.
7. Mair SD, Zarzour RH, Speer KP. Posterior labral injury in contact athletes. Am J Sports Med 1998;26(6):753–8.
8. Bottoni CR, Wilckens JH, DeBerardino TM, et al. A prospective, randomized evaluation of arthroscopic stabilization versus nonoperative treatment in patients with

acute, traumatic, first-time shoulder dislocations. Am J Sports Med 2002;30(4): 576–80.

9. Buss DD, Lynch GP, Meyer CP, et al. Nonoperative management for in-season athletes with anterior shoulder instability. Am J Sports Med 2004;32(6):1430–3.

10. Wheeler JH, Ryan JB, Arciero RA, et al. Arthroscopic versus nonoperative treatment of acute shoulder dislocations in young athletes. Arthroscopy 1989;5(3):213–7.

11. Brophy RH, Chehab EL, Barnes RP, et al. Predictive value of orthopedic evaluation and injury history at the NFL combine. Med Sci Sports Exerc 2008;40(8): 1368–72.

12. Brophy RH, Gill CS, Lyman S, et al. Effect of shoulder stabilization on career length in national football league athletes. Am J Sports Med 2011;39(4):704–9.

13. Brophy RH, Lyman S, Chehab EL, et al. Predictive value of prior injury on career in professional American football is affected by player position. Am J Sports Med 2009;37(4):768–75.

14. Altchek DW, Warren RF, Skyhar MJ, et al. T-plasty modification of the Bankart procedure for multidirectional instability of the anterior and inferior types. J Bone Joint Surg Am 1991;73(1):105–12.

15. Bigliani LU, Kurzweil PR, Schwartzbach CC, et al. Inferior capsular shift procedure for anterior-inferior shoulder instability in athletes. Am J Sports Med 1994; 22(5):578–84.

16. Gill TJ, Micheli LJ, Gebhard F, et al. Bankart repair for anterior instability of the shoulder. Long-term outcome. J Bone Joint Surg Am 1997;79(6):850–7.

17. Jobe FW, Giangarra CE, Kvitne RS, et al. Anterior capsulolabral reconstruction of the shoulder in athletes in overhand sports. Am J Sports Med 1991;19(5):428–34.

18. Pagnani MJ, Dome DC. Surgical treatment of traumatic anterior shoulder instability in American football players. J Bone Joint Surg Am 2002;84(5):711–5.

19. Uhorchak JM, Arciero RA, Huggard D, et al. Recurrent shoulder instability after open reconstruction in athletes involved in collision and contact sports. Am J Sports Med 2000;28(6):794–9.

20. Meller R, Krettek C, Gosling T, et al. Recurrent shoulder instability among athletes: changes in quality of life, sports activity, and muscle function following open repair. Knee Surg Sports Traumatol Arthrosc 2007;15(3):295–304.

21. Tjoumakaris FP, Bradley JP. The rationale for an arthroscopic approach to shoulder stabilization. Arthroscopy 2011;27(10):1422–33.

22. Brophy RH, Marx RG. The treatment of traumatic anterior instability of the shoulder: nonoperative and surgical treatment. Arthroscopy 2009;25(3):298–304.

23. Hobby J, Griffin D, Dunbar M, et al. Is arthroscopic surgery for stabilisation of chronic shoulder instability as effective as open surgery? A systematic review and meta-analysis of 62 studies including 3044 arthroscopic operations. J Bone Joint Surg Br 2007;89(9):1188–96.

24. Lenters TR, Franta AK, Wolf FM, et al. Arthroscopic compared with open repairs for recurrent anterior shoulder instability. A systematic review and meta-analysis of the literature. J Bone Joint Surg Am 2007;89(2):244–54.

25. DeBerardino TM, Arciero RA, Taylor DC, et al. Prospective evaluation of arthroscopic stabilization of acute, initial anterior shoulder dislocations in young athletes. Two- to five-year follow-up. Am J Sports Med 2001;29(5):586–92.

26. Ide J, Maeda S, Takagi K. Arthroscopic Bankart repair using suture anchors in athletes: patient selection and postoperative sports activity. Am J Sports Med 2004;32(8):1899–905.

27. Mazzocca AD, Brown FM Jr, Carreira DS, et al. Arthroscopic anterior shoulder stabilization of collision and contact athletes. Am J Sports Med 2005;33(1):52–60.

28. Larrain MV, Montenegro HJ, Mauas DM, et al. Arthroscopic management of traumatic anterior shoulder instability in collision athletes: analysis of 204 cases with a 4- to 9-year follow-up and results with the suture anchor technique. Arthroscopy 2006;22(12):1283–9.

29. Rhee YG, Ha JH, Cho NS. Anterior shoulder stabilization in collision athletes: arthroscopic versus open Bankart repair. Am J Sports Med 2006;34(6):979–85.

30. Neyton L, Young A, Dawidziak B, et al. Surgical treatment of anterior instability in rugby union players: clinical and radiographic results of the Latarjet-Patte procedure with minimum 5-year follow-up. J Shoulder Elbow Surg 2012;21(12):1721–7.

31. Allain J, Goutallier D, Glorion C. Long-term results of the Latarjet procedure for the treatment of anterior instability of the shoulder. J Bone Joint Surg Am 1998; 80(6):841–52.

32. Pollock RG, Bigliani LU. Recurrent posterior shoulder instability. Diagnosis and treatment. Clin Orthop Relat Res 1993;(291):85–96.

33. Burkhead WZ Jr, Rockwood CA Jr. Treatment of instability of the shoulder with an exercise program. J Bone Joint Surg Am 1992;74(6):890–6.

34. Hawkins RJ, Belle RM. Posterior instability of the shoulder. Instr Course Lect 1989;38:211–5.

35. Hawkins RJ, Koppert G, Johnston G. Recurrent posterior instability (subluxation) of the shoulder. J Bone Joint Surg Am 1984;66(2):169–74.

36. Hurley JA, Anderson TE, Dear W, et al. Posterior shoulder instability. Surgical versus conservative results with evaluation of glenoid version. Am J Sports Med 1992;20(4):396–400.

37. Tibone J, Ting A. Capsulorrhaphy with a staple for recurrent posterior subluxation of the shoulder. J Bone Joint Surg Am 1990;72(7):999–1002.

38. Tibone JE, Prietto C, Jobe FW, et al. Staple capsulorrhaphy for recurrent posterior shoulder dislocation. Am J Sports Med 1981;9(3):135–9.

39. Tibone JE, Bradley JP. The treatment of posterior subluxation in athletes. Clin Orthop Relat Res 1993;(291):124–37.

40. Misamore GW, Facibene WA. Posterior capsulorrhaphy for the treatment of traumatic recurrent posterior subluxations of the shoulder in athletes. J Shoulder Elbow Surg 2000;9(5):403–8.

41. Williams RJ 3rd, Strickland S, Cohen M, et al. Arthroscopic repair for traumatic posterior shoulder instability. Am J Sports Med 2003;31(2):203–9.

42. Kim SH, Ha KI, Park JH, et al. Arthroscopic posterior labral repair and capsular shift for traumatic unidirectional recurrent posterior subluxation of the shoulder. J Bone Joint Surg Am 2003;85(8):1479–87.

43. Bradley JP, Baker CL 3rd, Kline AJ, et al. Arthroscopic capsulolabral reconstruction for posterior instability of the shoulder: a prospective study of 100 shoulders. Am J Sports Med 2006;34(7):1061–71.

44. Radkowski CA, Chhabra A, Baker CL, et al. Arthroscopic capsulolabral repair for posterior shoulder instability in throwing athletes compared with nonthrowing athletes. Am J Sports Med 2008;36(4):693–9.

45. Pennington WT, Sytsma MA, Gibbons DJ, et al. Arthroscopic posterior labral repair in athletes: outcome analysis at 2-year follow-up. Arthroscopy 2010; 26(9):1162–71.

46. Badge R, Tambe A, Funk L. Arthroscopic isolated posterior labral repair in rugby players. Int J Shoulder Surg 2009;3(1):4–7.

Management of the Athlete with a Failed Shoulder Instability Procedure

F. Winston Gwathmey Jr, MD[a], Jon J.P. Warner, MD[b],*

KEYWORDS

- Shoulder instability • Recurrence • Athlete • Bankart • Latarjet

KEY POINTS

- The athlete requires a highly functional shoulder, but also routinely exposes his or her shoulder to excessive force and stress.
- High recurrence rates after arthroscopic stabilization have been reported in athletes.
- Risk factors for recurrence include age less than 20, contact/collision sports, higher level of competition, capsular laxity, glenoid bone loss, and engaging Hill-Sachs deformities.
- Fundamental to successful revision surgery is choosing the correct procedure and is based on careful analysis of etiology of failure and risk factors for recurrence.

INTRODUCTION

Athletes with shoulder instability represent a challenge for the shoulder surgeon. Not only do they require a highly functional shoulder in order to perform at a high level, but they also routinely expose their shoulders to demanding and potentially dangerous situations. An elite baseball pitcher's shoulder may exceed 165° of external rotation and generate 70 Nm of torque.[1] A rugby tackle generates forces approaching 2000 N at the shoulder joint.[2]

Conventional open Bankart repair historically was the gold standard for stabilization in athletes because of reported low recurrence rates and high rates of return to play.[3–5] Improving techniques and implants have influenced a paradigm shift toward arthroscopic repair, and now most surgeons recommend arthroscopic Bankart repair for the athlete with instability, citing equivalent results to open repair.[6–9]

However, when critically analyzed, the results of Bankart repair may not be as good as originally thought, especially in high-risk populations such as athletes (**Fig. 1**). Balg

[a] Orthopaedic Sports Medicine, Massachusetts General Hospital, 175 Cambridge Street, 4th Floor, Boston, MA 02114, USA; [b] The MGH Shoulder Service, The Boston Shoulder Institute, Massachusetts General Hospital, Harvard Medical School, 55 Fruit Street, Suite 3200, Boston, MA 02114, USA
* Corresponding author.
E-mail address: jwarner@partners.org

Clin Sports Med 32 (2013) 833–863
http://dx.doi.org/10.1016/j.csm.2013.07.016
0278-5919/13/$ – see front matter © 2013 Elsevier Inc. All rights reserved.

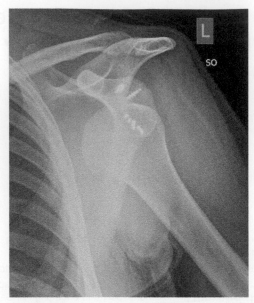

Fig. 1. Left shoulder anteroposterior (AP) radiograph of a 22-year-old ice hockey player with a recurrent anterior dislocation after 2 prior arthroscopic stabilization attempts. Note multiple metallic anchors placed during prior surgeries.

and Boileau[10] prospectively followed 131 patients after arthroscopic Bankart repair and found recurrence in 14.5%. Voos and colleagues[11] found a recurrence rate of 17.8% in a prospective cohort of 83 patients. In both studies, the rates were significantly higher in younger patients, those with ligamentous laxity, and those who participated in sports, all factors characteristic of athletes. One-third of athletes who returned to contact sports had a recurrence in the study by Balg and Boileau.[10] Such high recurrence rates have led some surgeons to recommend a bony procedure such as the Bristow or Latarjet coracoid transfer for stabilization in high-risk patients.[10,12,13]

Athletes who present with failed stabilization procedures are complicated. They have already endured an initial instability event, potentially multiple recurrences, missed playing time, at least one prior surgery, months of rehabilitation to get back to their sport, and now a recurrence after surgery. Not only must athletes face additional missed playing time and potentially more surgery and rehabilitation, they face an increased risk of another recurrence after revision and a substantial possibility of not returning to their sport.[14–20]

Appropriate management of the athlete after failed instability surgery requires careful analysis of the factors that contributed to recurrence, and successful revision surgery must address those factors to reliably achieve a stable shoulder and allow return to play. This article reviews failed surgical shoulder stabilization in athletes and outlines an algorithm for management.

OUTCOMES OF PRIMARY STABILIZATION

Open Bankart repair has been reported to have low recurrence rates and a reliable return to sport. In 1978, Rowe and colleagues[3] reported a rate of recurrent instability of 3.5% with 97% of athletes returning to sports after the procedure. Twenty-five years later, Pagnani and Dome[5] reported a 3.4% recurrence rate in American football players, with return to play in all of the college and professional players studied. In a direct comparison of open and arthroscopic Bankart repair in collision athletes, Rhee and colleagues[21] found that those who underwent arthroscopic repair had a recurrence rate twice that of the open repair group (25% vs 12.5%). In addition, 90% of the open repair group returned to sports at complete or near-complete preinjury levels of performance compared with 62.5% in the arthroscopic group.

Early experience with arthroscopic techniques did not match the results of open techniques. Arthroscopic repair with bioabsorbable tacks, widely used in the 1990s and initially claimed to be equivalent to open techniques, were abandoned because of unacceptably high recurrence rates, which approached 40% in several studies.[7,22–24] With the evolution of new devices and techniques, in particular the introduction of the arthroscopic suture anchor techniques, many now consider arthroscopic Bankart repair to be equivalent to open stabilization.[6,8,25–27] Kim and colleagues[28] studied 167 patients who underwent arthroscopic Bankart repair with suture anchors and found a recurrence rate of 4.2% at a mean of 44 months' follow-up. A recent meta-analysis of 26 studies of long-term outcomes in 1781 patients after Bankart repair showed an 11% recurrence rate after arthroscopic Bankart repair compared with 8% after open repair.[8] When only the arthroscopic suture anchor technique was considered, the rate of recurrence was 8.5%. The overall rate of return to sport was 87% for arthroscopic suture anchor Bankart repair and 89% for open Bankart repair.

Low recurrence rates have been shown with coracoid transfer for primary stabilization. In a long-term prospective study of 118 patients who underwent Bristow-Latarjet stabilization, Hovelius and colleagues[29] found postoperative dislocations in 4 (3.4%) and subluxations in 12 (10.2%) at a mean follow-up of 15.2 years. In a subsequent comparative study, Hovelius and colleagues[12] reported recurrent instability in 13.4% of patients who underwent Bristow-Latarjet versus 28.7% of those who underwent Bankart repair at a mean follow-up of 17 years. In a comparison of 102 patients who underwent primary stabilization, Bessiere and colleagues[13] found a 2-fold increase in recurrence after Bankart repair (23.5%) versus Latarjet (11.7%) at follow-up of at least 5 years. Neyton and colleagues[30] studied the Latarjet-Patte procedure in 34 rugby players and found no postoperative recurrences at a mean follow-up of 12 years. In that study, 65% of players were able to return to playing rugby.

APPROACH TO THE ATHLETE WITH FAILED STABILIZATION

Throughout the management of the athlete who has failed a prior instability surgery, the surgeon must maintain an open dialogue with the athletes as well as their families, coaches, and trainers. A potentially fulfilling or lucrative career is in jeopardy, and the surgeon should set realistic expectations. The nature of failure must be clearly defined for each patient. Failure in a collision athlete may manifest as a new dislocation, whereas pain, stiffness, or weakness may be perceived as failure in an overhead athlete. Athletes should be counseled on their individual risk factors, emphasizing those that may be mitigated by surgical technique and/or postoperative activity modification, so that they participate in the decision-making process.

The comprehensive evaluation of an athlete with a postoperative recurrence requires collection of key elements from a systematic history, physical examination, and imaging. Integration of these elements into the treatment algorithm establishes the indications to choose a successful revision surgery.

History

The history provides fundamental information about the cause of failure and insight into the potential for successful revision. Patient-specific risk factors that predict recurrence both in the primary and revision setting include younger age, male sex, hyperlaxity, participation in collision or contact sport (**Table 1**), and higher level of competition.[10,11,15,31–36] Some athletes, such as football linebackers and defensive backs, are at increased risk by virtue of the demands of the position in which they play.[37] Older athletes are at risk for rotator cuff injury after dislocation.[38] The surgeon should be wary of athletes with a history of multidirectional or voluntary instability because results after revision are less predictable.[19,39,40]

The surgeon should endeavor to obtain the operative report and arthroscopic photographs to review the technique and quality of the primary stabilization. The photographs may also provide insight into the status of the capsule, labrum, glenoid, and humeral head at the time of the first surgery. Some athletes have undergone multiple prior stabilization attempts, and consequently have higher risk for recurrence after revision.[19]

The rehabilitation after the initial surgery should be reviewed because persistent motion loss, deconditioning, or early return to play may have contributed to the reinjury.[11,41–43] Castagna and colleagues[43] found loss of greater than 15° of external rotation in 42.8% of athletes who experienced a postoperative instability event. Voos and colleagues[11] proposed that a young athlete should be restricted from return to sport for at least 9 months after surgery so that a thorough sport-specific rehabilitation protocol could be implemented.

The mechanism of reinjury provides key information because a recurrence from a high-energy mechanism may signify a retear of a well-fixed labrum, whereas a recurrence from minimal trauma may signify an inadequate repair. Recurrent subluxations or dislocations with progressive ease or with routine daily events indicate a significant bony injury.[44,45] The mechanism of reinjury may also predict potential for successful

Table 1		
Classification of sports by degree of contact		
Type	**Definition**	**Examples**
Collision	Athletes purposely hit or collide with each other or inanimate objects, including the ground, with great force	Football Ice hockey Wrestling Boxing
Contact	Athletes routinely make contact with each other or inanimate objects but usually with less force than in collision sports	Basketball Soccer Field hockey Lacrosse
Limited contact	Contact with other athletes or inanimate objects is infrequent and inadvertent	Baseball Softball Racquetball Skiing
Noncontact	No contact as part of sport	Golf Tennis Running Swimming

Adapted from Committee on Sports Medicine and Fitness. American Academy of Pediatrics: Medical conditions affecting sports participation. Pediatrics 2001;107(5):1205–9.

revision. Levine and colleagues[19] found excellent results after revision stabilization in all patients who had a redislocation with major trauma, whereas a third of patients had poor results when minimal trauma caused the recurrence.

Examination

The examination should start with the uninjured shoulder to establish a baseline for motion, strength, and stability. Hyperlaxity may be identified by passive external rotation of the shoulder with the arm at a neutral adduction of greater than 85° (**Fig. 2**).[10,39,46] In addition, evidence of generalized laxity may be seen in examination of other joints.[47]

The involved shoulder should be examined carefully for range of motion, strength, and positions of apprehension, noting side-to-side differences. Subscapularis dysfunction, most commonly encountered after open surgery, contributes to poor outcomes. Excessive passive external rotation or weakness in internal rotation is a harbinger of clinically significant subscapularis injury.[25,48,49] Loss of motion suggests capsular contracture and/or subscapularis scarring, which may complicate revision surgery.[46,50,51] Weakness in abduction or external rotation raises concern for rotator cuff disorders.[25] A careful neurologic examination helps to detect subtle deficits that may result from injury-related or iatrogenic injury to the brachial plexus or axial nerve.[52]

The direction and degree of instability should be characterized. Previously unrecognized posterior, inferior, or multidirectional instability that may have contributed to recurrence should not be missed. Apprehension with posteriorly directed force on the adducted arm is seen with posterior capsulolabral disorders, whereas a positive sulcus sign and/or hyperabduction in excess of 20° compared with the contralateral side occurs with injury to the inferior glenohumeral ligament.[33,46,53] Significant glenoid injury

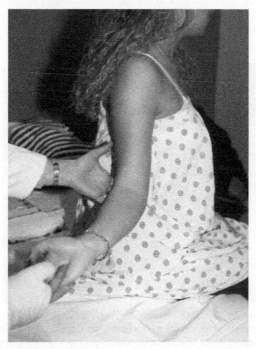

Fig. 2. External rotation of greater than 85° with the arm at the side of the body indicates baseline shoulder hyperlaxity.

or Hill-Sachs lesion may manifest as crepitus in positions of apprehension.[25,54] Concomitant injuries to the biceps anchor and/or tendon as well as the acromioclavicular joint should be assessed because they may require attention at revision surgery.[46,52]

Imaging

Comprehensive imaging is central to the understanding of the cause of recurrence as well as for the development of the preoperative plan. Baseline plain radiographs of the shoulder may reveal osseous anatomy or disorders characteristic of recurrent instability (**Fig. 3**). The relationship between the humeral head and the glenoid, the congruity of the articular surfaces, the presence and location of prior implants, and evidence of osteoarthritis should be noted. Anteroinferior glenoid fracture or blunting may be shown on standard anteroposterior (AP) or axillary lateral views.[10,55] More accurate calculation of bone loss is afforded by West Point or Bernageau views (**Fig. 4**).[56,57] Irregularities of the humeral head are commonly seen in recurrent instability, and a Hill-Sachs deformity visible on an AP radiograph with the arm in external rotation has been shown in cases of recurrent instability.[10,58]

Cross-sectional imaging is mandatory to delineate the anatomic factors leading to recurrence. Many athletes who are referred for failed stabilization have already undergone a standard magnetic resonance imaging (MRI) examination ordered by a well-meaning primary care provider. Standard, nonarthrogram MRI, although useful in showing the anatomy of the shoulder, has limited usefulness in detecting clinically significant capsulolabral disorders, in particular after previous repair.[59,60] In addition, MRI frequently underestimates glenoid bone loss.[61] The addition of intra-articular contrast improves diagnostic accuracy, and magnetic resonance arthrography can reliably show recurrent labral tears, anterior labral periosteal sleeve avulsion (ALPSA) lesions, humeral avulsion of the glenohumeral ligament (HAGL), Hill-Sachs lesions, and articular cartilage injuries (**Fig. 5**).[62–64]

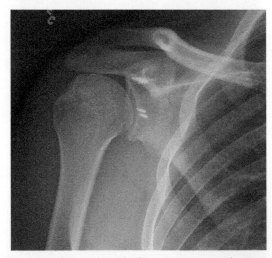

Fig. 3. Right shoulder AP radiograph with the arm in internal rotation of a 24-year-old professional soccer player with recurrent subluxations after a prior arthroscopic Bankart and superior labral repair. Note the metallic suture anchors in the glenoid, the anteroinferior glenoid irregularity, and impaction fracture of the posterolateral aspect of the humeral head.

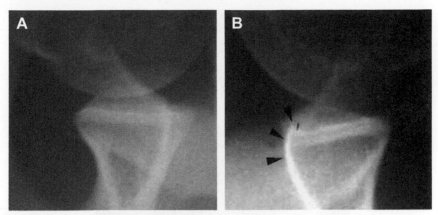

Fig. 4. (A) Bernageau glenoid profile view of the normal contralateral shoulder for comparison. (B) Bernageau view of the injured shoulder showing the blunted angle sign (*arrowheads*), which indicates glenoid bone loss. (*From* Edwards TB, Boulahia A, Walch G. Radiographic analysis of bone defects in chronic anterior shoulder instability. Arthroscopy 2003;19(7):737; with permission.)

With increasing recognition of the association between osseous disorders and recurrent instability, computed tomography (CT) has emerged as a key imaging modality. Conventional CT imaging supplements plain radiographs and allows accurate measurement of glenoid defects.[61] CT arthrography is comparable with magnetic resonance arthrography for assessing labral detachments and articular cartilage loss (**Fig. 6**).[65]

Three-dimensional (3D) CT imaging is superior to all other imaging modalities for showing bony anatomy and should be obtained when there is any concern for clinically

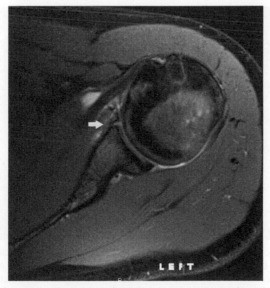

Fig. 5. Left shoulder MR arthrogram showing a recurrent Bankart lesion (*arrow*) in a 26-year-old recreational athlete who has failed a prior arthroscopic stabilization.

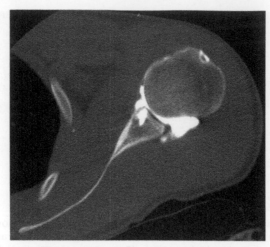

Fig. 6. Left shoulder CT arthrogram of a 24-year-old basketball player with recurrent post-operative instability reveals deficiency of the anterior glenoid and capsulolabral structures. Note the previously placed suture anchor in the glenoid. Arthroscopic revision Bankart repair in this patient may not be successful in restoring a stable shoulder.

significant osseous defect. Multiple studies have shown high accuracy and reliability of 3D CT and have supported its use in the imaging algorithm for recurrent insta-bility.[44,55,61,66,67] With reformatting, the humeral head can be subtracted, providing an unobstructed view of the glenoid for calculation of bone loss.[44,68] Application of a best-fit circle to the inferior aspect of the CT-reconstructed glenoid permits geometric calculation of the osseous defect (**Fig. 7**).[67,69,70] The volume, location, and orientation of a Hill-Sachs lesion also can be accurately shown by 3D CT, aiding in the identification of the potential for engagement.[58] Chuang and colleagues[71]

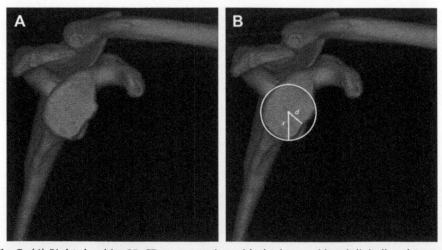

Fig. 7. (*A*) Right shoulder 3D CT reconstruction with the humeral head digitally subtracted shows a significant bony injury to the anterior glenoid. (*B*) Best-fit circle applied to the glenoid face centered on the inferior bare spot. The size of the glenoid defect can be calculated by comparing the radius of the circle with the distance between the center of the circle and edge of the defect.

recommended use of 3D CT as an essential preoperative assessment of bone loss to determine the need for a bone grafting procedure.

Arthroscopy

An examination of the shoulder under anesthesia is mandatory to obtain an objective understanding of the direction and degree of instability before starting the procedure. Although the surgical plan usually is clear before entering the operating room, arthroscopy can elucidate equivocal cases or show previously unrecognized disorders. The status of the previous repair can be ascertained as well as the position and location of the anchors (**Fig. 8**). In planned open cases, arthroscopy may also show important concomitant lesions that require intervention.[72]

The condition of the remaining labrum and capsule may prohibit an adequate revision arthroscopic Bankart repair or capsulorrhaphy. In one study of revision arthroscopic Bankart repair, the labrum was thinned or absent in 61% and the capsule thinned or patulous in 56%.[17] In cases of previous thermal capsulorrhaphy, the capsule may be severely attenuated or absent.[73] In many cases, the labrum scars to the glenoid neck and requires mobilization to restore it to its anatomic location on the face of the glenoid. The presence of an ALPSA lesion raises concerns about the ability to obtain a durable arthroscopic repair (**Fig. 9**). In one study, ALPSA lesions repaired arthroscopically had a recurrence rate of 19.2% compared with 7.4% for Bankart lesions.[74]

Bone loss may be underrepresented on preoperative imaging or new bone loss may have occurred before surgery, necessitating a careful arthroscopic assessment of the glenoid. The central bare spot of the inferior glenoid may be used as an arthroscopic reference point to gauge bone loss. Burkhart and colleagues[75] described a method in which the arthroscope is placed in the anterosuperior portal and the distance from the anterior and posterior rim to the bare spot is measured using a calibrated probe inserted through the posterior portal.

Shoulder stability testing may be performed under arthroscopy. An arthroscopic load and shift may provide a clearer idea of the degree of humeral translation.[15] Placing the arm into an abducted and externally rotated position can show a clinically significant engaging Hill-Sachs that may need attention (**Fig. 10**).[76]

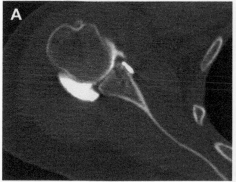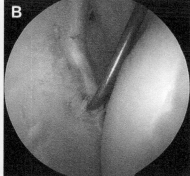

Fig. 8. (*A*) Right shoulder CT arthrogram of a 22-year-old athlete who has had recurrent dislocations after a prior arthroscopic Bankart repair. (*B*) Arthroscopy viewing from the posterior portal shows failed anterior labral repair with loose sutures and attenuated capsulolabral tissue. Caused by the poor tissue quality, revision arthroscopic stabilization was not pursued and this patient underwent a Latarjet procedure.

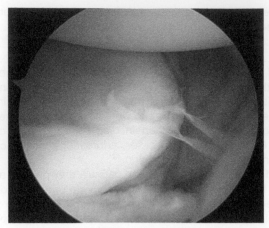

Fig. 9. Arthroscopic view from the anterosuperior portal of the anterior glenoid with an ALPSA lesion. The labrum has been torn from the glenoid face and is scarred medially.

The surgeon should incorporate the arthroscopic findings into the treatment algorithm and must be prepared to perform an alternative surgery if the preponderance of factors contradicts arthroscopic revision stabilization.

WHY DID IT FAIL?

The surgeon managing a failed shoulder stabilization procedure in an athlete should investigate the potential causes of failure to prevent it from occurring again. In addition, the athlete may be frustrated or disillusioned by the poor outcome and may question why the surgery failed and what can be done to prevent another failure.

New Trauma

As anticipated in this population, returning to the activity responsible for the initial dislocation is the major contributor to recurrence. A recent epidemiologic study of

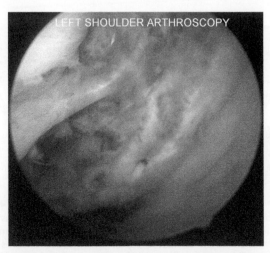

Fig. 10. Arthroscopic view of a large Hill-Sachs lesion that engages the anterior glenoid with anteriorly directed force on the humeral head.

more than 3600 shoulder dislocations showed that sports injuries were responsible for 85% of dislocations in patients less than 30 years of age.[52] Most recurrent dislocations after stabilization are therefore from new athletic trauma.[45] In one study of 8 recurrent dislocations after open Bankart repair in a cohort of 49 rugby players at an average follow-up of 28 years, all were from new trauma sustained by the athlete after return to playing rugby.[77] In separate studies by Gill and colleagues[4] and Uhorchak and colleagues,[78] significant trauma was responsible in all patients who had recurrence after open Bankart repair. Significant new trauma has been implicated in recurrence after arthroscopic Bankart repair, as reported by Owens and colleagues[24] who found that all of their recurrent dislocations and subluxations occurred with athletic trauma.

As a result, athletes with the most routine exposure to significant trauma, such as collision and contact athletes, have the highest risk of reinjury after stabilization. Cho and colleagues showed a recurrence rate of 28.6% in collision athletes after arthroscopic Bankart repair compared with 6.7% in noncollision athletes. Balg and Boileau[10] found that contact athletes had an almost 2-fold increase risk of recurrence, and Stein and colleagues[79] found a more than 3-fold increased risk.

Functional Deficit

Failure of surgical stabilization in an athlete does not always manifest as a recurrent instability event. Loss of motion, weakness, or persistent apprehension may prevent an athlete from returning to the prior level of performance.[80] Overhead athletes consistently have lower rates of return to sport than other athletes, likely because of greater functional and range-of-motion demands on the repaired shoulder.[81–83] Patients often lose some motion after surgery, particularly external rotation, which may impair shoulder function.[3,4,21,26,43] Ide[81] found that only 68% of the overhead athletes studied could return to the previous level of sport after arthroscopic Bankart repair compared with 85.7% of contact athletes. In the study by Rowe and colleagues,[3] only 33% of athletes could throw a baseball with the same velocity as before surgery. Stein and colleagues[79] found that overhead and martial arts athletes took significantly longer to return to their prior levels of performance and had persistent significant impairments for sport ability and reattained proficiency compared with other athletes.

Patient Factors

Age is the most well-defined patient factor, and adolescent athletes have a 2-fold to 4-fold greater risk of recurrence than their adult counterparts.[10,11,36,84] In a study of adolescent athletes between the ages of 13 and 18 years, Castagna and colleagues[84] found a recurrence rate of 21.5% after arthroscopic Bankart repair using suture anchors. Voos and colleagues[11] showed recurrence in 37.5% of patients younger than 20 years of age compared with 15.3% in older patients. The reasons behind the increased risk are multifactorial and possibly related to increased capsulolabral compliance in younger athletes, decreased muscular bulk, less athletic experience in proper technique, and the increased number of potential exposures over the course of their remaining athletic careers.

Higher rates of failure have also been shown in patients with hyperlaxity. Voos and colleagues[11] found that a third of their patients who had recurrence after stabilization showed ligamentous laxity, and Balg and Boileau[10] reported a recurrence rate of 18.9% in patients with hyperlaxity compared with 4.9% in those without. In a review of failed stabilization procedures, Rowe and colleagues[85] found excessive laxity of the capsule in 83% of cases.

Glenoid

The glenohumeral joint is frequently described as a golf ball (humeral head) on a tee (glenoid). A significant chip off of the tee results in the golf ball falling to the ground. Without a competent glenoid, the joint remains unstable regardless of which soft tissue stabilization technique is chosen. Glenoid damage is common in patients with instability. Sugaya and colleagues[67] used 3D CT to determine that 90 of 100 patients with instability had an abnormal glenoid. A fracture involving at least 5% of the glenoid was seen in 28 cases, whereas an impacted or rounded anteroinferior rim was seen in another 40 cases.

Determining the critical size for a glenoid bone defect has been a frequent subject of inquiry. In a cadaver study, Itoi and colleagues[86] investigated stability and motion after Bankart repair, and an osseous defect of 21% caused significant instability and loss of external rotation. Burkhart and DeBeer[87] coined the term inverted pear to describe a glenoid in which the normal pear-shaped configuration has been reversed because of anteroinferior bone loss. Lo and colleagues[88] showed that the mean amount of bone loss needed to create the inverted pear appearance of the glenoid in a cadaver was 7.5 mm or at least 25% to 27% of the inferior glenoid width.

Significant glenoid bone loss has consistently been shown to be a substantial cause for failure of soft tissue anterior shoulder stabilization (**Fig. 11**). Burkhart and DeBeer[87] cited a 67% recurrence risk with the inverted-pear glenoid compared with 4% in those with no bone loss. In contact athletes with bone loss, the risk of recurrence was 89%. Ahmed and colleagues[42] found percentage of bone loss to predict failure after arthroscopic Bankart repair, reporting a 3-fold increased risk with greater than 25% bone loss. In a study of patients who underwent revision for failed anterior repair, Tauber and colleagues[45] found a significant glenoid defect in 56%.

However, it should be noted that a reparable bony fragment should be differentiated from attritional bone loss. Mologne and colleagues[89] reported successful arthroscopic repair in all cases in which a bony Bankart fragment was incorporated into the repair, whereas 3 of 10 patients with attritional bone loss experienced recurrent instability. Porcellini and colleagues[90] found low recurrence rates with arthroscopic repair of acute (2.4%) and chronic (4.2%) bony Bankart injuries.

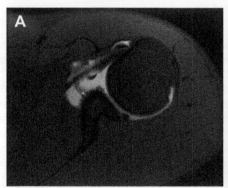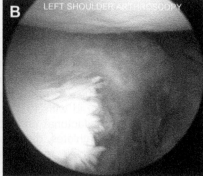

Fig. 11. (*A*) Left shoulder CT arthrogram of a 17-year-old right-hand-dominant high school quarterback who sustained a traumatic redislocation after a prior arthroscopic Bankart repair. A significant osseous defect is shown in the anterior glenoid and the deficient anterior labral tissue has scarred medially. (*B*) Arthroscopic view from an anterosuperior portal confirms greater than 25% bone loss and no reparable labrum. This patient underwent open stabilization with a Latarjet procedure.

Humeral Head

The Hill-Sachs lesion, an impaction fracture involving the posterosuperior humeral head as a result of impact against the anterior glenoid during dislocation or subluxation, is frequently found in recurrent instability.[58] One recent study reported a Hill-Sachs lesion in 88% of shoulders with shoulder instability.[91] The engaging Hill-Sachs, as defined by Burkhart and DeBeer,[87] presents the long axis of its defect parallel to the anterior glenoid with the shoulder in a functional position of abduction and external rotation, so that the Hill-Sachs lesion engages the anteroinferior corner of the glenoid (**Fig. 12**).[87]

Yamamoto and colleagues[92] introduced the glenoid track by marking the humeral head contact on the glenoid through an arc of abduction with the arm in maximum external rotation. They concluded that orientation and location are more important than size, and a linear defect medial to the medial margin of the track is at high risk of engagement with the anterior glenoid. In a subsequent study, Kurokawa and colleagues observed features of an engaging Hill-Sachs in 7 of 100 consecutive patients with shoulder instability.[93]

Hill-Sachs lesions are commonly seen in failed stabilization procedures. Rowe and colleagues[85] analyzed a series of failed anterior stabilizations and found a Hill-Sachs lesion in 76%. The presence of a nonengaging Hill-Sachs does not necessarily cause a recurrence, but a Hill-Sachs that engages the anterior glenoid has been shown to increase the risk significantly. In Burkhart and De Beer's[87] study, recurrence was seen in all 3 cases of engaging Hill-Sachs.[87] Ahmad and colleagues[42] found an engaging Hill-Sachs in 65% of recurrences. Citing these high recurrence rates, several investigators discourage Bankart repair in selected cases, instead recommending a primary bony procedure to increase the glenoid arc, or soft tissue filling (remplissage) of the humeral head defect to prevent Hill-Sachs engagement.[10,25,42,58,94]

Surgical Factors

Error in indication

The surgical technique for primary stabilization must be evaluated critically to understand the cause of recurrence. In one study of revision stabilization, suboptimal surgical technique was found in 75% of primary failures.[15] Before scrutinizing the technique, it is important to ensure that the proper primary surgery was selected for

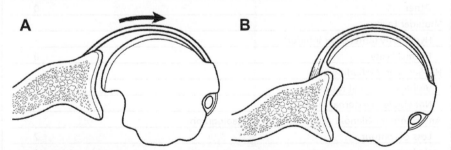

A **B**

Fig. 12. (*A*) Engaging Hill-Sachs lesion. (*B*) With the arm in abduction and external rotation, the humeral head defect engages the anterior glenoid, predisposing the shoulder to recurrent instability. (*From* Burkhart SS, De Beer JF. Traumatic glenohumeral bone defects and their relationship to failure of arthroscopic Bankart repairs: significance of the inverted pear glenoid and the humeral engaging Hill-Sachs lesion. Arthroscopy 2000;16(7):681; with permission.)

the athlete. Good technique cannot overcome poor indications, and some patients may be condemned to failure if the wrong surgery is performed.

Although some cases have clear contraindications to arthroscopic repair, such as excessive glenoid bone loss, many cases may multiple features that complicate the algorithm. Balg and Boileau[10] attempted to elucidate this algorithm by stratifying risk factors responsible for recurrence after arthroscopic Bankart procedure.[10] Analyzing characteristics shared by 19 patients (out of 131) who failed stabilization, they identified patient age less than 20 years, involvement in contact or overhead sports, shoulder hyperlaxity, significant Hill-Sachs lesion, and loss of the sclerotic inferior glenoid contour as risk factors for recurrence. Each of these factors was assigned a relative risk value from 0 to 2 and then summed to calculate the instability severity index score (**Table 2**). When applied to the cohort, a patient score of 3 or less had a recurrence rate of 5%, whereas a recurrence rate of 70% was found in those with a score of more than 6. They concluded that an arthroscopic Bankart is appropriate in low-risk patients, but a Latarjet should be considered in those with high instability scores.

Errors in technique

A poorly executed Bankart repair may be the principal cause of failure because inadequate restoration of the anatomy undermines the stability of the joint. If the labrum and attached capsule are not sufficiently mobilized and anatomically reduced to the glenoid face, the resulting repair does not recreate the glenoid concavity compression

Table 2 Instability severity index score	
Prognostic Factor	**Points**
Age at Surgery (y)	
≤20	2
>20	0
Level of Sport (Preoperative)	
Competitive	2
Recreational/none	0
Type of Sport (Preoperative)	
Contact or overhead	1
Other	0
Shoulder Laxity	
Hyperlaxity (anterior or inferior)	1
Normal laxity	0
Hill-Sachs on AP Radiograph	
Visible in external rotation	2
Not visible in external rotation	0
Anteroinferior Glenoid Appearance on AP Radiograph	
Loss of contour	2
No lesion	0
Total possible points	10[a]

[a] Recurrence rate by instability severity index score: 5% (≤3); 10% (<6); 70% (>6).
Data from Balg F, Boileau P. The instability severity index score. A simple pre-operative score to select patients for arthroscopic or open shoulder stabilisation. J Bone Joint Surg Br 2007; 89(11):1470–7. doi:10.1302/0301-620X.89B11.18962.

or properly tension the capsule.[41,54,95] Misplacement of anchor medially on the glenoid neck malreduces the capsulolabral complex and compromises the stability of the repair construct.[17]

The durability of the repair is conferred by securing the critical injured anteroinferior capsulolabral complex. Fixation strength may be inadequate if fewer than 3 anchors are used, and several studies cite insufficient anchors in the inferior glenoid as a contributor to recurrence.[9,17,41,96–99] The ability of arthroscopic technique to achieve fixation in the inferior glenoid has been questioned. One study reported that 87% of failed arthroscopic cases had no anchors inferior to the 4 o'clock position.[99]

Reducing capsular volume is key to restoring stability, and redundant capsule from inadequate plication and advancement of the anterior capsule is frequently seen in revision cases.[17–19,85] Failure to address rotator interval or posterior capsular laxity permits residual instability after Bankart repair.[96] Asymmetric capsular repair that fails to address a stretched inferior glenohumeral ligament and capsule may lead to overconstraint anteriorly and superiorly but persistent inferior instability.[19,32] Thermal capsulorrhaphy, used frequently in the past to reduce capsular volume, has been associated with severe capsular damage.[73] A humeral avulsion of the capsule (HAGL lesion) may lead to recurrent instability if neglected.[45,100]

Poor technique during open repair may result in structural damage or alteration of anatomy that contributes to failure. Approach-related morbidity to the subscapularis is frequently implicated in failure after open stabilization. In one study, clinical subscapularis muscle insufficiency was present after 53.8% of primary cases and 91.6% of revision cases.[49] Subscapularis scarring causes loss of motion, contributes to recurrent instability, and may complicate revision surgery.[19,46,51,85,101]

REVISION STABILIZATION

The surgeon planning revision stabilization must address the factors that caused the initial stabilization to fail as well as any new disorders caused by the reinjury. In addition to the previously described risk factors for recurrent instability, the athlete who presents for revision stabilization possesses the most fundamental risk factor for recurrence after revision: a failed primary stabilization. As a result, recurrence in athletes after revision stabilization tends to be higher than that after primary stabilization. Possible reasons include continued exposure of the surgically repaired shoulder to trauma, the additive damage of multiple injuries to the labrum and capsule, further bone loss to the glenoid and humeral head, and anatomic changes and scarring from the multiple operations on the shoulder.

Fundamental to the revision stabilization process is choosing the correct revision surgery. It is irresponsible to deem an athlete who needs revision stabilization as being comparable with a primary instability case. Revision Bankart repair may be appropriate in some revision situations but should be considered with caution. An athlete who has failed one arthroscopic stabilization is at risk to fail another. Performing the same surgery in the revision setting that failed in the primary setting is destined for failure unless there exists a clear technical reason for failure of primary repair that can be corrected in the revision setting or the athlete has sustained a significant trauma and now has a distinct new injury that is amenable to repair. The surgeon must assess the cause of failure to determine whether the athlete may be better served with a more robust stabilization.

Revision Bankart Repair

Although some consider open revision Bankart repair to be the gold standard for post-stabilization recurrence, several studies support the equivalence of arthroscopic revision for the appropriate indications.[14–18,33,46,75,76,85,97,99,102,103] However, revision Bankart repair should only be used in athletes with minimal risk factors for recurrence, and must not be used in the presence of significant glenoid bone loss and/or engaging Hill-Sachs lesion.

The Bankart repair attempts to return the injured capsulolabral structures to preinjury positions so that they may resume their stabilizing functions. The revision setting is frequently complicated by prior hardware, altered anatomy, glenoid bone loss, capsular attenuation, and scar tissue. Essential to the repair is the restoration of the anteroinferior labral bumper. Even with intensive mobilization of scarred capsulolabral tissue from the glenoid neck, a robust labrum frequently cannot be restored.[97] Attachment of the plicated capsule to the glenoid face may serve to replicate the labral bumper in cases of labral deficiency.[15,46,97] Nonetheless, ALPSA lesions and labral deficiency are associated with significant recurrence rates and should compel the surgeon to consider converting to a stabilization such as a Latarjet.[16,97]

Multiple anchors below the glenoid equator are recommended to secure the anteroinferior labrum, and some investigators recommend a low anteroinferior portal (5:00 or 5:30 position) through the subscapularis to facilitate anchor placement in the inferior glenoid.[16,46,96,97,104] Orthogonal placement of the anchor into the glenoid improves pullout strength.[105] Double-loaded suture anchors have higher tensile strength than single-loaded anchors.[106]

In the revision setting, the anterior capsule is frequently stretched, thinned, and/or patulous and emphasis should be placed on sufficient plication and superior advancement of the anterior capsule.[17,45,46,85] Proper tensioning to prevent postoperative loss of motion may be achieved by tightening the inferior capsule with the shoulder positioned in abduction and external rotation and the superior capsule with the shoulder in adduction and external rotation.[107] After repair of the Bankart lesion and plication of the anterior capsule, persistent anterior laxity may be addressed with a rotator interval closure, whereas inferior or posterior laxity may require inferior or posterior capsular plication to reduce the volume of the axillary pouch and inferior capsule.[15,16,46,108]

Revision Bankart repair generally has poorer results than primary stabilization, with higher recurrence rates, lower return-to-sports rates, and lower clinical outcome measures (**Table 3**). Conventional opinion supported open revision for failed shoulder stabilization because of a perceived improved ability to accurately restore the anatomy needed to confer stability.[33,40,85,98,99,109] Levine and colleagues[19] reported good or excellent results in 39 of 50 shoulders treated with open revision stabilization, with 78% return to previous level of sport at a mean follow-up of 4.7 years. Recurrent dislocation occurred in 9 patients (18%) and subluxation in 2 patients (4%). Patients who had undergone multiple prior stabilization attempts had a recurrence rate of 44%. Cho and colleagues[33] evaluated 26 patients who underwent open revision of a failed arthroscopic Bankart repair and found good or excellent clinical outcome in 88.5% and a recurrence rate of 11.5% at an average of 42 months' follow-up. Sisto[99] revised 30 arthroscopic failures with open stabilization and reported no postoperative recurrences and 86.7% good or excellent results.

The proliferation of arthroscopic shoulder stabilization has expanded to the revision setting. Kim and colleagues[17] studied 23 patients who underwent arthroscopic revision stabilization of a prior open or arthroscopic failure and found a rate of recurrent instability of 13%. In that study, 78.3% of athletes had complete or near-complete return to sport. A higher rate of instability was found by Neri and colleagues,[18] who reported postoperative instability in 3 of 11 patients (27.2%) who underwent revision arthroscopic Bankart repair. Subsequent studies have shown recurrence rates after arthroscopic revision stabilization between 6.3% and 18.8%.[15,16,97,108] The largest series of arthroscopic revision Bankart repair was reported by Bartl and colleagues,[97] who found a recurrence rate of 10.7% in 56 patients at a mean follow-up of 37 months. Age predicted recurrence, and the mean age of patients with recurrent instability was 22.6 years, compared with 30.8 years in those with stable shoulders.

Boileau and colleagues[46] published their results of arthroscopic revision of 22 patients who had failed a variety of open procedures that included 17 Latarjet procedures and 5 Eden-Hybbinette procedures. Five patients in this series had undergone multiple prior stabilization attempts. At a mean follow-up of 43 months, a recurrent subluxation event had occurred in only 1 patient. Twenty of 22 patients were satisfied with their outcomes. However, only 47% of athletes were able to return to their prior levels of sport and 32% had persistent pain. The investigators concluded that arthroscopic revision stabilization provides "satisfactory results in a selected patient population."[46]

Two recent studies compared revision with primary arthroscopic Bankart repair. Krueger and colleagues[103] compared a cohort of 20 patients who underwent revision arthroscopic Bankart repair with a matched cohort of 20 primary patients. At final follow-up at greater than 2 years after surgery, the revision group had worse clinical outcomes than the primary group according to Rowe score (81.8 vs 89), Walch-Duplay score (75.5 vs 85.3), Melbourne instability shoulder score (73.7 vs 90.2), Western Ontario shoulder instability index (68.9 vs 89.8), and subjective shoulder value (69.3 vs 91.8). Although no patients in either group had a recurrent dislocation or subluxation, 2 patients in the revision group had positive apprehension sign. In addition, only 6 patients in the revision group could return to the same level of sport, compared with 15 in the primary group. Seven patients who underwent revision had to change sports or stop playing.

In a similar study of 10 revision arthroscopic repairs compared with a matched cohort of 15 primary repairs, Millar and Murrell[14] found more encouraging results for revision surgery. At a mean follow-up of more than 3 years, they found no significant differences between the groups in terms of pain, function, range of motion, strength, and UCLA and Rowe shoulder scores, reporting good or excellent outcomes according to Rowe score in all but 2 patients in each group. However, in the revision group, 2 of 10 patients (20%) had a recurrent dislocation compared with 1 of 15 (6.7%) in the primary group. The investigators concluded that revision stabilization is as effective as primary stabilization.

Coracoid Transfer

The coracoid transfer, described in the 1950s by both Helfet[110] and Latarjet,[111] involves grafting the tip (Bristow) or body (Latarjet) of the coracoid to the anteroinferior glenoid (**Fig. 13**). The stabilizing effects of the transferred coracoid are both static and dynamic. The bone block statically restores the glenoid depth and width, increasing the glenoid contact surface area, and the transferred conjoint tendon serves as a buttress against anterior humeral head translation when the arm in a position of abduction and external rotation.[110] Capsular augmentation and tightening can be performed by suturing the capsule to the stump of the coracoacromial ligament left attached to the coracoid graft.[55,112] As an alternative, the capsule may be shifted superiorly and the graft may be placed in an extra-articular position.[113,114]

The coracoid transfer possesses numerous advantages for athletes in the revision setting (**Fig. 14**). The multifactorial stabilizing effect of the transfer obviates the robust labral or capsular repair that is often difficult to achieve with the revision Bankart repair. The grafted coracoid process addresses the anteroinferior glenoid deficiency commonly encountered in recurrent instability, restoring the articular surface and

Table 3
Results of revision stabilization

Study	n	Revision Surgery	Primary Surgery	Mean Age (y)	Follow-up (mo)	Recurrence Rate (Dislocation/ Subluxation)	Return to Play	Note
Arce et al,[15] 2012	16	Arthroscopic	Open or arthroscopic	26.8	30.9	18.8% (2/1)	50% full return 37.5% lower level 12.5% no return	
Krueger et al,[103] 2011	20	Arthroscopic	Open or arthroscopic	29	24.7	0**	30% same level 35% decreased level 20% changed sport 15% stopped sport	*Matched to primary cohort (n = 20) **Apprehension in 2
Bartl et al,[97] 2011	56	Arthroscopic	Open or arthroscopic	29.4	37	10.7% (4/2)	76% prior level* 24% lower level or changed sport	*1 of 3 professional athletes returned at prior level
Boileau et al,[46] 2009	22	Arthroscopic	Open*	31	43	1 (4.5%) (0/1)*	47% to prior level	*18/22 had prior bony stabilization (Latarjet or Eden-Hybbinette) and 5/22 had multiple prior stabilization attempts **Apprehension in 2
Barnes et al,[108] 2009	17	Arthroscopic	Open or arthroscopic	30	38	6.3% (1/0)*	NR	*Apprehension in 3
Patel et al,[76] 2008	40	Arthroscopic	Open or arthroscopic	33.1	36	4 (10%)	80% (most similar to that achieved when their shoulder was stable)	—

Millar & Murrell,[14] 2008	10	Arthroscopic*	Open	35	37	20% (2/0)**	NR	*Matched to primary cohort (n = 15) **Apprehension in 1
Franceschi et al,[127] 2008	10	Arthroscopic	Arthroscopic	25.6	68	10% (1/0)	All returned to previous sports levels*	*Return to play not specifically reported in results
Creighton et al,[16] 2007	18	Arthroscopic	Open or arthroscopic	28.6	29.7	16.7% (1/2)	NR	—
Neri et al,[18] 2003	11	Arthroscopic	Open or arthroscopic	28	34.4	27.2% (2/1)	64% return to sport (most at same level)	—
Kim et al,[17] 2002	23	Arthroscopic	Open or arthroscopic	24	36	13.0% (1/2)	78.3% complete or near-complete return to preinjury level	*Apprehension in 2
Cho et al,[33] 2009	26	Open	Arthroscopic	24	42	11.5% (3/0)	84.7% complete or near-complete return to preinjury level	Constant score increased from 65.1 to 86.7 Rowe score increased from 39 to 81
Sisto,[99] 2007	30	Open	Arthroscopic	24	46	0*	87% to previous level 13% no return**	*Negative apprehension in all patients **All overhead athletes
Meehan & Petersen,[109] 2005	25	Open	Open or arthroscopic	31.7	60	16% (4 total)	NR	—
Levine et al,[19] 2000	50	Open	Open or arthroscopic	27	56.4	22% (9/2)*	78% return to desired level of sport	*7 patients with recurrent instability later discovered to be voluntary dislocators
Schmid et al,[116] 2012	49	Latarjet	Open or arthroscopic	29	38	4.1% (0/2)*	NR	*Apprehension in 5

Abbreviation: NR, not reported.

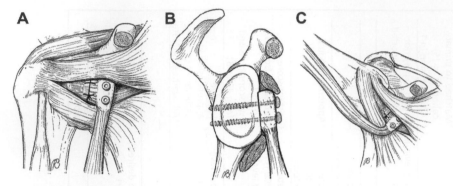

Fig. 13. The Latarjet procedure. (*A*) The osteotomized coracoid process and attached conjoint tendon is transferred through a split in the subscapularis to the anterior glenoid flush with the articular surface. (*B*) Proper graft position at the anteroinferior glenoid provides static stability by addressing the bony defect and extending the glenoid arc. Two screws drilled parallel to the articular surface secure the graft. (*C*) The conjoint tendon acts as a dynamic buttress when the arm is abducted and externally rotated. (*From* Edwards TB, Walch G. The Latarjet procedure for recurrent anterior shoulder instability: rationale and technique. Oper Tech Sports Med 2002;10:30; with permission.)

normalizing the glenohumeral contact pressures.[25,55,115] Hill-Sachs engagement is eliminated by widening of the glenoid and extension of the glenoid arc.[114] The transferred conjoint tendon provides dynamic stability for athletes in the main position of apprehension.[110] The postoperative rehabilitation can be accelerated with no external rotation restrictions because the rigid fixation of the bone graft allows early motion, and the surgeon can have confidence in returning the athlete to play with radiographic union shown on CT (**Fig. 15**).[30]

Coracoid transfer requires careful technique to ensure good results, the most important of which is the placement of the graft.[46,113,116] The ideal position for the transferred coracoid is flush with the glenoid rim at or below the glenoid equator.[46] Hovelius and colleagues[113] found an 83% recurrence rate after Bristow-Latarjet when the graft was positioned more than 1 cm from the glenoid rim. A graft placed too far laterally may restrict motion and precipitate arthrosis.[116,117]

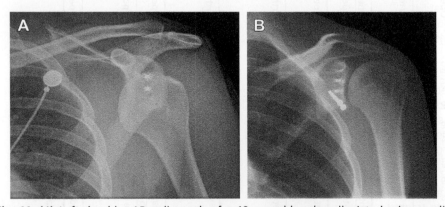

Fig. 14. (*A*) Left shoulder AP radiograph of a 19-year-old male collegiate hockey goalie revealing a postoperative dislocation after a previous arthroscopic Bankart repair. (*B*) Postoperative radiograph after revision stabilization with Latarjet procedure.

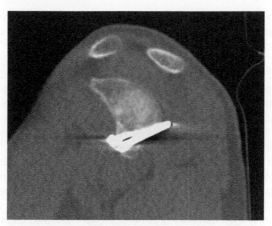

Fig. 15. Oblique sagittal CT image in the plane of the glenoid 5 months after Latarjet procedure reveals union of the coracoid bone graft.

Schmid and colleagues[116] retrospectively evaluated 49 patients who underwent the Latarjet procedure for failed stabilization. In this series, no patients redislocated after revision surgery and only 2 patients (4.1%) experienced subluxation events. Subjective good or excellent results were reported in 87.8% and the mean subjective shoulder value increased from 53% before surgery to 79% after surgery. Preoperative pain predicted postoperative pain. Hovelius and colleagues[113] recently published long-term follow-up results from 319 consecutive Bristow-Latarjet procedures performed between 1980 and 2004, of which 23 were revisions of prior failed stabilizations. At final follow-up, the overall recurrent instability rate was 17.9% (16 dislocations, 41 subluxations), and 307 of 319 (96.2%) were satisfied or very satisfied with their results. The recurrence rate in the revision group was 26.1% (1 dislocation, 5 subluxations) but, despite this high rate, 22 of 23 (95.7%) were satisfied with the result. Bony union of the coracoid graft was associated with the best results.

Several complications specific to coracoid transfer have been reported.[46,118,119] Intraoperative fracture of the coracoid compromises its function as an anterior bone block. Screw breakage, loss of fixation, and graft migration may result in postoperative instability.[118,119] Cannulated screws have been implicated in cases of hardware failure.[119] Postoperative pain is common in patients with graft or hardware problems.[46] Neurovascular injury during the procedure may impair shoulder function.[119]

Glenoid Bone Grafting

Glenoid bone loss may be addressed by structural bone grafting of the anterior glenoid. In a study of 11 cases in which autogenous tricortical iliac crest bone graft was used to reconstruct the deficient anterior glenoid, Warner and colleagues[120] found no recurrent instability and 100% return to play at a mean of 33 months after surgery. Auffarth and colleagues[121] reported no recurrent instability and excellent clinical outcomes in 47 patients treated with anatomic bone grafting using autogenous iliac crest shaped into a J configuration and impacted into the anterior glenoid. At a mean follow-up of 9.3 years, Steffen and Hertel[122] found 1 dislocation among 43 patients treated with iliac crest bone grafting. Lunn and colleagues[123] recommended consideration of iliac crest bone grafting to salvage a failed Latarjet procedure, reporting a 12% recurrence rate and 68% return to predislocation level of sport. Distal tibia allograft has also been proposed in the setting of significant glenoid deficiency because of its anatomic similarity to the glenoid articular surface, conformity to the humeral head, and capacity for secure fixation and incorporation.[124]

Hill-Sachs Management

Most Hill-Sachs lesions can be rendered inconsequential with an adequate anterior repair and capsular plication.[75] In large lesions that threaten stability, engagement may be eliminated with restoration of the articular arc through coracoid transfer or bone grafting.[114] Some investigators have recommended filling the defect with an osteochondral allograft to correct the humeral head deformity.[125,126] The defect may also be filled with the posterior capsule and the adjacent infraspinatus tendon to prevent engagement and limit anterior translation of the humeral head. Termed remplissage, for the French word for "filling," this technique has been proposed for large engaging Hill-Sachs lesions as a potential augmentation to Bankart repair in the absence of bone loss. Boileau and colleagues[94] showed high healing rates of the remplissage and a recurrence rate of 2.1% in 47 cases. Loss of motion is an expected consequence, although it may not significantly affect return to sports.[94]

SUMMARY

The athlete with a failed instability procedure requires a thoughtful and systematic approach to achieve a good outcome. Goals of treatment should be defined and realistic expectations should be set. Revision stabilization has a high rate of recurrent instability, low rates of return to play, and low clinical outcome scores. Fundamental to successful revision surgery is choosing the correct procedure. The decision is straightforward in athletes with clear factors that predict recurrence (significant glenoid bone loss, engaging Hill-Sachs lesions) because only a bony procedure can restore the articular arc of the glenoid. Arthroscopic revision Bankart repair may be appropriate in those athletes who have an obvious Bankart tear and no bone loss after a traumatic reinjury.

The challenge for the shoulder surgeon is identifying the best surgery for the athlete who does not have such clear-cut indications. Each factor that has the potential to lead to a poor outcome needs to be collected and calculated. Patient factors (age, laxity, type and level of sport), injury factors (mechanism of injury, capsulolabral injury, glenoid bone loss, Hill-Sachs lesion), and technical factors (previous surgery performed, integrity of repair, scarring) must be integrated into the treatment algorithm. Based on this collection of factors, the shoulder surgeon should be prepared to provide the athlete with the surgery that provides the best chance to return to playing sports and the lowest risk of recurrent instability.

REFERENCES

1. Fleisig GS, Andrews JR, Dillman CJ, et al. Kinetics of baseball pitching with implications about injury mechanisms. Am J Sports Med 1995;23(2):233–9. Available at: http://www.ncbi.nlm.nih.gov/pubmed/7778711. Accessed March 10, 2013.
2. Usman J, McIntosh AS, Fréchède B. An investigation of shoulder forces in active shoulder tackles in rugby union football. J Sci Med Sport 2011;14(6):547–52. http://dx.doi.org/10.1016/j.jsams.2011.05.006.
3. Rowe CR, Patel D, Southmayd WW. The Bankart procedure: a long-term end-result study. J Bone Joint Surg Am 1978;60(1):1–16. Available at: http://www.ncbi.nlm.nih.gov/pubmed/624747. Accessed March 4, 2013.

4. Gill TJ, Micheli LJ, Gebhard F, et al. Bankart repair for anterior instability of the shoulder. Long-term outcome. J Bone Joint Surg Am 1997;79(6):850–7. Available at: http://www.ncbi.nlm.nih.gov/pubmed/9199382. Accessed February 17, 2013.

5. Pagnani MJ, Dome DC. Surgical treatment of traumatic anterior shoulder instability in American football players. J Bone Joint Surg Am 2002;84-A(5):711–5. Available at: http://www.ncbi.nlm.nih.gov/pubmed/12004010. Accessed March 4, 2013.

6. Kropf EJ, Tjoumakaris FP, Sekiya JK. Arthroscopic shoulder stabilization: is there ever a need to open? Arthroscopy 2007;23(7):779–84. http://dx.doi.org/10.1016/j.arthro.2007.03.004.

7. Kartus C, Kartus J, Matis N, et al. Long-term independent evaluation after arthroscopic extra-articular Bankart repair with absorbable tacks. A clinical and radiographic study with a seven to ten-year follow-up. J Bone Joint Surg Am 2007;89(7):1442–8. http://dx.doi.org/10.2106/JBJS.F.00363.

8. Harris JD, Gupta AK, Mall NA, et al. Long-term outcomes after Bankart shoulder stabilization. Arthroscopy 2013;1–14. http://dx.doi.org/10.1016/j.arthro.2012.11.010.

9. Cole BJ, L'Insalata J, Irrgang J, et al. Comparison of arthroscopic and open anterior shoulder stabilization. A two to six-year follow-up study. J Bone Joint Surg Am 2000;82-A(8):1108–14. Available at: http://www.ncbi.nlm.nih.gov/pubmed/10954100. Accessed March 18, 2013.

10. Balg F, Boileau P. The instability severity index score. A simple pre-operative score to select patients for arthroscopic or open shoulder stabilisation. J Bone Joint Surg Br 2007;89(11):1470–7. http://dx.doi.org/10.1302/0301-620X.89B11.18962.

11. Voos JE, Livermore RW, Feeley BT, et al. Prospective evaluation of arthroscopic Bankart repairs for anterior instability. Am J Sports Med 2010;38(2):302–7. http://dx.doi.org/10.1177/0363546509348049.

12. Hovelius L, Vikerfors O, Olofsson A, et al. Bristow-Latarjet and Bankart: a comparative study of shoulder stabilization in 185 shoulders during a seventeen-year follow-up. J Shoulder Elbow Surg 2011;20(7):1095–101. http://dx.doi.org/10.1016/j.jse.2011.02.005.

13. Bessiere C, Trojani C, Pélégri C, et al. Coracoid bone block versus arthroscopic Bankart repair: a comparative paired study with 5-year follow-up. Orthop Traumatol Surg Res 2013. http://dx.doi.org/10.1016/j.otsr.2012.12.010.

14. Millar NL, Murrell GA. The effectiveness of arthroscopic stabilisation for failed open shoulder instability surgery. J Bone Joint Surg Br 2008;90(6):745–50. http://dx.doi.org/10.1302/0301-620X.90B6.20018.

15. Arce G, Arcuri F, Ferro D, et al. Is selective arthroscopic revision beneficial for treating recurrent anterior shoulder instability? Clin Orthop Relat Res 2012; 470(4):965–71. http://dx.doi.org/10.1007/s11999-011-2001-0.

16. Creighton RA, Romeo AA, Brown FM, et al. Revision arthroscopic shoulder instability repair. Arthroscopy 2007;23(7):703–9. http://dx.doi.org/10.1016/j.arthro.2007.01.021.

17. Kim SH, Ha KI, Kim YM. Arthroscopic revision Bankart repair: a prospective outcome study. Arthroscopy 2002;18(5):469–82. http://dx.doi.org/10.1053/jars.2002.32230.

18. Neri BR, Tuckman DV, Bravman JT, et al. Arthroscopic revision of Bankart repair. J Shoulder Elbow Surg 2003;16(4):419–24. http://dx.doi.org/10.1016/j.jse.2006.05.016.

19. Levine WN, Arroyo JS, Pollock RG, et al. Open revision stabilization surgery for recurrent anterior glenohumeral instability. Am J Sports Med 2000;28(2):156–60.

Available at: http://www.ncbi.nlm.nih.gov/pubmed/10750990. Accessed March 4, 2013.

20. Marquardt B, Garmann S, Schulte T, et al. Outcome after failed traumatic anterior shoulder instability repair with and without surgical revision. J Shoulder Elbow Surg 2007;16(6):742–7. http://dx.doi.org/10.1016/j.jse.2007.02.132.

21. Rhee YG, Ha JH, Cho NS. Anterior shoulder stabilization in collision athletes: arthroscopic versus open Bankart repair. Am J Sports Med 2006;34(6): 979–85. http://dx.doi.org/10.1177/0363546505283267.

22. Arciero RA, Taylor DC, Snyder RJ, et al. Arthroscopic bioabsorbable tack stabilization of initial anterior shoulder dislocations: a preliminary report. Arthroscopy 1995;11(4):410–7. Available at: http://www.ncbi.nlm.nih.gov/pubmed/7575872. Accessed March 9, 2013.

23. Privitera DM, Bisson LJ, Marzo JM. Minimum 10-year follow-up of arthroscopic intra-articular Bankart repair using bioabsorbable tacks. Am J Sports Med 2012; 40(1):100–7. http://dx.doi.org/10.1177/0363546511425891.

24. Owens BD, DeBerardino TM, Nelson BJ, et al. Long-term follow-up of acute arthroscopic Bankart repair for initial anterior shoulder dislocations in young athletes. Am J Sports Med 2009;37(4):669–73. http://dx.doi.org/10.1177/0363546508328416.

25. Millett PJ, Clavert P, Warner JJ. Open operative treatment for anterior shoulder instability: when and why? J Bone Joint Surg Am 2005;87(2):419–32. http://dx. doi.org/10.2106/JBJS.D.01921.

26. Bottoni CR, Smith EL, Berkowitz MJ, et al. Arthroscopic versus open shoulder stabilization for recurrent anterior instability: a prospective randomized clinical trial. Am J Sports Med 2006;34(11):1730–7. http://dx.doi.org/10. 1177/0363546506288239.

27. Kim SJ, Jung M, Moon HK, et al. Is the transglenoid suture technique recommendable for recurrent shoulder dislocation? A minimum 5-year follow-up in 59 non-athletic shoulders. Knee Surg Sports Traumatol Arthrosc 2009;17(12): 1458–62. http://dx.doi.org/10.1007/s00167-009-0748-6.

28. Kim SH, Ha KI, Cho YB, et al. Arthroscopic anterior stabilization of the shoulder: two to six-year follow-up. J Bone Joint Surg Am 2003;85-A(8):1511–8. Available at: http://www.ncbi.nlm.nih.gov/pubmed/12925631. Accessed February 26, 2013.

29. Hovelius L, Sandström B, Sundgren K, et al. One hundred eighteen Bristow-Latarjet repairs for recurrent anterior dislocation of the shoulder prospectively followed for fifteen years: study I—clinical results. J Shoulder Elbow Surg 2004;13(5):509–16. http://dx.doi.org/10.1016/j.jse.2004.02.013.

30. Neyton L, Young A, Dawidziak B, et al. Surgical treatment of anterior instability in rugby union players: clinical and radiographic results of the Latarjet-Patte procedure with minimum 5-year follow-up. J Shoulder Elbow Surg 2012;21(12): 1721–7. http://dx.doi.org/10.1016/j.jse.2012.01.023.

31. Cho NS, Hwang JC, Rhee YG. Arthroscopic stabilization in anterior shoulder instability: collision athletes versus noncollision athletes. Arthroscopy 2006; 22(9):947–53. http://dx.doi.org/10.1016/j.arthro.2006.05.015.

32. Boone JL, Arciero RA. Management of failed instability surgery: how to get it right the next time. Orthop Clin North Am 2010;41(3):367–79. http://dx.doi.org/ 10.1016/j.ocl.2010.02.009.

33. Cho NS, Yi JW, Lee BG, et al. Revision open Bankart surgery after arthroscopic repair for traumatic anterior shoulder instability. Am J Sports Med 2009;37(11): 2158–64. http://dx.doi.org/10.1177/0363546509339015.

34. O'Driscoll SW, Evans DC. Contralateral shoulder instability following anterior repair. An epidemiological investigation. J Bone Joint Surg Br 1991;73(6):

941–6. Available at: http://www.ncbi.nlm.nih.gov/pubmed/1955441. Accessed March 11, 2013.

35. Randelli P, Ragone V, Carminati S, et al. Risk factors for recurrence after Bankart repair a systematic review. Knee Surg Sports Traumatol Arthrosc 2012;20(11): 2129–38. http://dx.doi.org/10.1007/s00167-012-2140-1.

36. Porcellini G, Campi F, Pegreffi F, et al. Predisposing factors for recurrent shoulder dislocation after arthroscopic treatment. J Bone Joint Surg Am 2009;91(11): 2537–42. http://dx.doi.org/10.2106/JBJS.H.01126.

37. Kaplan LD, Flanigan DC, Norwig J, et al. Prevalence and variance of shoulder injuries in elite collegiate football players. Am J Sports Med 2005;33(8): 1142–6. http://dx.doi.org/10.1177/0363546505274718.

38. Berbig R, Weishaupt D, Prim J, et al. Primary anterior shoulder dislocation and rotator cuff tears. J Shoulder Elbow Surg 1999;8(3):220–5. Available at: http://www.ncbi.nlm.nih.gov/pubmed/10389076. Accessed March 12, 2013.

39. Gerber C, Nyffeler RW. Classification of glenohumeral joint instability. Clin Orthop Relat Res 2002;400:65–76. Available at: http://www.ncbi.nlm.nih.gov/pubmed/12072747. Accessed March 4, 2013.

40. Zabinski SJ, Callaway GH, Cohen S, et al. Revision shoulder stabilization: 2- to 10-year results. J Shoulder Elbow Surg 1999;8(1):58–65. Available at: http://www.ncbi.nlm.nih.gov/pubmed/10077799. Accessed March 19, 2013.

41. Boileau P, Villalba M, Héry J, et al. Risk factors for recurrence of shoulder instability after arthroscopic Bankart repair. J Bone Joint Surg Am 2006;1755–63. Available at: http://jbjs.org/article.aspx?articleID=27609&atab=7. Accessed January 6, 2013.

42. Ahmed I, Ashton F, Robinson C. Arthroscopic Bankart repair and capsular shift for recurrent anterior shoulder instability functional outcomes and identification of risk factors for recurrence. J Bone Joint Surg Am 2012;1308–15. Available at: http://jbjs.org/article.aspx?articleID=1216206. Accessed January 6, 2013.

43. Castagna A, Markopoulos N, Conti M, et al. Arthroscopic Bankart suture-anchor repair: radiological and clinical outcome at minimum 10 years of follow-up. Am J Sports Med 2010;38(10):2012–6. http://dx.doi.org/10.1177/0363546510372614.

44. Provencher MT, Bhatia S, Ghodadra NS, et al. Recurrent shoulder instability: current concepts for evaluation and management of glenoid bone loss. J Bone Joint Surg Am 2010;92(Suppl 2):133–51. http://dx.doi.org/10.2106/JBJS.J.00906.

45. Tauber M, Resch H, Forstner R, et al. Reasons for failure after surgical repair of anterior shoulder instability. J Shoulder Elbow Surg 2004;13(3):279–85. http://dx.doi.org/10.1016/S1058274604000254.

46. Boileau P, Richou J, Lisai A, et al. The role of arthroscopy in revision of failed open anterior stabilization of the shoulder. Arthroscopy 2009;25(10):1075–84. http://dx.doi.org/10.1016/j.arthro.2009.04.073.

47. Beighton P, Horan F. Orthopaedic aspects of the Ehlers-Danlos syndrome. J Bone Joint Surg Br 1969;51(3):444–53. Available at: http://www.ncbi.nlm.nih.gov/pubmed/5820785. Accessed March 10, 2013.

48. Sachs RA, Williams B, Stone ML, et al. Open Bankart repair: correlation of results with postoperative subscapularis function. Am J Sports Med 2005; 33(10):1458–62. http://dx.doi.org/10.1177/0363546505275350.

49. Scheibel M, Tsynman A, Magosch P, et al. Postoperative subscapularis muscle insufficiency after primary and revision open shoulder stabilization. Am J Sports Med 2006;34(10):1586–93. http://dx.doi.org/10.1177/0363546506288852.

50. Lusardi DA, Wirth MA, Wurtz D, et al. Loss of external rotation following anterior capsulorrhaphy of the shoulder. J Bone Joint Surg Am 1993;75(8):1185–92.

Available at: http://www.ncbi.nlm.nih.gov/pubmed/8354677. Accessed March 12, 2013.

51. Vezeridis PS, Goel DP, Shah AA, et al. Postarthroscopic arthrofibrosis of the shoulder. Sports Med Arthrosc 2010;18(3):198–206. http://dx.doi.org/10.1097/JSA.0b013e3181ec84a5.

52. Robinson CM, Shur N, Sharpe T, et al. Injuries associated with traumatic anterior glenohumeral dislocations. J Bone Joint Surg Am 2012;94(1):18–26. http://dx.doi.org/10.2106/JBJS.J.01795.

53. Gagey O, Gagey N. The hyperabduction test. An assessment of the laxity of the inferior glenohumeral ligament. J Bone Joint Surg Br 2001;83(1):69–74. Available at: http://www.bjj.boneandjoint.org.uk/content/83-B/1/69.abstract. Accessed March 22, 2013.

54. Bedi A, Ryu RK. Revision arthroscopic Bankart repair. Sports Med Arthrosc 2010;18(3):130–9. http://dx.doi.org/10.1097/JSA.0b013e3181ec8484.

55. Piasecki DP, Verma NN, Romeo AA, et al. Glenoid bone deficiency in recurrent anterior shoulder instability: diagnosis and management. J Am Acad Orthop Surg 2009;17(8):482–93. Available at: http://www.ncbi.nlm.nih.gov/pubmed/19652030. Accessed March 4, 2013.

56. Itoi E, Lee SB, Amrami KK, et al. Quantitative assessment of classic anteroinferior bony Bankart lesions by radiography and computed tomography. Am J Sports Med 2003;31(1):112–8. Available at: http://www.ncbi.nlm.nih.gov/pubmed/12531767. Accessed March 4, 2013.

57. Murachovsky J, Bueno RS, Nascimento LG, et al. Calculating anterior glenoid bone loss using the Bernageau profile view. Skeletal Radiol 2012;41(10): 1231–7. http://dx.doi.org/10.1007/s00256-012-1439-9.

58. Provencher MT, Frank RM, Leclere LE, et al. The Hill-Sachs lesion: diagnosis, classification, and management. J Am Acad Orthop Surg 2012;20(4):242–52. http://dx.doi.org/10.5435/JAAOS-20-04-242.

59. Suder PA, Frich LH, Hougaard K, et al. Magnetic resonance imaging evaluation of capsulolabral tears after traumatic primary anterior shoulder dislocation. A prospective comparison with arthroscopy of 25 cases. J Shoulder Elbow Surg 1995;4(6):419–28. Available at: http://www.ncbi.nlm.nih.gov/pubmed/8665286. Accessed March 13, 2013.

60. Kirkley A, Litchfield R, Thain L, et al. Agreement between magnetic resonance imaging and arthroscopic evaluation of the shoulder joint in primary anterior dislocation of the shoulder. Clin J Sport Med 2003;13(3):148–51. Available at: http://www.ncbi.nlm.nih.gov/pubmed/12792208. Accessed March 13, 2013.

61. Rerko MA, Pan X, Donaldson C, et al. Comparison of various imaging techniques to quantify glenoid bone loss in shoulder instability. J Shoulder Elbow Surg 2012;1–7. http://dx.doi.org/10.1016/j.jse.2012.05.034.

62. Woertler K, Waldt S. MR imaging in sports-related glenohumeral instability. Eur Radiol 2006;16(12):2622–36. http://dx.doi.org/10.1007/s00330-006-0258-6.

63. Beltran J, Rosenberg ZS, Chandnani VP, et al. Glenohumeral instability: evaluation with MR arthrography. Radiographics 1997;17(3):657–73. Available at: http://www.ncbi.nlm.nih.gov/pubmed/9153704. Accessed March 13, 2013.

64. Volpi D, Olivetti L, Budassi P, et al. Capsulo-labro-ligamentous lesions of the shoulder: evaluation with MR arthrography. Radiol Med 2003;105(3):162–70. Available at: http://www.ncbi.nlm.nih.gov/pubmed/12835639. Accessed March 13, 2013.

65. Oh JH, Kim JY, Choi JA, et al. Effectiveness of multidetector computed tomography arthrography for the diagnosis of shoulder pathology: comparison with

magnetic resonance imaging with arthroscopic correlation. J Shoulder Elbow Surg 2010;19(1):14–20. http://dx.doi.org/10.1016/j.jse.2009.04.012.

66. Bishop JY, Jones GL, Rerko MA, et al. 3-D CT is the most reliable imaging modality when quantifying glenoid bone loss. Clin Orthop Relat Res 2013;471(4): 1251–6. http://dx.doi.org/10.1007/s11999-012-2607-x.

67. Sugaya H, Moriishi J, Dohi M, et al. Glenoid rim morphology in recurrent anterior glenohumeral instability. J Bone Joint Surg Am 2003;85–A(5):878–84. Available at: http://www.ncbi.nlm.nih.gov/pubmed/12728039. Accessed January 8, 2013.

68. Provencher MT, Detterline AJ, Ghodadra N, et al. Measurement of glenoid bone loss: a comparison of measurement error between 45 degrees and 0 degrees bone loss models and with different posterior arthroscopy portal locations. Am J Sports Med 2008;36(6):1132–8. http://dx.doi.org/10.1177/0363546508316041.

69. Nofsinger C, Browning B, Burkhart SS, et al. Objective preoperative measurement of anterior glenoid bone loss: a pilot study of a computer-based method using unilateral 3-dimensional computed tomography. Arthroscopy 2011; 27(3):322–9. http://dx.doi.org/10.1016/j.arthro.2010.09.007.

70. Barchilon VS, Kotz E, Barchilon Ben-Av M, et al. A simple method for quantitative evaluation of the missing area of the anterior glenoid in anterior instability of the glenohumeral joint. Skeletal Radiol 2008;37(8):731–6. http://dx.doi.org/10.1007/s00256-008-0506-8.

71. Chuang TY, Adams CR, Burkhart SS. Use of preoperative three-dimensional computed tomography to quantify glenoid bone loss in shoulder instability. Arthroscopy 2008;24(4):376–82. http://dx.doi.org/10.1016/j.arthro.2007.10.008.

72. Arrigoni P, Huberty D, Brady PC, et al. The value of arthroscopy before an open modified Latarjet reconstruction. Arthroscopy 2008;24(5):514–9. http://dx.doi.org/10.1016/j.arthro.2007.11.021.

73. Park HB, Yokota A, Gill HS, et al. Revision surgery for failed thermal capsulorrhaphy. Am J Sports Med 2005;33(9):1321–6. http://dx.doi.org/10.1177/0363546504273048.

74. Ozbaydar M, Elhassan B, Diller D, et al. Results of arthroscopic capsulolabral repair: Bankart lesion versus anterior labroligamentous periosteal sleeve avulsion lesion. Arthroscopy 2008;24(11):1277–83. http://dx.doi.org/10.1016/j.arthro.2008.01.017.

75. Burkhart SS, Debeer JF, Tehrany AM, et al. Quantifying glenoid bone loss arthroscopically in shoulder instability. Arthroscopy 2002;18(5):488–91. http://dx.doi.org/10.1053/jars.2002.32212.

76. Patel RV, Apostle K, Leith JM, et al. Revision arthroscopic capsulolabral reconstruction for recurrent instability of the shoulder. J Bone Joint Surg Br 2008; 90(11):1462–7. http://dx.doi.org/10.1302/0301-620X.90B11.21072.

77. Fabre T, Abi-Chahla ML, Billaud A, et al. Long-term results with Bankart procedure: a 26-year follow-up study of 50 cases. J Shoulder Elbow Surg 2010;19(2): 318–23. http://dx.doi.org/10.1016/j.jse.2009.06.010.

78. Uhorchak JM, Arciero RA, Huggard D, et al. Recurrent shoulder instability after open reconstruction in athletes involved in collision and contact sports. Am J Sports Med 2000;28(6):794–9. Available at: http://www.ncbi.nlm.nih.gov/pubmed/11101100. Accessed March 4, 2013.

79. Stein T, Linke RD, Buckup J, et al. Shoulder sport-specific impairments after arthroscopic Bankart repair: a prospective longitudinal assessment. Am J Sports Med 2011;39(11):2404–14. http://dx.doi.org/10.1177/0363546511417407.

80. Pavlik A, Csépai D, Hidas P, et al. Sports ability after Bankart procedure in professional athletes. Knee Surg Sports Traumatol Arthrosc 1996;4(2):116–20. Available at: http://www.ncbi.nlm.nih.gov/pubmed/8884733. Accessed March 13, 2013.

81. Ide J. Arthroscopic Bankart repair using suture anchors in athletes: patient selection and postoperative sports activity. Am J Sports Med 2004;32(8): 1899–905. http://dx.doi.org/10.1177/0363546504265264.

82. Bigliani LU, Kurzweil PR, Schwartzbach CC, et al. Inferior capsular shift procedure for anterior-inferior shoulder instability in athletes. Am J Sports Med 1994; 22(5):578–84. Available at: http://www.ncbi.nlm.nih.gov/pubmed/7810778. Accessed March 13, 2013.

83. Franceschi F, Papalia R, Del Buono A, et al. Glenohumeral osteoarthritis after arthroscopic Bankart repair for anterior instability. Am J Sports Med 2011; 39(8):1653–9. http://dx.doi.org/10.1177/0363546511404207.

84. Castagna A, Delle Rose G, Borroni M, et al. Arthroscopic stabilization of the shoulder in adolescent athletes participating in overhead or contact sports. Arthroscopy 2012;28(3):309–15. http://dx.doi.org/10.1016/j.arthro.2011.08.302.

85. Rowe CR, Zarins B, Ciullo JV. Recurrent anterior dislocation of the shoulder after surgical repair. Apparent causes of failure and treatment. J Bone Joint Surg Am 1984;66(2):159–68. Available at: http://www.ncbi.nlm.nih.gov/pubmed/6693441. Accessed March 14, 2013.

86. Itoi E, Lee SB, Berglund LJ, et al. The effect of a glenoid defect on anteroinferior stability of the shoulder after Bankart repair: a cadaveric study. J Bone Joint Surg Am 2000;82(1):35–46. Available at: http://www.ncbi.nlm.nih.gov/pubmed/ 10653082. Accessed March 4, 2013.

87. Burkhart SS, De Beer JF. Traumatic glenohumeral bone defects and their relationship to failure of arthroscopic Bankart repairs. Arthroscopy 2000;16(7): 677–94. http://dx.doi.org/10.1053/jars.2000.17715.

88. Lo IK, Parten PM, Burkhart SS. The inverted pear glenoid: an indicator of significant glenoid bone loss. Arthroscopy 2004;20(2):169–74. http://dx.doi.org/10. 1016/j.arthro.2003.11.036.

89. Mologne TS, Provencher MT, Menzel KA, et al. Arthroscopic stabilization in patients with an inverted pear glenoid: results in patients with bone loss of the anterior glenoid. Am J Sports Med 2007;35(8):1276–83. http://dx.doi.org/10. 1177/0363546507300262.

90. Porcellini G, Paladini P, Campi F, et al. Long-term outcome of acute versus chronic bony Bankart lesions managed arthroscopically. Am J Sports Med 2007;35(12):2067–72. http://dx.doi.org/10.1177/0363546507305011.

91. Yiannakopoulos CK, Mataragas E, Antonogiannakis E. A comparison of the spectrum of intra-articular lesions in acute and chronic anterior shoulder instability. Arthroscopy 2007;23(9):985–90. http://dx.doi.org/10.1016/j.arthro.2007. 05.009.

92. Yamamoto N, Itoi E, Abe H, et al. Contact between the glenoid and the humeral head in abduction, external rotation, and horizontal extension: a new concept of glenoid track. J Shoulder Elbow Surg 2007;16(5):649–56. http://dx.doi.org/10. 1016/j.jse.2006.12.012.

93. Kurokawa D, Yamamoto N, Nagamoto H, et al. The prevalence of a large Hill-Sachs lesion that needs to be treated. J Shoulder Elbow Surg 2013. http://dx. doi.org/10.1016/j.jse.2012.12.033.

94. Boileau P, O'Shea K, Vargas P, et al. Anatomical and functional results after arthroscopic Hill-Sachs remplissage. J Bone Joint Surg Am 2012;94(7): 618–26. http://dx.doi.org/10.2106/JBJS.K.00101.

95. Cole BJ, Romeo AA. Arthroscopic shoulder stabilization with suture anchors: technique, technology, and pitfalls. Clin Orthop Relat Res 2001;(390):17–30. Available at: http://www.ncbi.nlm.nih.gov/pubmed/11550863. Accessed March 19, 2013.

96. Mazzocca AD, Brown FM, Carreira DS, et al. Arthroscopic anterior shoulder stabilization of collision and contact athletes. Am J Sports Med 2005;33(1):52–60. http://dx.doi.org/10.1177/0363546504268037.

97. Bartl C, Schumann K, Paul J, et al. Arthroscopic capsulolabral revision repair for recurrent anterior shoulder instability. Am J Sports Med 2011;39(3):511–8. http://dx.doi.org/10.1177/0363546510388909.

98. Levine WN, Richmond JC, Donaldson WR. Use of the suture anchor in open Bankart reconstruction. A follow-up report. Am J Sports Med 1994;22(5):723–6. Available at: http://www.ncbi.nlm.nih.gov/pubmed/7810801. Accessed March 19, 2013.

99. Sisto DJ. Revision of failed arthroscopic Bankart repairs. Am J Sports Med 2007; 35(4):537–41. http://dx.doi.org/10.1177/0363546506296520.

100. Rhee YG, Cho NS. Anterior shoulder instability with humeral avulsion of the glenohumeral ligament lesion. J Shoulder Elbow Surg 2007;16(2):188–92. http://dx.doi.org/10.1016/j.jse.2006.06.017.

101. Dewing CB, Horan MP, Millett PJ. Two-year outcomes of open shoulder anterior capsular reconstruction for instability from severe capsular deficiency. Arthroscopy 2012;28(1):43–51. http://dx.doi.org/10.1016/j.arthro.2011.07.002.

102. Brophy RH, Gill CS, Lyman S, et al. Effect of shoulder stabilization on career length in national football league athletes. Am J Sports Med 2011;39(4): 704–9. http://dx.doi.org/10.1177/0363546510382887.

103. Krueger D, Kraus N, Pauly S, et al. Subjective and objective outcome after revision arthroscopic stabilization for recurrent anterior instability versus initial shoulder stabilization. Am J Sports Med 2011;39(1):71–7. http://dx.doi.org/10.1177/0363546510379336.

104. Carreira DS, Mazzocca AD, Oryhon J, et al. A prospective outcome evaluation of arthroscopic Bankart repairs: minimum 2-year follow-up. Am J Sports Med 2006;34(5):771–7. http://dx.doi.org/10.1177/0363546505283259.

105. Ilahi OA, Al-Fahl T, Bahrani H, et al. Glenoid suture anchor fixation strength: effect of insertion angle. Arthroscopy 2004;20(6):609–13. Available at: http://www.ncbi.nlm.nih.gov/pubmed/15241312. Accessed March 21, 2013.

106. Kamath GV, Hoover S, Creighton RA, et al. Biomechanical analysis of a double-loaded glenoid anchor configuration: can fewer anchors provide equivalent fixation? Am J Sports Med 2013;41(1):163–8. http://dx.doi.org/10.1177/0363546512469090.

107. Warner JJ, Johnson D, Miller M, et al. Technique for selecting capsular tightness in repair of anterior-inferior shoulder instability. J Shoulder Elbow Surg 1995;4(5): 352–64. Available at: http://www.ncbi.nlm.nih.gov/pubmed/8548438. Accessed March 21, 2013.

108. Barnes CJ, Getelman MH, Snyder SJ. Results of arthroscopic revision anterior shoulder reconstruction. Am J Sports Med 2009;37(4):715–9. http://dx.doi.org/10.1177/0363546508328411.

109. Meehan RE, Petersen SA. Results and factors affecting outcome of revision surgery for shoulder instability. J Shoulder Elbow Surg 2005;14(1):31–7. http://dx.doi.org/10.1016/j.jse.2004.05.005.

110. Helfet AJ. Coracoid transplantation for recurring dislocation of the shoulder. J Bone Joint Surg Br 1958;40-B(2):198–202. Available at: http://www.ncbi.nlm.nih.gov/pubmed/13539102. Accessed February 28, 2013.

111. Latarjet M. Treatment of recurrent dislocation of the shoulder. Lyon Chir 1954; 49(8):994–7. Available at: http://www.ncbi.nlm.nih.gov/pubmed/13234709. Accessed February 17, 2013.

112. Wellmann M, De Ferrari H, Smith T, et al. Biomechanical investigation of the stabilization principle of the Latarjet procedure. Arch Orthop Trauma Surg 2012; 132(3):377–86. http://dx.doi.org/10.1007/s00402-011-1425-z.

113. Hovelius L, Sandström B, Olofsson A, et al. The effect of capsular repair, bone block healing, and position on the results of the Bristow-Latarjet procedure (study III): long-term follow-up in 319 shoulders. J Shoulder Elbow Surg 2012; 21(5):647–60. http://dx.doi.org/10.1016/j.jse.2011.03.020.

114. Burkhart SS, De Beer JF, Barth JR, et al. Results of modified Latarjet reconstruction in patients with anteroinferior instability and significant bone loss. Arthroscopy 2007;23(10):1033–41. http://dx.doi.org/10.1016/j.arthro.2007.08.009.

115. Ghodadra N, Gupta A, Romeo AA, et al. Normalization of glenohumeral articular contact pressures after Latarjet or iliac crest bone-grafting. J Bone Joint Surg Am 2010;92(6):1478–89. http://dx.doi.org/10.2106/JBJS.I.00220.

116. Schmid SL, Farshad M, Catanzaro S, et al. The Latarjet procedure for the treatment of recurrence of anterior instability of the shoulder after operative repair: a retrospective case series of forty-nine consecutive patients. J Bone Joint Surg Am 2012;94(11):e75. http://dx.doi.org/10.2106/JBJS.K.00380.

117. Allain J, Goutallier D, Glorion C. Long-term results of the Latarjet procedure for the treatment of anterior instability of the shoulder. J Bone Joint Surg Am 1998; 80(6):841–52. Available at: http://www.ncbi.nlm.nih.gov/pubmed/9655102. Accessed March 19, 2013.

118. Butt U, Charalambous CP. Complications associated with open coracoid transfer procedures for shoulder instability. J Shoulder Elbow Surg 2012;21(8): 1110–9. http://dx.doi.org/10.1016/j.jse.2012.02.008.

119. Shah AA, Butler RB, Romanowski J, et al. Short-term complications of the Latarjet procedure. J Bone Joint Surg Am 2012;94(6):495–501. http://dx.doi.org/10. 2106/JBJS.J.01830.

120. Warner JJ, Gill TJ, O'hollerhan JD, et al. Anatomical glenoid reconstruction for recurrent anterior glenohumeral instability with glenoid deficiency using an autogenous tricortical iliac crest bone graft. Am J Sports Med 2006;34(2): 205–12. http://dx.doi.org/10.1177/0363546505281798.

121. Auffarth A, Schauer J, Matis N, et al. The J-bone graft for anatomical glenoid reconstruction in recurrent posttraumatic anterior shoulder dislocation. Am J Sports Med 2008;36(4):638–47. http://dx.doi.org/10.1177/0363546507309672.

122. Steffen V, Hertel R. Rim reconstruction with autogenous iliac crest for anterior glenoid deficiency: forty-three instability cases followed for 5-19 years. J Shoulder Elbow Surg 2012;22(4):550–9. http://dx.doi.org/10.1016/j.jse.2012.05.038.

123. Lunn JV, Castellano-Rosa J, Walch G. Recurrent anterior dislocation after the Latarjet procedure: outcome after revision using a modified Eden-Hybinette operation. J Shoulder Elbow Surg 2008;17(5):744–50. http://dx.doi.org/10.1016/j.jse. 2008.03.002.

124. Provencher MT, Ghodadra N, LeClere L, et al. Anatomic osteochondral glenoid reconstruction for recurrent glenohumeral instability with glenoid deficiency using a distal tibia allograft. Arthroscopy 2009;25(4):446–52. http://dx.doi.org/10. 1016/j.arthro.2008.10.017.

125. Kropf EJ, Sekiya JK. Osteoarticular allograft transplantation for large humeral head defects in glenohumeral instability. Arthroscopy 2007;23(3):322.e1–5. http://dx.doi.org/10.1016/j.arthro.2006.07.032.

126. Chapovsky F, Kelly JD. Osteochondral allograft transplantation for treatment of glenohumeral instability. Arthroscopy 2005;21(8):1007. http://dx.doi.org/10.1016/j.arthro.2005.04.005.

127. Franceschi F, Longo UG, Ruzzini L, et al. Arthroscopic salvage of failed arthroscopic Bankart repair: a prospective study with a minimum follow-up of 4 years. Am J Sports Med 2008;36(7):1330–6. http://dx.doi.org/10.1177/0363546508314403.

Nonoperative and Postoperative Rehabilitation for Glenohumeral Instability

Kevin E. Wilk, PT, DPT, FAPTA[a,b,c,*], Leonard C. Macrina, MSPT, SCS, CSCS[a,c]

KEYWORDS

- Proprioception • Shoulder instability • Rehabilitation • Return to function

KEY POINTS

- The glenohumeral joint relies on the dynamic stabilizers and neuromuscular control system to provide functional stability.
- Non-operative rehabilitation should be employed for most patients with glenohumeral instability, especially with multidirectional instability.
- The focus of the rehabilitation should be to maximize muscular strength, endurance while improving dynamic stability, proprioception and neuromuscular control.

INTRODUCTION

Shoulder instability is a common abnormality often seen in the orthopedic and sports medicine setting. An appropriate rehabilitation program plays a vital role in the successful outcome following an episode of shoulder instability. The glenohumeral joint allows a tremendous amount of mobility to function, thus making it inherently unstable and the most frequently dislocated joint in the body.[1] Because of the joint's poor osseous congruence and capsular laxity, it greatly relies on the dynamic stabilizers and neuromuscular system to provide functional stability.[2] Therefore, differentiation between normal translation and pathologic instability is often difficult to determine. There exists a wide range of shoulder instabilities, from subtle subluxations (as seen in overhead athletes) to gross instability. Acquired instability, often seen in the overhead thrower, is another type of shoulder abnormality. Often the success of the

[a] Champion Sports Medicine, A Physiotherapy Associates Clinic, Birmingham, AL, USA; [b] Tampa Bay Rays Baseball Team, Tampa Bay, FL, USA; [c] American Sports Medicine Institute, Birmingham, AL, USA
* Corresponding author. Champion Sports Medicine, 805 Saint Vincent's Drive, Suite G100, Birmingham, AL 35205.
E-mail address: Kwilkpt@hotmail.com

Clin Sports Med 32 (2013) 865–914
http://dx.doi.org/10.1016/j.csm.2013.07.017
0278-5919/13/$ – see front matter © 2013 Elsevier Inc. All rights reserved.

rehabilitation program is based on accurate recognition and a well-designed treatment program for the specific type of instability present.

Nonoperative rehabilitation is often implemented for patients diagnosed with a variety of shoulder instabilities. Based on the classification system of glenohumeral instability as well as several key factors (**Box 1**),[3] a nonoperative rehabilitation program may be developed. This article discusses and outlines these factors, along with the nonoperative rehabilitation and postoperative programs for various types of shoulder instability that are intended to return patients to their previous level of function.

NONOPERATIVE REHABILITATION GUIDELINES

Specific guidelines to consider in the rehabilitation of a patient with traumatic instability are outlined in this section. A 4-phase rehabilitation program is discussed, followed by an overview of variations and key rehabilitation principles for congenital and acquired laxity.

Phase I: Acute Phase

The first-time episode of dislocation is generally more painful than the recurrent episodes. The 3 most common forms of instability are anterior, posterior, and multidirectional. Anterior instability is the most common traumatic type of instability seen in the general orthopedic population. It has been reported that this type of instability represents approximately 95% of all traumatic shoulder instabilities.[4] Conversely, a patient presenting with atraumatic or congenital instability often presents with a history of repetitive injuries and symptomatic complaints, owing to the unique characteristic of excessive capsular laxity and capsular redundancy in this patient population. Often the patient does not complain of a single instability episode but rather a feeling of shoulder laxity or an inability to perform specific tasks. These patients often experience episodes of traumatic subluxations rather than dislocations. Varying degrees of shoulder instability exist, ranging from a subtle subluxation to gross (uncontrollable) instability. The term subluxation refers to the complete separation of the articular surfaces with spontaneous reduction.[5] By contrast, a dislocation is a complete separation of the articular surfaces, and requires a specific movement or manual reduction to relocate the joint.[5]

Acutely dislocated patients usually self-limit their motion by guarding the injured extremity in an internally rotated and adducted position against the side of their

---

Box 1
Seven key factors to consider in the rehabilitation of the unstable shoulder

1. Onset of the abnormality

2. Degree of instability: subluxation versus dislocation

3. Frequency of dislocation: chronic versus acute

4. Direction of instability: anterior, posterior, multidirectional

5. Concomitant abnormalities

6. End-range neuromuscular control

7. Premorbid activity level

body to protect the injured shoulder. The goals of the acute phase are to: (1) diminish pain, inflammation, and muscle guarding; (2) promote and protect healing soft tissues; (3) prevent the negative effects of immobilization; (4) reestablish baseline dynamic joint stability; and (5) prevent further damage to the glenohumeral joint capsule (**Appendix 1**, Protocol).

The authors allow immediate limited and controlled motion following a traumatic dislocation in some patients (age 18–30 years) but immobilize patients between the ages of 30 and 55 years old. However, motion is restricted so as not to cause further tissue attenuation. A short period of immobilization in a sling to control pain and allow scar tissue to form for enhanced stability may be necessary for 7 to 14 days. Paterson and colleagues,[6] in a systematic review and meta-analysis of 6 articles, reported no long-term benefit from immobilization for longer than 1 week in patients younger than 30 years. Hovelius and colleagues[7–10] have demonstrated that the rate of recurrent dislocations is based on the patient's age and is not affected by the length of postinjury immobilization. Individuals between the ages of 19 and 29 years are the most likely to experience multiple episodes of instability. Hovelius and colleagues[7–10] noted that patients in their 20s exhibited a recurrence rate of 60%, whereas patients in their 30s to 40s had a recurrence rate of less than 20%. The incidence of recurrent dislocation ranges from 17% to 96%, with a mean of 67% in patient populations between the ages of 21 and 30 years.[1,4,6,9,11–19] Therefore, the rehabilitation program should progress cautiously in young athletic individuals. In adolescents the recurrence rate is as high as 92%[20] and is 100% with open physes,[21] although no long-term benefits regarding recurrence rates and immobilization have been observed in younger patients between the ages of 17 and 29 years.[9,22] Individuals older than 29 years are usually immobilized for 2 to 4 weeks to allow scarring of the injured capsule.

The ideal position to immobilize the glenohumeral joint has traditionally been in internal rotation (IR) with the arm close to the body. Studies by Itoi and colleagues[23–26] examined positional differences of immobilization and compared the rates of recurrent dislocations. The investigators concluded that immobilization in external rotation (ER) significantly reduced the recurrence rate of instability in chronic and first-time dislocations. Itoi and colleagues[25] have recommended immobilization with the arm in 30° of abduction and ER, compared with a group of patients immobilized in IR. The results indicated a 0% recurrence rate in ER and 30% incidence of instability in the group immobilized in IR. The investigators stated that the resultant Bankart lesion had improved coaptation to the glenoid rim with immobilization in ER versus conventional immobilization in a sling. Several investigators[27,28] have reported no improved stability and outcomes with immobilization in ER; thus the current consensus as stated by Paterson and colleagues[6] is that there seems to be no benefit in immobilizing the shoulder in ER following anterior dislocation. Furthermore, potential complications with immobilization may include a decrease in joint proprioception, muscle disuse, and atrophy, and a loss of range of motion (ROM) in specific age groups. Therefore, prolonged use of immobilization following a traumatic dislocation may not be recommended in all patients. The authors recommend a short period of immobilization for young active individuals for 1 week in an IR traditional sling; conversely for patients older than 30, especially if an anterior labral periosteal sleeve avulsion (ALPSA) lesion is identified, immobilization for 3 weeks in a traditional IR sling is recommended.

Passive ROM (PROM) is initiated in a restricted and protected range based on the patient's symptoms. The early motion is intended to promote healing, enhance collagen organization, stimulate joint mechanoreceptors, and aid in decreasing the patient's pain through neuromuscular modulation.[18,29–31] Pain-free active assisted

ROM (AAROM) exercises such as pendulums and ER/IR at 45° of abduction using an L-bar or golf club may also be initiated, in addition to PROM exercises performed in a pain-free arc of motion, and passive/active joint positioning in a restricted motion. Modalities such as ice, laser therapy and transcutaneous electrical nerve stimulation (TENS) may also be beneficial in decreasing pain, inflammation, and muscle guarding.

Strengthening exercises are initially performed through submaximal, pain-free isometric contractions to initiate muscle recruitment and retard muscle atrophy. Electrical stimulation of the posterior cuff musculature may also be incorporated to enhance this muscle-fiber recruitment process early on in the rehabilitation process, and also in the next phase when the patient initiates isotonic strengthening activities. Reinold and colleagues[32] reported that the use of electrical stimulation improved force production of the rotator cuff, particularly the external rotators, immediately after surgery.

Dynamic stabilization exercises are also performed to reestablish dynamic joint stability. The patient maintains a static position as the rehabilitation specialist performs manual rhythmic stabilization drills to facilitate muscular cocontractions. These manual rhythmic stabilization drills are performed for the shoulder internal and external rotators in the scapular plane at 30° of abduction, and are performed at pain-free angles that do not compromise the healing capsule. Rhythmic stabilizations for flexion and extension may also be performed with the shoulder at 100° flexion and 10° of horizontal abduction. Strengthening exercises are also performed for the scapular retractors and depressors to re-position the scapula in its proper position, and are critical for successful rehabilitation.

Closed kinetic chain exercises such as weight shifting against the wall or onto a ta-ble are performed to produce a cocontraction of the surrounding glenohumeral musculature and to facilitate joint mechanoreceptors to enhance proprioception. Weight shifts are usually performed immediately following the injury unless posterior instability or an articular cartilage lesion is present.

Phase II: Intermediate Phase

During the intermediate phase, the program emphasizes regaining full ROM along with progressing strengthening exercises of the rotator cuff, thus reestablishing the muscular balance of the glenohumeral joint, scapular stabilizers, and surrounding shoulder muscles. Before the patient enters Phase II certain criteria must be met, which include diminishing pain and inflammation, satisfactory static stability, and adequate neuromuscular control.

To achieve the desired goals of this phase, passive ROM is performed to the pa-tient's tolerance with the goal of attaining nearly full ROM. AAROM exercises using a rope and pulley along with flexion and ER/IR exercises at 90° of abduction using an L-bar may be progressed to tolerance without stressing the involved tissues. ER at 90° of abduction is generally limited to 65° to 70° to avoid overstressing the healing anterior capsuloligamentous structures. These restrictions are typically maintained for approximately 4 to 8 weeks, but eventually increase to full ROM as tolerated by the patient.

Isotonic strengthening exercises are also initiated during this phase. Emphasis is placed on increasing the strength of the internal and external rotators and scapular muscles to maximize dynamic stability. The ultimate goal of the strengthening phase is to reestablish muscular balance following the injury. Kibler[1] noted that scapular position and strength deficits have been shown to contribute to glenohumeral joint instability. Exercises initially include ER and IR with exercise tubing at 0° of abduction along with side-lying ER and prone rowing. During the latter part of this phase, exercises are progressed to include the "Thrower's Ten" strengthening program (**Appendix 2**) to emphasize rotator cuff and scapulothoracic muscle strength. Manual resistive exercises such as side-lying ER and prone rowing may also prove beneficial by having the clinician vary the resistance throughout the ROM. Incorporating manual concentric and eccentric manual exercises and rhythmic stabilization drills at end range to enhance neuromuscular control and dynamic stability is also recommended.

Closed kinetic chain exercises are progressed to include a hand-on-the-wall stabilization drill in the plane of the scapular at shoulder height as far as is tolerated by the patient (**Fig. 1**). Push-ups are performed first with hands on a table, then progressed to a push-up on a ball or unstable surface while the rehabilitation specialist performs rhythmic stabilizations to the involved and uninvolved upper extremity along with the trunk, to integrate dynamic stability and core strengthening (tilt board, ball, and so forth). Caution should be exercised while performing closed kinetic chain exercises in patients with posterior instability for 6 to 8 weeks to allow for adequate tissue healing and strength gains. Furthermore, patients with significant scapular winging should perform push-ups with a plus[33] until adequate scapular strength is accomplished. Core stabilization drills should also be performed to enhance scapular control. In addition, strengthening exercises may be advanced in regards of resistance, repetitions, and sets as the patient improves. End-range rhythmic stabilization drills with the arm at 45° of abduction are also performed. The authors refer to these exercises as perturbation drills. Exercises such as tubing with manual resistance and end-range rhythmic stabilization drills are also performed (**Fig. 2**). The goal of these exercise drills is to improve proprioception and neuromuscular control at end range. Often these exercises are performed seated on a stability ball to recruit core, hip, and scapular muscles as the patient attempts to maintain good stability and posture.

Phase III: Advanced Strengthening

In the advanced strengthening phase the focus is on improving strength, dynamic stability, and neuromuscular control near end range through a series of progressive

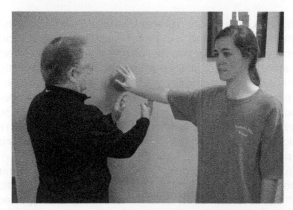

Fig. 1. Hand onto a ball on the wall in the plane of the scapula to promote joint dynamic stabilization through coactivation and compressive forces in the glenohumeral joint.

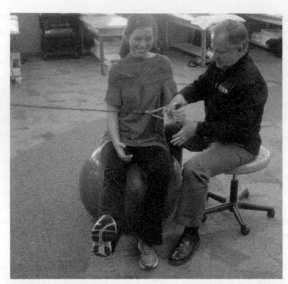

Fig. 2. Seated tubing with manual resistance by the rehabilitation specialist to promote dynamic stability and neuromuscular control, and enhance proprioception.

strengthening exercises, leading to a gradual return to activity. Criteria to enter this phase include: (1) minimal pain and tenderness; (2) full ROM; (3) symmetric capsular mobility; and (4) good (at least 4/5 manual muscle test) strength, endurance, and dynamic stability of the scapulothoracic and upper extremity musculature.

Neuromuscular control may be defined as the efferent or motor output in reaction to an afferent or sensory input.[2,15] The afferent input is the ability to detect the glenohumeral joint position and motion in space, with resultant efferent response by the dynamic stabilizers as they blend with the joint capsule to assist in stabilization of the humeral head. Injury with resultant insufficient neuromuscular control could result in deleterious effects to the patient. As a result, the humeral head may not center itself within the glenoid, thereby compromising the surrounding static stabilizers. The patient with poor neuromuscular control may exhibit excessive humeral head migration with the potential for injury, an inflammatory response, and reflexive inhibition of the dynamic stabilizers.

Several investigators have reported that neuromuscular control of the glenohumeral joint may be negatively affected by joint instability. Lephart and colleagues[15] compared the ability to detect passive motion and the ability to reproduce joint positions in normal, unstable, and surgically repaired shoulders. The investigators reported a significant decrease in proprioception and kinesthesia in the shoulders with instability when compared with normal shoulders and with shoulders undergoing surgical stabilization procedures. Smith and Brunolli[34] reported a significant decrease in proprioception following a shoulder dislocation. Blasier and colleagues[35] reported that individuals with significant capsular laxity showed a decrease in proprioception when compared with patients with normal laxity.

Muscle fatigue has also been associated with a decrease in neuromuscular control. Carpenter and colleagues[36] observed the ability to detect passive motion of shoulders positioned at 90° of abduction and 90° of ER. The investigators reported a decrease in both the detection of ER and IR movement following an isokinetic fatigue protocol. Thus, exercises designed to enhance endurance in the upper extremity, such as low resistance and high repetitions (20–30 repetitions per set), are incorporated during this phase. Also, exercise sets using time may be incorporated, such as 30-second or 60-second exercise bouts. To this end a program has been developed to enhance cocontraction and dynamic stabilization and to improve endurance. This program is referred to as the Advanced Throwers Ten Program (**Appendix 3**).[37]

Aggressive upper body strengthening through the continuation of a progressive isotonic resistance program is recommended. A gradual increase in resistance as well as a progression to a more functional position by performing tubing exercises at 90° of abduction to strengthen the external and internal rotators is also recommended. In addition, more aggressive isotonic strengthening exercises such as bench press, seated row, and latissimus pull-downs may be incorporated in a protected ROM during this phase. During bench press and seated rows, the patient is instructed to not extend the upper extremities beyond the plane of the body during the descending phase to minimize stress on the shoulder capsule. Latissimus pull-downs are performed in front of the head, and the patient is instructed to avoid full extension of the arms to minimize the amount of traction force applied to the shoulder joint. Also during this phase perturbation training is performed, particularly at end ROM. This technique involves postural and positional disturbances by the rehabilitation specialist to create apprehension and to train the patient to stabilize the humeral head. The authors consider it essential that the patient has adequate dynamic stability before returning to functional activities that invoke stresses at extremes of motion.

A patient wishing to return to athletic participation may be instructed to perform plyometric exercises for the upper extremity. These activities are incorporated to regain any remaining functional ROM as well as to improve neuromuscular control, and to train the extremity to produce and dissipate forces. Initially, 2-handed drills close to the body such as chest pass, and side-to-side and overhead soccer throws using a 3- to 5-lb medicine ball may be performed to enhance dynamic stabilization of the glenohumeral joint. Exercises are initiated with 2 hand drills close to the center of gravity and gradually progress to longer lever arms away from the patient's body. Drills are progressed to challenge the dynamic stabilizers of the shoulder.

After approximately 2 weeks of pain-free 2-handed drills, the athlete progresses to 1-handed plyometric drills using a small medicine ball (1–2 lb) while throwing into a trampoline. Wall dribbles in the 90/90 position to improve overhead muscle endurance may also be incorporated.

Phase IV: Return to Activity Phase

In the return to activity phase the goal is to increase, gradually and progressively, the functional demands on the shoulder in order for the patient to return to unrestricted sport or daily activities. Other goals of this phase are to maintain the patient's muscular strength and endurance, dynamic stability, and functional ROM. The criteria to progress into this phase include: (1) full functional ROM; (2) adequate static stability; (3) satisfactory muscular strength and endurance; (4) adequate dynamic stability; and (5) a satisfactory clinical examination.

The general orthopedic patient continues to perform a maintenance program to improve strength, dynamic stability, and neuromuscular control as well as maintaining full, functional, and pain-free ROM. The athlete continues to perform aggressive strengthening exercises such as plyometrics, proprioceptive neuromuscular facilitation drills, and isotonic strengthening. In addition, the athlete may begin functional sport activities through an interval return to sport program.[38] These activities are designed to gradually return motion, function, and confidence in the upper extremity by progressing through graduated sport-specific activities.[38–40] These interval sport programs are set up to minimize the chance of re-injury while training the patient for the demands of each individual sport. Each program should be individualized based on the patient's injury, skill level, and goals. The duration of each program is based on several factors including the extent of the injury, the sport, and level of play, along with the time of season. The athlete is allowed to return to unrestricted sports activities after completion of an appropriately designed rehabilitation program and a successful clinical examination including full ROM, strength, and adequate dynamic stability and neuromuscular control. The authors routinely perform a combination of isokinetic testing for overhead athletes, referred to as the Thrower's Series.[41,42] Criteria to begin an interval sport program includes an ER/IR strength ratio of 66% to 76% or higher at 180° per second, and an ER to abduction ratio of 67% to 75% or higher at 180° per second.[41,42] Patients returning to contact sports such as hockey, football, or rugby may be required to wear a shoulder-stability brace for the initiation of the return to sport.

NONOPERATIVE REHABILITATION OF POSTERIOR INSTABILITY

The nonoperative treatment of recurrent posterior shoulder instability is designed to alleviate the initial symptoms of the current episode and improve dynamic stability to minimize the recurrence of the condition. The authors follow several guidelines when the rehabilitation program is initiated. First, the patient is instructed to avoid aggravating activities, which may include pushing motions, horizontal adductions, and excessive IR. Football players are instructed not to perform bench press, push-ups, or any blocking drills until cleared by the physician. In baseball players, no throwing or hitting (especially if the lead shoulder) is permitted until medical clearance by the treating physician. The second rehabilitation goal is to establish good scapula control and base from which the arm can function. Thus the program focuses on postural corrections, scapular muscular strengthening, and scapular neuromuscular control. Specific exercises include prone horizontal abduction on a stability ball, lower trapezius robbery movement,[43] wall slides,[44] prone rowing into ER on the stability ball,[45] and scapula neuromuscular control drills.[46]

In addition, the authors emphasize rotator-cuff muscle strengthening, specifically the external rotators and the posterior deltoid. Specific exercises routinely performed are rhythmic stabilization (ER/IR), side-lying ER,[47] standing ER with resistance bands or a cable column, prone rowing at 90° of abduction- and prone horizontal abduction with full ER.

Once the strengthening and posture goals are met, the emphasis changes to end-range stabilization through perturbation training, end-range stabilization, and endurance. A side-lying plank position on a plinth while performing side-lying ER is beneficial for restoring core strength while working the posterior rotator cuff. Progression of the plank position onto a stability ball further challenges the core musculature. During the advanced phase, endurance training is emphasized and gradually progressed with increased repetitions, time-bout exercises, and sustained-hold exercises, similarly to the principles of the advanced throwing program.[37]

Once the nonoperative goals are accomplished, the athlete initiates a gradual return-to-sport program. During this phase the athlete's signs and symptoms are monitored carefully and progressed accordingly. The authors have not found glenohumeral joint stabilization braces to be of benefit during this phase, but scapular control has been shown to be extremely beneficial.

REHABILITATION OF ATRAUMATIC SHOULDER INSTABILITY

Rehabilitation of the patient with congenital shoulder instability poses a significant challenge for the rehabilitation specialist. Patients typically presents with several episodes of instability, which limits them from performing certain tasks that may include daily work tasks as well as recreational or sports activities. This type of instability may arise from several factors, including excessive capsular redundancy and capsular laxity, poor osseous configuration such as a flattened glenoid fossa, or weakness in the glenohumeral and scapular musculature resulting in poor neuromuscular control. Any of these factors, individually or in combination, may contribute to pathologic glenohumeral instability.

Multidirectional instability (MDI) or multidirectional laxity (MDL) can be identified as shoulder instability in more than 1 plane of motion. Patients with MDL have a congenital predisposition and exhibit ligamentous laxity caused by excessive collagen elasticity of the capsule. Rodeo and colleagues[48] reported such patients exhibit a greater concentration of elastin than collagen, as well as collagen fibrils of smaller diameter. The authors consider an inferior displacement of greater than 8 to 10 mm during the sulcus sign (**Fig. 3**) with the arm adducted to the side as significant hypermobility, thus suggesting significant congenital laxity.[2]

The goals of the rehabilitation program for the patient with atraumatic instability are to improve proprioception, dynamic stability, and neuromuscular control; increase muscle tone, and optimize scapular position and muscle strength to gradually return the patient to functional activities without limitations. As previously mentioned, the early phase of rehabilitation involves reducing shoulder pain and muscular inhibition while abstaining from activities that cause apprehension.

Shoulder muscle activation in patients with congenital laxity has been shown to differ from that in a normal, stable shoulder.[49–54] Normal force coupling that exists to dynamically stabilize the glenohumeral joint is altered, resulting in excessive humeral head migration and a feeling of subluxation by the patient. Burkhead and Rockwood[55] found that an exercise program was effective in the management of 80% of patients with atraumatic instability. Misamore and colleagues[56] reported improved results in 28 of 59 patients in a long-term follow-up study of atraumatic athletic patients.

The rehabilitation program (**Appendix 4**) for the patient with atraumatic instability involves slowly regaining motion without excessive stress to the involved tissues. The patient often presents with excessive ROM, therefore PROM activities are not

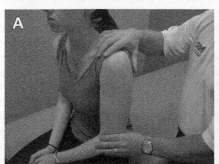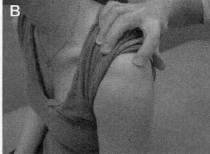

Fig. 3. Sulcus sign to assess glenohumeral laxity. (*A*) Position to assess a sulcus sign in a patient with suspected MDI. (*B*) Patient demonstrating a positive sulcus sign as noted by the amount of inferior translation of the humerus within the glenoid.

the focus of the rehabilitation program. Special attention is placed to avoid positions, movements, or stretches to the involved tissues that may place the shoulder in an unstable position. Modalities such as cryotherapy, iontophoresis, laser therapy, and TENS may be used to minimize pain and inflammation. Reducing shoulder pain may also be accomplished through gentle motion activities to neuromodulate pain, nonsteroidal anti-inflammatories prescribed by the physician, and abstention from painful arcs of active and passive ROM.

The primary focus of the early phase of the rehabilitation program is to minimize any further muscle atrophy and reflexive inhibition resulting from disuse, repeated subluxation episodes, and pain. Exercises are focused on creating dynamic stability, improved scapular position, enhanced proprioception, and increased muscle tone throughout the body. Isometric contraction exercises may be performed for the glenohumeral muscles, particularly the rotator cuff. Rhythmic stabilization drills may also be performed to facilitate a muscular cocontraction/coactivation to improve neuromuscular control and enhance the sensitivity of the afferent mechanoreceptors.[15] The goal is to create a more efficient agonist/antagonist cocontraction, thus to improve force coupling and joint stability during active movements.

The authors believe that exercises such as rhythmic stabilization drills and weight-bearing exercises to promote a cocontraction and an improvement in proprioception are beneficial in this patient population. Axial compression or weight-bearing exercises are progressed from standing weight shifts on a table top to hand-on-wall with the shoulder in the scapular plane. Rhythmic stabilizations of the involved extremity as well as at the core and trunk may be applied during these weight-bearing drills to further challenge the patient's dynamic stability and neuromuscular control. The patient may be placed in a plank position (prone on elbows) and on the knees to enhance cocontraction at the shoulder joint and enhance core stability. The authors prefer the plank position to the push-up position because of the scapula position that exists in the latter. In the push-up position the scapula is internally rotated, protracted, and anteriorly tilted, all undesirable positions. The plank position is progressed from planks on the wall, to planks on knees, to planks on feet, and finally to planks on unstable surfaces. Unstable surfaces such as tilt boards, foam, and large exercise balls may be incorporated to further challenge the patient's dynamic stability while in the closed chain position, while further promoting a coactivation or cocontraction of the surrounding musculature.

Patients with congenital laxity often present with significant rotator-cuff and scapular strength deficits, particularly the external rotators, scapular retractors, and scapular depressors. A progressive isotonic strengthening program may be initiated to improve rotator-cuff and scapular musculature strength, endurance, and dynamic stability. Proper scapula stability and movement is vital for asymptomatic function. Scapula strengthening will improve proximal stability and will therefore enable distal-segment mobility during the patient's functional tasks. These exercises may include ER at 0° of abduction, side-lying ER, standing ER at 90° of abduction, prone ER, prone rowing, prone extension, and prone horizontal abduction at 100° with ER. Other scapular training exercises commonly incorporated include serratus wall slides[44] and a dynamic hug for serratus anterior strengthening.[33] Bilateral ER with scapular retraction and table press-downs with scapular retraction may also be performed to strengthen the lower trapezius. Neuromuscular control drills are performed for the scapula musculature by having the rehabilitation specialist manually resist scapula movements.[46] The goal of these drills is to enhance strength and endurance, and to improve scapula proprioception.

The function of the neuromuscular control system must not be overlooked in this patient population. Functional exercise drills that include positions of instability to induce a reflexive muscular response[2,57,58] may protect against future injury or recurring episodes of instability. Active joint-repositioning tasks, proprioceptive neuromuscular facilitation (PNF), and plyometric exercises may be beneficial and may evoke a neuromuscular response. The authors encourage exercises to be performed on a stability ball. By performing these exercises on an unstable surface, these drills increase the demands on the glenohumeral and scapular muscles. Often these exercises are performed on a stability ball with one foot on the floor and the opposite arm keeping a sustained hold on a dumbbell, a principle from the Advanced Thrower's Ten Program.[37] All of these techniques are used to enhance core activation and the overall tone within the body to improve overall stability.

Once sufficient strength of the scapular stabilizers and posterior rotator cuff has been achieved, the patient is encouraged to use the shoulder only in the most stable positions: those in the plane of the scapular during humeral elevation. Activities that promote a feeling of joint instability, with or without subluxation or dislocation, should be avoided. Only when coordination and confidence are achieved through progressive strengthening should the patient attempt activities in an intrinsically unstable position. Bracing of the glenohumeral joint for return to sporting activities may also be necessary to provide immobilization or controlled ROM to protect against further injury.

The primary focus of the rehabilitation program for the patient with a congenitally unstable shoulder is to enhance strength and balance in the rotator cuff, improve scapular position and core stability, and improve proprioception and neuromuscular control. Once symptoms have subsided and sufficient strength has been achieved the patient may resume normal shoulder function, which may include most sporting activities.

ACQUIRED INSTABILITY

The throwing shoulder, especially in baseball pitchers, consistently demands a considerable amount of attention in the orthopedic and sports medicine community because of the frequency with which it is injured.[57,59–65] The pitcher exhibits unique ROM characteristics, which are often important to consider when evaluating and treating the thrower's shoulder. Therefore the clinical and rehabilitation specialist should have an accurate understanding of the typical variations in motion and strength within the overhead thrower to prevent, evaluate, or treat the athlete.[46,65–68]

The shoulder joint is frequently injured in the overhead-throwing athlete. Conte and colleagues[69] reported that 28% of all injuries sustained to professional baseball pitchers occur within the shoulder. McFarland and Wasik[70] reported that upper extremity injuries in collegiate baseball players accounted for 75% of the time lost from the sport as a result of injury. In fact, the pitcher was the most commonly injured position (69%), and rotator-cuff tendonitis was the most common type of reported injury. Several investigations have documented that shoulder injuries are more common in pitchers than in position players.[69,70]

The ROM changes observed in the overhead thrower may contribute to the injuries observed in this population. The changes in ER and IR ROM are initially due to the osseous adaptations, which represents a change in side-to-side ROM by approximately 12°.[67] Other factors such as muscular tightness,[65,66,71] posterior capsular tightness,[72,73] and scapular position[74,75] are superimposed onto the osseous adaptations and may contribute to an injury. Further research is needed to determine the exact risk factors for shoulder injuries in the thrower, and the other structures that contribute to the loss of shoulder IR and the increase in ER.

Numerous investigators have documented a difference between IR motion of the throwing and nonthrowing shoulders in throwing athletes.[61,75–78] This disparity in IR of the throwing shoulder when compared with the nonthrowing side has been referred to as glenohumeral joint IR deficit (GIRD).[76] Most recently defined by Kibler and colleagues,[79] GIRD occurs when there is a 15° or greater loss in IR measurements when the throwing shoulder is compared with the nonthrowing shoulder. Some clinicians[77,80,81] have suggested GIRD as a cause of specific shoulder injuries in throwing athletes. Wilk and colleagues[65] proposed the total rotational motion (TRM) concept of glenohumeral mobility in the throwing shoulder, in which the amount of ER and IR measured at 90° of abduction are added together to calculate a total rotational arc of motion. The investigators reported that the TRM in the throwing shoulders of professional baseball pitchers should be within 5° of the nonthrowing shoulder, and a TRM arc greater than 5° may be a contributing factor to shoulder injuries in throwers.[65,81] The investigators went on to conclude that there is a higher incidence in shoulder injuries when the TRM is outside the 5° window.

Based on the aforementioned articles, the authors believe it is necessary to perform stretching and ROM exercises on pitchers who exhibit ROM characteristics that may predispose them to injury. The ROM values that make the thrower more susceptible to injury are: (1) side-to-side TRM differences greater than 5°; and (2) GIRD of 12° or more compared with the contralateral shoulder. Several investigators have reported stretching programs in college players[82] and professional baseball pitchers,[83] which were effective in maintaining or improving shoulder IR ROM.

Based on these data, the authors have developed a new stretching program for the posterior shoulder soft tissue. These stretches include the traditional sleeper stretch (**Fig. 4**), sleeper stretch with a lift (**Fig. 5**), sleeper stretch in the scapula plane (**Fig. 6**), and side lying in the scapula plane/horizontal adduction (cross-body stretch with IR) (**Fig. 7**), which can be performed alone or with a rehabilitation specialist.[84] A horizontal adduction stretch is also incorporated, with the patient assisting into IR (**Fig. 8**). The stretches are often performed in the side-lying position to stabilize the scapula, but a modified side-lying position is recommended (**Fig. 9**) to position the patient/athlete in the scapular plane, thus minimizing shoulder impingement. These exercises are performed to improve the flexibility of the posterior musculature, which

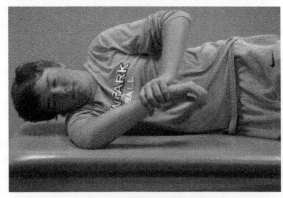

Fig. 4. Sleeper stretch designed to improve internal rotation range of motion through stretching the posterior musculature and capsule.

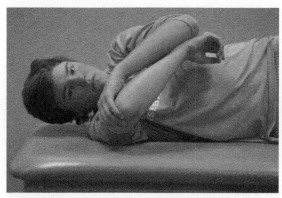

Fig. 5. Sleeper stretch with a lift to pretension the posterior soft tissue and localize the stretch.

may become tight as a result of the high eccentric muscle contractions and forces (repetitive microtrauma) during the deceleration phase of the throwing motion. The ultimate goal of stretching is to restore IR PROM to within approximately 10° to 12° of the nondominant side. The clinical and rehabilitation specialist should also consider regaining TRM to within 5° of the opposite shoulder.

Another structure to consider when improving IR in the baseball pitcher is the posterior capsule. Although this structure is rarely found to become excessively tight on clinical examination, it should be noted as a possible limitation to shoulder IR in some individuals. The rehabilitation technique used by the authors to improve the posterior capsular mobility is joint mobilization. It is important that the rehabilitation specialist performs the glide in a posterolateral direction (**Fig. 10**) that is perpendicular to the glenoid face, to avoid abutting the humeral head with the glenoid rim.

The overhead thrower is a unique athlete with unique physical demands and injury risks. Restoring glenohumeral PROM in the overhead athlete is critical in preventing

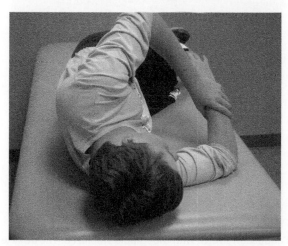

Fig. 6. Sleeper stretch in the scapula plane to decrease stress on the subacromial structures and place the shoulder in a more functional and comfortable position.

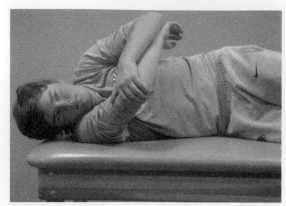

Fig. 7. Side-lying cross-body stretch as the athlete progressively pushes the shoulder into internal rotation.

future injury and the potential need for surgery. The clinical and rehabilitation specialist should have a clear understanding of proper measurement and treatment techniques for the overhead-throwing athlete. In fact, the rehabilitation efforts should attempt to maximize results in the thrower through the following goals: (1) IR of the dominant arm within 12° of the opposite arm; (2) TRM within 5° of the opposite side; and (3) postural correction exercises to stretch tight structures and strengthen the weak scapula stabilizers. The authors believe that these critical factors can decrease the risk of injury in overhead throwers.

Internal impingement has been described in the literature by Walch and associates.[85] Andrews and Meister[86] originally identified the lesion in the overhead thrower.

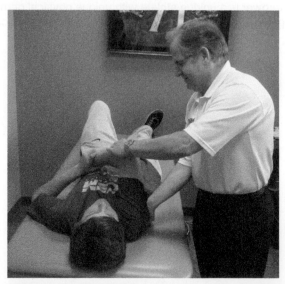

Fig. 8. Horizontal adduction stretch with the scapula stabilized. The athlete assists by gently pushing the involved shoulder into further internal rotation to enhance the stretch on the posterior structures.

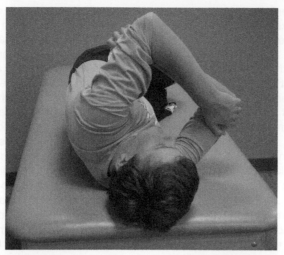

Fig. 9. Modified side-lying self-horizontal/internal rotation stretch to decrease stress on the subacromial structures and place the shoulder in the scapula plane.

This cuff lesion develops when the arm is abducted and externally rotated, such as in the cocking phase of throwing. During this movement, the humeral head tends to glide anteriorly (especially when the anterior capsule is hypermobile). As this motion occurs, the supraspinatus and infraspinatus impinge (or produce friction) on the posterosuperior edge of the glenoid rim, resulting in an undersurface tearing of the rotator cuff and fraying of the posterosuperior glenoid labrum. This lesion is extremely common in athletes using overhead movements.

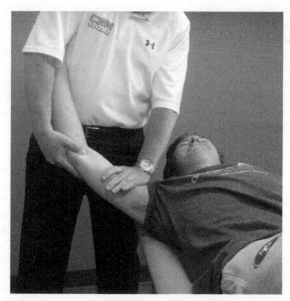

Fig. 10. Joint mobilization in a posterolateral direction to improve posterior capsular mobility.

Often the underlying cause of symptomatic internal impingement is excessive anterior shoulder laxity. One of the primary goals of the rehabilitation program is to enhance the athlete's dynamic stabilization capacity, thus controlling anterior humeral head translation. Another essential goal is to restore flexibility to the posterior rotator-cuff muscles of the glenohumeral joint. The authors strongly caution against aggressive stretching of the anterior and inferior glenohumeral structures, as this may result in increased anterior translation. In addition, the program should emphasize muscular strengthening of the posterior rotator cuff to reestablish muscular balance and improve joint-compression abilities. The scapular muscles must also be an area of increased focus, to restore proper scapula position and motion. Restoring dynamic stabilization is an essential goal in minimizing the anterior translation of the humeral head during the late cocking and early acceleration phases of throwing.

Exercise drills such as PNF patterns with rhythmic stabilization are incorporated.[40,46,57] Stabilization drills performed at the end range of ER are beneficial in enhancing dynamic stabilization. Perturbation training to the shoulder joint is performed to enhance proprioception, dynamic stabilization, and neuromuscular control during this phase. In the authors' opinion, this form of training has been extremely effective in treating the thrower with posterior/superior impingement.

REHABILITATION FOLLOWING ANTERIOR BANKART REPAIR

Rehabilitation following arthroscopic Bankart repair involves gradually restoring glenohumeral PROM while respecting the constraints of the healing tissues. Many investigators advocate postoperative immobilization for 4 to 6 weeks and a guarded motion program. Wickiewicz and colleagues[87] suggested 4 weeks of immobilization followed by AAROM and PROM exercises from week 4 and full motion by approximately 8 to 10 weeks. Various investigators have suggested several time frames for immobilization. Some suggested 3 weeks of immobilization after arthroscopic stabilization,[88,89] others 4 weeks, and yet others 6 weeks. Grana and colleagues[89] noted that some patients may not comply with long periods of strict immobilization because of the minimal pain and less operative morbidity following the arthroscopic approach. These patients may return to some activities prematurely.

The rehabilitation program is divided into 4 specific phases (**Appendix 5**). The first phase is considered the maximal protection phase or restricted motion phase. Immediately after surgery, the patient's shoulder is placed in an abduction brace (**Fig. 11**); this brace is used consistently for the first 2 to 4 weeks and is worn during sleep for 4 to 6 weeks after surgery. During the first 2 weeks, the patient is allowed to perform AAROM and PROM exercises. The active-assisted motion is restricted to 60° of forward flexion, 45° of IR, and 5° to 10° of ER with the arm placed in 45° of abduction. In addition, PROM is performed for shoulder flexion to a maximum of 90° and IR and ER, with the arm at 45° of abduction. These ranges are strictly enforced to prevent potentially deleterious forces on the anteroinferior aspect of the glenohumeral capsule where the surgical procedure has been performed. During this phase, the patient also performs submaximal and subpainful isometrics for the shoulder musculature. In addition, cryotherapy and other modalities may be used to reduce postoperative pain and inflammation.

At 3 to 4 weeks, ROM is increased but restricted. PROM and AAROM flexion is allowed to 90°, while ER ROM is limited to 20° to 30°. In addition, the patient performs light strengthening exercises to restore dynamic joint stability, such as rhythmic stabilization exercises for the ER/IR muscles and submaximal isometrics for all the shoulder musculature. At week 4 the sling is usually discontinued, based on the clinical

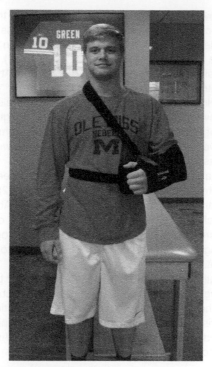

Fig. 11. Ultrasling abduction pillow (DJO Global, Vista, CA) used postoperatively to protect the healing tissues.

assessment of the stability of the joint and the patient's response to surgery and pain level. Occasionally the patient is encouraged to continue use of the abduction pillow while sleeping, to restrict excessive uncontrolled shoulder motions and positioning. At this time, AAROM and PROM exercises are continued gradually to improve abduction and ER, as well as flexion and IR.

During the first 6 weeks, the authors restrict motion to prevent overloading or overstressing the repaired capsule. Furthermore, an attempt is made to gradually restore motion, which helps to prevent the negative effects of immobilization and assists in collagen formation and organization. During these first 6 weeks, care must be taken by the clinician not to overstress the healing tissue and the soft-tissue fixation.

At approximately week 6 after the surgery, the goal is to gradually restore motion and initiate light isotonic strengthening of the rotator cuff and scapula stabilizers. The ER/IR stretching and motion exercises are performed at 45° of abduction, which produces a mild stretch on the inferior capsule (during ER motion). The patient is encouraged to gradually improve shoulder flexion, progressing to approximately 140°. Also at this time, the patient is allowed to begin light-resistance isotonic strengthening exercises. The ER/IR muscles are exercised using exercise tubing. In addition, a light weight (1–2 lb) can be used to perform abduction to 90°, flexion to 90°, and scapular musculature strengthening such as prone rowing and prone extension.

Phase II, the moderate protection phase, begins at week 6 and progresses to week 14. The goals of this phase are to: (1) gradually restore full, nonpainful ROM; (2) preserve the integrity of the surgical repair; (3) restore muscular strength and endurance; and (4) allow some functional activities. During this phase, all motions gradually progress. Shoulder flexion and abduction progress to 180°. Shoulder IR and ER motion exercises are performed at 90° of abduction, and at 7 to 8 weeks the patient should have 75° to 80° of ER and full IR (70°–75°). At weeks 9 to 10, full ROM is expected; ER should be approximately 85° to 90°. At week 12, the authors begin aggressively to stretch the thrower's shoulder past 90° or ER with the goal of 115° to 125° of ER. During this phase, all strengthening exercises gradually progress with the goal of improving rotator-cuff and scapular strength, restoring muscular balance, and enhancing dynamic stabilization of the glenohumeral joint complex. The patient is not allowed to perform isotonic exercises on weight-lifting equipment such as the bench press, pullovers, and so forth.

Phase III is the minimal protection phase, extending from weeks 14 through 22. The goals of this phase are to: (1) establish or maintain full ROM; (2) improve strength and endurance; and (3) initiate functional activities gradually. At approximately 14 to 16 weeks, activities such as light swimming exercises at 90° of abduction, plyometrics, and golf swings are permitted. An interval throwing program (**Appendix 6**) or other interval sport programs may be initiated at weeks 16 to 18 if the criteria have been met by the patient.

The advanced strengthening phase extends from weeks 22 through 26. This phase is characterized by aggressive strengthening exercises such as plyometrics, PNF drills, isotonic strengthening, and functional sports activities. In the overhead-throwing athlete, throwing from the pitching mound may be initiated. Contact sports may also be permitted during this period. Competitive throwing is usually not permitted until 7 to 9 months after surgery.

REHABILITATION FOLLOWING POSTERIOR REPAIR AND/OR STABILIZATION

The rehabilitation program following posterior shoulder stabilization and/or posterior labrum repair is more conservative than that following an anterior stabilization procedure. The rehabilitation program following posterior stabilization surgery is much slower, with more restrictions and precautions. The most significant differences are the type of postoperative brace used, length of time in the postoperative brace, restrictions of shoulder motion, and length of recovery time before returning to sports.

Following surgery, the patient is placed into a shoulder immobilizer brace with the arm positioned in either neutral rotation or slight ER, thus minimizing tension on the posterior capsule (**Fig. 12**). The postoperative shoulder immobilizer is worn for 6 weeks, and the patient is instructed to wear the brace all day and sleep in the brace as well. The only time the brace is not worn is when the patient is performing exercises and showering. The authors allow early but restricted PROM exercises immediately following surgery. PROM is initiated with the shoulder abducted to 45°, and IR is performed to neutral and ER to approximately 20° to 25° (**Fig. 13**). PROM for shoulder flexion is to 90° in the scapular plane. Isometrics and rhythmic stabilization exercises (**Fig. 14**) for the scapula and rotator-cuff muscles are also performed. All of the strengthening exercises are performed at a pain-free level and with the shoulder in neutral rotation.

During the first 8 weeks of recovery, the focus is to gradually increase the patient's PROM without causing excessive and unwanted posterior shoulder laxity, while gradually enhancing the patient's strength and dynamic stabilization. During this time frame, the authors restrict excessive shoulder IR, horizontal adduction beyond neutral for 8 weeks, and no pushing motions for 8 to 12 weeks. By weeks 10 to 12 postoperatively, the patient should exhibit nearly full PROM; usually 90° of ER at 90° of

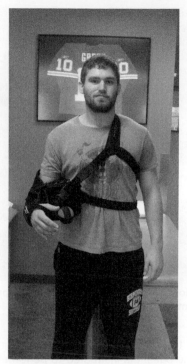

Fig. 12. Ultrasling II abduction pillow (DJO Global, Vista, CA) maintains the shoulder in an externally rotated position to reduce stress on the posterior structures.

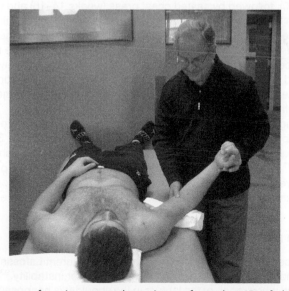

Fig. 13. Passive range of motion external rotation performed at 45° of abduction immediately following surgery to neuromodulate pain, assist in healing, and improve range of motion.

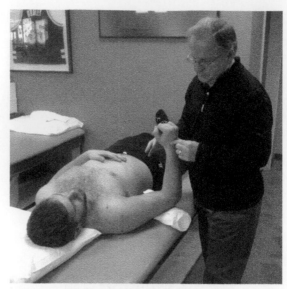

Fig. 14. Rhythmic stabilization exercises in the scapula plane to promote rotator cuff activation and neuromuscular control.

abduction, flexion to 165° to 170°, and IR at 90° of abduction to approximately 45° to 50°. During this phase, the patient is instructed to perform rotator-cuff and scapula strengthening exercises as described earlier to improve neuromuscular control, and exercises to enhance dynamic stabilization.

During weeks 12 to 26, the strengthening and dynamic stabilization exercises are increased. In addition, isotonic strengthening exercises such as seated rowing are initiated (week 10), followed by seated chest press (weeks 14–16) and two-hand plyometrics at weeks 12 to 16. A gradual return to sports-specific drills is initiated when the patient fulfills specific criteria, depending on the sport and position they are returning to. For overhead-throwing athletes, gradual return to sports would be initiated at 6 to 7 months postoperatively with a return to competition at approximately 9 months. For athletes involved in contact sports, the return to competition is approximately 7 to 9 months, but depends on the position that they play. Football linemen usually may return to competition at 7 to 9 months following surgery.

Several investigators have reported excellent results following arthroscopic surgery for shoulder stabilization. Provencher and colleagues[90] reported on 33 consecutive patients with a follow-up at 39 months, of whom 83% had a stable shoulder. Savoie and colleagues[91] reported on 131 patients with an average follow-up of 28 months, of whom 97% were stable. Lenart and colleagues[92] reported on 34 consecutive patients following arthroscopic repair, of whom 94% had a stable shoulder at 36 months.

REHABILITATION FOLLOWING ANTERIOR LATARJET PROCEDURE

The Latarjet procedure was developed in France by Dr Laurent Lafosse approximately 60 years ago, and has been used to treat chronic shoulder instability.[93–95] This procedure is performed when repair of the labrum in the shoulder is not possible. Indications for this procedure are a shoulder dislocation associated with a glenoid bone fracture, a large Hill-Sachs lesion, or an engaging Hill-Sachs lesion with continued instability and loss of function. In addition, the patient may have had a previous shoulder reconstruction, labral repair, or stabilization surgery with continued shoulder instability.

Immediately postoperatively, the patient presents to rehabilitation with the arm in an abduction pillow. The rehabilitation specialist should gradually restore PROM for the first 8 weeks. Owing to the nature of the surgery, the early postoperative therapy must protect the subscapularis and the developing bony merging of the coracoid process. Therefore, ER PROM at 30° of abduction is limited to 20° to 30° for the first 2 to 4 weeks. Slowly reestablishing full ER PROM by 8 to 10 weeks after the surgery will enable good healing while not compromising the integrity of the muscle.

Strengthening of the surrounding shoulder musculature may be initiated with submaximal and pain-free isometrics. IR strengthening should be limited for the first 6 weeks to allow adequate healing to occur. Light isotonic strengthening, as described previously, may be initiated 6 to 8 weeks postoperatively. Again the goals are to improve strength, dynamic stability, and neuromuscular control before returning to a sport-specific training program at approximately 16 weeks after surgery. Excellent results have been reported throughout the literature for return to sports, including contact-type sports, with very few complications.[93,96,97]

REHABILITATION FOLLOWING STABILIZATION PROCEDURES
Capsular Shift or Plication

Surgical management for patients with MDI often consists of reducing the excessive capsular volume that surrounds the glenohumeral joint in an effort to provide improved static stability. In this group of patients, a positive sulcus sign reveals an abundance of inferior humeral translation caused by an excessive rotator interval and inferior capsule. Ultimately the goal is to restore normal joint biomechanics and arthrokinematics, which will enable the patient to return to normal function without further onset of instability episodes. This procedure remains a viable option to return patients to their prior level of function, with good to excellent results expected.[98,99]

Immediately postoperatively, the primary goal is to protect the healing tissues through the use of an immobilizer or abduction pillow for at least 6 weeks. The rehabilitation specialist may apply controlled stresses through gentle PROM and AAROM to 90° to 100° of elevation for the first 4 to 6 weeks. Gentle isometric strengthening activities are also initiated to prevent atrophy of the surrounding musculature. At 6 weeks after surgery, PROM and AAROM are progressed until full motion is achieved by approximately 10 to 12 weeks. Special consideration should be given to avoiding stretching of the tissue, which may result in excessive humeral translation and poor outcomes. The slow ROM progression is critical in achieving good long-term outcomes. An isotonic strengthening program for the rotator-cuff and scapula stabilizers may be initiated to improve dynamic stability and neuromuscular control, as described in previous sections. There should be a concerted effort to improve proprioception and correct postural abnormalities in this subpopulation of unstable shoulders. In the authors' opinion, these simple corrections are vital to regaining full function without further episodes of instability.

SUMMARY

The glenohumeral joint is an inherently unstable joint that relies on the interaction of the dynamic and static stabilizers to maintain stability. Disruption of this interplay or poor development of any of these factors may result in instability, pain, and a loss of function. Rehabilitation will vary based on the type of instability present and the key principles described. Whether a course of nonoperative rehabilitation is followed or the patient presents postoperatively, a comprehensive program designed to establish full ROM and balance capsular mobility, in addition to maximizing muscular strength, endurance, proprioception, dynamic stability, and neuromuscular control is essential. A functional approach to rehabilitation using movement patterns and sport-specific positions along with an interval sport program will allow a gradual return to athletics. The focus of the program should minimize the risk of recurrence and ensure that the patient can safely return to functional activities.

REFERENCES

1. Kibler WB. The role of the scapula in athletic shoulder function. Am J Sports Med 1998;26(2):325–37.
2. Wilk KE, Arrigo CA, Andrews JR. Current concepts: the stabilizing structures of the glenohumeral joint. J Orthop Sports Phys Ther 1997;25(6):364–79.
3. Wilk KE, Macrina LC, Reinold MM. Non-operative rehabilitation for traumatic and atraumatic glenohumeral instability. N Am J Sports Phys Ther 2006;1:16–31.
4. Rowe CR. Prognosis in dislocations of the shoulder. J Bone Joint Surg Am 1956; 38(5):957–77.
5. Rockwood CA, Matsen FA, Wirth MA, et al. The shoulder. 2nd edition. Philadelphia: Saunders; 1998.
6. Paterson WH, Throckmorton TW, Koester M, et al. Position and duration of immobilization after primary anterior shoulder dislocation: a systematic review and meta-analysis of the literature. J Bone Joint Surg Am 2010;92(18):2924–33.
7. Hovelius L, Eriksson K, Fredin H, et al. Recurrences after initial dislocation of the shoulder. Results of a prospective study of treatment. J Bone Joint Surg Am 1983;65(3):343–9.
8. Hovelius L. Anterior dislocation of the shoulder in teen-agers and young adults. Five-year prognosis. J Bone Joint Surg Am 1987;69(3):393–9.
9. Hovelius L, Augustini BG, Fredin H, et al. Primary anterior dislocation of the shoulder in young patients. A ten-year prospective study. J Bone Joint Surg Am 1996;78(11):1677–84.
10. Hovelius L, Nilsson JA, Nordqvist A. Increased mortality after anterior shoulder dislocation: 255 patients aged 12-40 years followed for 25 years. Acta Orthop 2007;78(6):822–6.
11. Aronen JG, Regan K. Decreasing the incidence of recurrence of first time anterior shoulder dislocations with rehabilitation. Am J Sports Med 1984;12(4): 283–91.
12. Henry JH, Genung JA. Natural history of glenohumeral dislocation—revisited. Am J Sports Med 1982;10(3):135–7.
13. Hoelen MA, Burgers AM, Rozing PM. Prognosis of primary anterior shoulder dislocation in young adults. Arch Orthop Trauma Surg 1990;110(1):51–4.
14. Kazar B, Relovszky E. Prognosis of primary dislocation of the shoulder. Acta Orthop Scand 1969;40(2):216–24.
15. Lephart SM, Warner JP, Borsa PA, et al. Proprioception of the shoulder joint in healthy, unstable, and surgically repaired shoulders. J Shoulder Elbow Surg 1994;3:371–80.
16. McLaughlin HL, MacLellan DI. Recurrent anterior dislocation of the shoulder. II. A comparative study. J Trauma 1967;7(2):191–201.
17. Simonet WT, Cofield RH. Prognosis in anterior shoulder dislocation. Am J Sports Med 1984;12(1):19–24.

18. Tipton CM, Matthes RD, Maynard JA, et al. The influence of physical activity on ligaments and tendons. Med Sci Sports 1975;7(3):165–75.
19. Yoneda B, Welsh RP, Macintosh DL. Conservative treatment of shoulder dislocation in young males. J Bone Joint Surg Br 1982;64:254–5.
20. Postacchini F, Gumina S, Cinotti G. Anterior shoulder dislocation in adolescents. J Shoulder Elbow Surg 2000;9(6):470–4.
21. Marans HJ, Angel KR, Schemitsch EH, et al. The fate of traumatic anterior dislocation of the shoulder in children. J Bone Joint Surg Am 1992;74(8):1242–4.
22. Kiviluoto O, Pasila M, Jaroma H, et al. Immobilization after primary dislocation of the shoulder. Acta Orthop Scand 1980;51(6):915–9.
23. Itoi E, Hatakeyama Y, Urayama M, et al. Position of immobilization after dislocation of the shoulder. A cadaveric study. J Bone Joint Surg Am 1999;81(3):385–90.
24. Itoi E, Sashi R, Minagawa H, et al. Position of immobilization after dislocation of the glenohumeral joint. A study with use of magnetic resonance imaging. J Bone Joint Surg Am 2001;83(5):661–7.
25. Itoi E, Hatakeyama Y, Kido T, et al. A new method of immobilization after traumatic anterior dislocation of the shoulder: a preliminary study. J Shoulder Elbow Surg 2003;12(5):413–5.
26. Itoi E, Hatakeyama Y, Sato T, et al. Immobilization in external rotation after shoulder dislocation reduces the risk of recurrence. A randomized controlled trial. J Bone Joint Surg Am 2007;89(10):2124–31.
27. Finestone A, Milgrom C, Radeva-Petrova DR, et al. Bracing in external rotation for traumatic anterior dislocation of the shoulder. J Bone Joint Surg Br 2009;91(7):918–21.
28. Liavaag S, Brox JI, Pripp AH, et al. Immobilization in external rotation after primary shoulder dislocation did not reduce the risk of recurrence: a randomized controlled trial. J Bone Joint Surg Am 2011;93(10):897–904.
29. Dehne E, Torp RP. Treatment of joint injuries by immediate mobilization. Based upon the spinal adaptation concept. Clin Orthop Relat Res 1971;77:218–32.
30. Haggmark T, Eriksson E, Jansson E. Muscle fiber type changes in human skeletal muscle after injuries and immobilization. Orthopedics 1986;9(2):181–5.
31. Salter RB, Hamilton HW, Wedge JH, et al. Clinical application of basic research on continuous passive motion for disorders and injuries of synovial joints: a preliminary report of a feasibility study. J Orthop Res 1984;1(3):325–42.
32. Reinold MM, Macrina LC, Wilk KE, et al. The effect of neuromuscular electrical stimulation of the infraspinatus on shoulder external rotation force production after rotator cuff repair surgery. Am J Sports Med 2008;36(12):2317–21.
33. Decker MJ, Hintermeister RA, Faber KJ, et al. Serratus anterior muscle activity during selected rehabilitation exercises. Am J Sports Med 1999;27(6):784–91.
34. Smith RL, Brunolli J. Shoulder kinesthesia after anterior glenohumeral joint dislocation. Phys Ther 1989;69(2):106–12.
35. Blasier RB, Carpenter JE, Huston LJ. Shoulder proprioception. Effect of joint laxity, joint position, and direction of motion. Orthop Rev 1994;23(1):45–50.
36. Carpenter JE, Blasier RB, Pellizzon GG. The effects of muscle fatigue on shoulder joint position sense. Am J Sports Med 1998;26(2):262–5.
37. Wilk KE, Yenchak AJ, Arrigo CA, et al. The advanced throwers ten exercise program: a new exercise series for enhanced dynamic shoulder control in the overhead throwing athlete. Phys Sportsmed 2011;39(4):90–7.
38. Reinold MM, Wilk KE, Reed J, et al. Interval sport programs: guidelines for baseball, tennis, and golf. J Orthop Sports Phys Ther 2002;32(6):293–8.
39. Ellenbecker TS, Mattalino AJ. The elbow in sport: injury, treatment, and rehabilitation. Champaign (IL): Human Kinetics; 1997.

40. Wilk KE, Reinold MM, Andrews JR. Postoperative treatment principles in the throwing athlete. Sports Med Arthrosc Rev 2001;9(1):69–95.
41. Wilk KE, Andrews JR, Arrigo CA, et al. The strength characteristics of internal and external rotator muscles in professional baseball pitchers. Am J Sports Med 1993;21(1):61–6.
42. Wilk KE, Andrews JR, Arrigo CA. The abductor and adductor strength characteristics of professional baseball pitchers. Am J Sports Med 1995;23(6):778.
43. Kibler WB, Sciascia AD, Uhl TL, et al. Electromyographic analysis of specific exercises for scapular control in early phases of shoulder rehabilitation. Am J Sports Med 2008;36(9):1789–98.
44. Hardwick DH, Beebe JA, McDonnell MK, et al. A comparison of serratus anterior muscle activation during a wall slide exercise and other traditional exercises. J Orthop Sports Phys Ther 2006;36(12):903–10.
45. Blackburn TA, McLeod WD, White B. Electromyographic analysis of posterior rotator cuff exercises. J Athl Train 1990;25:40–5.
46. Wilk KE, Obma P, Simpson CD, et al. Shoulder injuries in the overhead athlete. J Orthop Sports Phys Ther 2009;39(2):38–54.
47. Reinold MM, Wilk KE, Fleisig GS, et al. Electromyographic analysis of the rotator cuff and deltoid musculature during common shoulder external rotation exercises. J Orthop Sports Phys Ther 2004;34(7):385–94.
48. Rodeo SA, Suzuki K, Yamauchi M, et al. Analysis of collagen and elastic fibers in shoulder capsule in patients with shoulder instability. Am J Sports Med 1998; 26(5):634–43.
49. Barden JM, Balyk R, Raso VJ, et al. Atypical shoulder muscle activation in multidirectional instability. Clin Neurophysiol 2005;116(8):1846–57.
50. Kronberg M, Nemeth G, Brostrom LA. Muscle activity and coordination in the normal shoulder. An electromyographic study. Clin Orthop Relat Res 1990;(257):76–85.
51. Kronberg M, Brostrom LA, Nemeth G. Differences in shoulder muscle activity between patients with generalized joint laxity and normal controls. Clin Orthop Relat Res 1991;(269):181–92.
52. Morris AD, Kemp GJ, Frostick SP. Shoulder electromyography in multidirectional instability. J Shoulder Elbow Surg 2004;13(1):24–9.
53. Myers JB, Ju YY, Hwang JH, et al. Reflexive muscle activation alterations in shoulders with anterior glenohumeral instability. Am J Sports Med 2004;32(4):1013–21.
54. von Eisenhart-Rothe RM, Jager A, Englmeier KH, et al. Relevance of arm position and muscle activity on three-dimensional glenohumeral translation in patients with traumatic and atraumatic shoulder instability. Am J Sports Med 2002;30(4):514–22.
55. Burkhead WZ Jr, Rockwood CA Jr. Treatment of instability of the shoulder with an exercise program. J Bone Joint Surg Am 1992;74(6):890–6.
56. Misamore GW, Sallay PI, Didelot W. A longitudinal study of patients with multidirectional instability of the shoulder with seven- to ten-year follow-up. J Shoulder Elbow Surg 2005;14(5):466–70.
57. Wilk KE, Arrigo C. Current concepts in the rehabilitation of the athletic shoulder. J Orthop Sports Phys Ther 1993;18(1):365–78.
58. Wilk KE, Voight ML, Keirns MA, et al. Stretch-shortening drills for the upper extremities: theory and clinical application. J Orthop Sports Phys Ther 1993;17(5): 225–39.
59. Andrews JR, Casey PJ. Internal impingement. In: Krishnan SG, Hawkins RJ, Warren RF, editors. The shoulder and the overhead athlete. Philadelphia: Lippincott, Williams and Wilkins; 2004. p. 125–34.

60. Bigliani LU, Codd TP, Connor PM, et al. Shoulder motion and laxity in the professional baseball player. Am J Sports Med 1997;25(5):609–13.
61. Burkhart SS, Morgan CD, Kibler WB. The disabled throwing shoulder: spectrum of pathology part I: pathoanatomy and biomechanics. Arthroscopy 2003;19(4):404–20.
62. Jazrawi LM, McCluskey GM 3rd, Andrews JR. Superior labral anterior and posterior lesions and internal impingement in the overhead athlete. Instr Course Lect 2003;52:43–63.
63. Kibler WB. Role of the scapula in the overhead throwing motion. Contemp Orthop 1991;22:525–32.
64. Litchfield R, Hawkins R, Dillman CJ, et al. Rehabilitation for the overhead athlete. J Orthop Sports Phys Ther 1993;18(2):433–41.
65. Wilk KE, Meister K, Andrews JR. Current concepts in the rehabilitation of the overhead throwing athlete. Am J Sports Med 2002;30(1):136–51.
66. Reinold MM, Wilk KE, Macrina LC, et al. Changes in shoulder and elbow passive range of motion after pitching in professional baseball players. Am J Sports Med 2008;36(3):523–7.
67. Wilk KE, Macrina LC, Arrigo C. Passive range of motion characteristics in the overhead baseball pitcher and their implications for rehabilitation. Clin Orthop Relat Res 2012;470(6):1586–94.
68. Wilk KE, Macrina LC, Cain EL, et al. Rehabilitation of the overhead athlete's elbow. Sports Health 2012;4(5):404–14.
69. Conte S, Requa RK, Garrick JG. Disability days in major league baseball. Am J Sports Med 2001;29(4):431–6.
70. McFarland EG, Wasik M. Epidemiology of collegiate baseball injuries. Clin J Sport Med 1998;8(1):10–3.
71. Borsa PA, Wilk KE, Jacobson JA, et al. Correlation of range of motion and glenohumeral translation in professional baseball pitchers. Am J Sports Med 2005; 33(9):1392–9.
72. Burkhart SS, Morgan CD, Kibler WB. The disabled throwing shoulder: spectrum of pathology part III: the SICK scapula, scapular dyskinesis, the kinetic chain, and rehabilitation. Arthroscopy 2003;19(6):641–61.
73. Thomas SJ, Swanik CB, Higginson JS, et al. A bilateral comparison of posterior capsule thickness and its correlation with glenohumeral range of motion and scapular upward rotation in collegiate baseball players. J Shoulder Elbow Surg 2011;20(5):708–16.
74. Borich MR, Bright JM, Lorello DJ, et al. Scapular angular positioning at end range internal rotation in cases of glenohumeral internal rotation deficit. J Orthop Sports Phys Ther 2006;36(12):926–34.
75. Torres RR, Gomes JL. Measurement of glenohumeral internal rotation in asymptomatic tennis players and swimmers. Am J Sports Med 2009;37(5):1017–23.
76. Burkhart SS, Morgan CD, Kibler WB. The disabled throwing shoulder: spectrum of pathology. Part II: evaluation and treatment of SLAP lesions in throwers. Arthroscopy 2003;19(5):531–9.
77. Dines JS, Frank JB, Akerman M, et al. Glenohumeral internal rotation deficits in baseball players with ulnar collateral ligament insufficiency. Am J Sports Med 2009;37(3):566–70.
78. Ellenbecker TS, Roetert EP, Bailie DS, et al. Glenohumeral joint total rotation range of motion in elite tennis players and baseball pitchers. Med Sci Sports Exerc 2002;34(12):2052–6.
79. Kibler WB, Kuhn JE, Wilk K, et al. The disabled throwing shoulder: spectrum of pathology—10-year update. Arthroscopy 2013;29(1):141–61.e26.

80. Myers JB, Laudner KG, Pasquale MR, et al. Glenohumeral range of motion deficits and posterior shoulder tightness in throwers with pathologic internal impingement. Am J Sports Med 2006;34(3):385–91.
81. Wilk KE, Macrina LC, Fleisig GS, et al. Correlation of glenohumeral internal rotation deficit and total rotational motion to shoulder injuries in professional baseball pitchers. Am J Sports Med 2011;39(2):329–35.
82. Laudner KG, Sipes RC, Wilson JT. The acute effects of sleeper stretches on shoulder range of motion. J Athl Train 2008;43(4):359–63.
83. Lintner D, Mayol M, Uzodinma O, et al. Glenohumeral internal rotation deficits in professional pitchers enrolled in an internal rotation stretching program. Am J Sports Med 2007;35(4):617–21.
84. McClure P, Balaicuis J, Heiland D, et al. A randomized controlled comparison of stretching procedures for posterior shoulder tightness. J Orthop Sports Phys Ther 2007;37(3):108–14.
85. Walch G, Boileau P, Noel E, et al. Impingement of the deep surface of the infraspinatus tendon on the posterior glenoid rim. An arthroscopic study. J Shoulder Elbow Surg 1992;1:238–45.
86. Meister K, Andrews JR. Classification and treatment of rotator cuff injuries in the overhand athlete. J Orthop Sports Phys Ther 1993;18(2):413–21.
87. Wickiewicz TL, Pagnani MJ, Kennedy K. Rehabilitation of the unstable shoulder. Sports Med Arthrosc Rev 1993;1:227–35.
88. Arciero RA, Wheeler JH, Ryan JB, et al. Arthroscopic Bankart repair versus nonoperative treatment for acute, initial anterior shoulder dislocations. Am J Sports Med 1994;22(5):589–94.
89. Grana WA, Buckley PD, Yates CK. Arthroscopic Bankart suture repair. Am J Sports Med 1993;21(3):348–53.
90. Provencher MT, Bell SJ, Menzel KA, et al. Arthroscopic treatment of posterior shoulder instability: results in 33 patients. Am J Sports Med 2005;33(10):1463–71.
91. Savoie FH 3rd, Holt MS, Field LD, et al. Arthroscopic management of posterior instability: evolution of technique and results. Arthroscopy 2008;24(4):389–96.
92. Lenart BA, Sherman SL, Mall NA, et al. Arthroscopic repair for posterior shoulder instability. Arthroscopy 2012;28(10):1337–43.
93. Lafosse L, Boyle S, Gutierrez-Aramberri M, et al. Arthroscopic Latarjet procedure. Orthop Clin North Am 2010;41(3):393–405.
94. Lafosse L, Boyle S. Arthroscopic Latarjet procedure. J Shoulder Elbow Surg 2010;19(Suppl 2):2–12.
95. Lafosse L, Lejeune E, Bouchard A, et al. The arthroscopic Latarjet procedure for the treatment of anterior shoulder instability. Arthroscopy 2007;23(11):1242.e1–5.
96. Schmid SL, Farshad M, Catanzaro S, et al. The Latarjet procedure for the treatment of recurrence of anterior instability of the shoulder after operative repair: a retrospective case series of forty-nine consecutive patients. J Bone Joint Surg Am 2012;94(11):e75.
97. Schroder DT, Provencher MT, Mologne TS, et al. The modified Bristow procedure for anterior shoulder instability: 26-year outcomes in Naval Academy midshipmen. Am J Sports Med 2006;34(5):778–86.
98. Pollock RG, Owens JM, Flatow EL, et al. Operative results of the inferior capsular shift procedure for multidirectional instability of the shoulder. J Bone Joint Surg Am 2000;82(7):919–28.
99. Jacobson ME, Riggenbach M, Wooldridge AN, et al. Open capsular shift and arthroscopic capsular plication for treatment of multidirectional instability. Arthroscopy 2012;28(7):1010–7.

NON-OPERATIVE REHABILITATION
TRAUMATIC ANTERIOR SHOULDER INSTABILITY

The program will vary in length for each individual depending on several factors:

1. Severity of dislocation
2. Number of previous dislocations
3. Associated pathologies/lesions
4. Presence of bony lesions
5. Desired Goals and activities (sport, position, arm dominance)

I.   **PHASE I - ACUTE MOTION PHASE**

Goals: Diminish pain and inflammation
        Establish voluntary muscle activity /Diminish muscular spasm
        Retard muscular atrophy
        Initiate gentle ROM
        Initiate muscular control-prevent atrophy

** Note: During the early rehabilitation program, caution must be applied in placing the capsule under stress (i.e. stretching into ABD, ER) until dynamic joint stability is restored. It is important to refrain from activities in extreme ranges of motion early in the rehabilitation process.

- **Decrease Pain/Inflammation:**

  - Sling for comfort as needed (approx. 10-14 days
  - Therapeutic modalities (ice, electrotherapy, etc.)
  - NSAID's

- **Range of Motion Exercises:**

  - Gentle ROM only, no stretching
  - Pendulums
  - Rope & Pulley
    - Elevation in scapular plane to tolerance
  - Active-assisted ROM L-Bar to tolerance of pain
    - Flexion to tolerance/mid range only
    - IR with arm in scapular plane at 30° abduction to
    - ER with arm in scapular plane at 30° abduction to neutral

** DO NOT PUSH INTO ER OR HORIZONTAL ABDUCTION **

(continued on next page)

- **Strengthening/Proprioception Exercises:**

- Isometrics (performed with arm at side)(w/ EMS to posterior shoulder)
    - Flexion
    - Abduction
    - Extension
    - Internal Rotation (multi-angles)
    - External Rotation (scapular plane)
    - Biceps
    - Scapular retract/protract, elevate/depress

- Rhythmic Stabilizations
- ER/IR in scapular plane
- Flex/Ext at 90° abduction, 20° horizontal abduction
- Weight Shifts (CKC Exercises) – scapular plane
- Joint reproduction proprioceptive drills

II.   **PHASE II - INTERMEDIATE PHASE (STABILIZATION PHASE)**

Goals: Regain and improve muscular strength
Normalize ROM
Enhance proprioception
Improve neuromuscular control of shoulder complex

Criteria to Progress to Phase II:
1. Full Passive ROM (except ER)
2. Minimal Pain or Tenderness
3. "Good" MMT of IR, ER, Flexion, and Abduction
4. Baseline proprioception and dynamic stability **(light)**

- **Initiate Isotonic Strengthening**
- **Emphasis on External Rotation and Scapular Strengthening**
    - ER/IR Tubing
    - Scaption with ER (Full Can)
    - Abduction to 90 degrees
    - Side lying external rotation to 45 degrees w/ dumb-bell
    - Prone Extension to Neutral
    - Prone Horizontal Adduction
    - Prone Rowing
    - Lower trapezius
    - Biceps
    - Table Push-ups
    - Triceps

- **Improve Neuromuscular control of Shoulder Complex**
    - Initiation of proprioceptive neuromuscular facilitation
    - Scapular neuro-muscular control exercises (seated and side-lying)
    - Rhythmic stabilization drills
        - ER/IR at 90 degrees abduction
        - Flexion/Extension/Horizontal at 100° Flexion, 20° horizontal abduction
        - Progress to mid and end range of motion
    - Progress OKC program
        - PNF w/ rhythmic stabilization @ 90°, 125°, 145°

(*continued on next page*)

Appendix 1
(*continued*)

- Manual resistance ER (supine → sidelying), prone row
- ER/IR tubing with stabilization
  - Progress CKC exercises with rhythmic stabilizations
    - Wall stabilization on ball
    - Static holds in push-up position on ball
    - Push-ups on tilt board
  - Core
    - Abdominal strengthening
    - Trunk strengthening/Low back
    - Gluteal strengthening

- **Continue Use of Modalities** (as needed)
  - Ice, electrotherapy modalities

III.   **PHASE III - ADVANCED STRENGTHENING PHASE**

Goals: Improve strength/power/endurance
Improve neuromuscular control
Enhance dynamic stabilizations
Prepare patient/athlete for activity

Criteria to Progress to Phase III:
1. Full non-painful range of motion
2. No palpable tenderness
3. Continued progression of resistive exercises
4. Good – normal muscle strength

- **Continue use of modalities (as needed)**
- **Continue isotonic strengthening (PRE's)**
- Continue all exercises listed above
- Initiate T-band er w/ end ROM rhythmic stabilization
  - Progress to end range stabilization
  - Progress to full ROM strengthening
  - Progress to bench press in restricted ROM
  - Program to seated rowing and lat pull down in restricted ROM

- **Emphasize PNF**

- **Advanced neuromuscular control drills (for athletes)**
  - Ball flips on table
  - End range RS with tubing
  - Push-ups on ball/rocker board with rhythmic stabilizations
  - Manual scapular control drills

(*continued on next page*)

Appendix 1
(continued)

- **Endurance training**

  - Timed bouts of exercises – 30-60 seconds
  - Increase number of repetitions
  - Multiple bouts throughout day (3x)

- **Initiate plyometric training**
      2-hand drills:
  - Chest pass
  - Side to side
  - Overhead
  - Progress to 1-hand drills:
  - 90/90 throws
  - Wall dribbles

    ** PRECAUTION IS AVOIDING EXCESSIVE STRESS ON CAPSULE **

IV.   **PHASE IV - RETURN TO ACTIVITY PHASE**

     <u>Goals</u> Maintain optimal level of strength/power/endurance
     Progressively increase activity level to prepare patient/athlete for full
     functional return to activity/sport

     Criteria to Progress to Phase IV:
         1. Full ROM
         2. No pain or palpable tenderness
         3. Satisfactory isokinetic test
         4. Satisfactory clinical exam

- **Continue all exercises as in Phase III**
- **Initiate Interval Sport Program (As appropriate)**
- **Continue Modalities** (as needed)
- **Shoulder brace**

  - **FOLLOW-UP**

- Isokinetic Test
- Progress Interval Program
- Maintenance of Exercise Program

Appendix 2

Throwers Ten Exercise Program

The Thrower's Ten Program is designed to exercise the major muscles necessary for throwing. The Program's goal is to be an organized and concise exercise program. In addition, all exercises included are specific to the thrower and are designed to improve strength, power and endurance of the shoulder complex musculature.

1A. **Diagonal Pattern D2 Extension:** Involved hand will grip tubing handle overhead and out to the side. Pull tubing down and across your body to the opposite side of leg. During the motion, lead with your thumb. Perform _____ sets of _____ repetitions _____ daily.

1B. **Diagonal Pattern D2 Flexion:** Gripping tubing handle in hand of involved arm, begin with arm out from side 45° and palm facing backward. After turning palm forward, proceed to flex elbow and bring arm up and over involved shoulder. Turn palm down and reverse to take arm to starting position. Exercise should be performed _____ sets of _____ repetitions _____ daily.

2A. **External Rotation at 0° Abduction:** Stand with involved elbow fixed at side, elbow at 90° and involved arm across front of body. Grip tubing handle while the other end of tubing is fixed. Pull out arm, keeping elbow at side. Return tubing slowly and controlled. Perform _____ sets of _____ repetitions _____ times daily.

2B. **Internal Rotation at 0° Abduction:** Standing with elbow at side fixed at 90° and shoulder rotated out. Grip tubing handle while other end of tubing is fixed. Pull arm across body keeping elbow at side. Return tubing slowly and controlled. Perform _____ sets of _____ repetitions _____ times daily.

2C. (Optional) **External Rotation at 90° Abduction:** Stand with shoulder abducted 90°. Grip tubing handle while the other end is fixed straight ahead, slightly lower than the shoulder. Keeping shoulder abducted, rotate shoulder back keeping elbow at 90°. Return tubing and hand to start position.
I. Slow Speed Sets: (Slow and Controlled) Perform _____ sets of _____ repetitions _____ times daily.
II. Fast Speed Sets: Perform _____ sets of _____ repetitions _____ times daily.

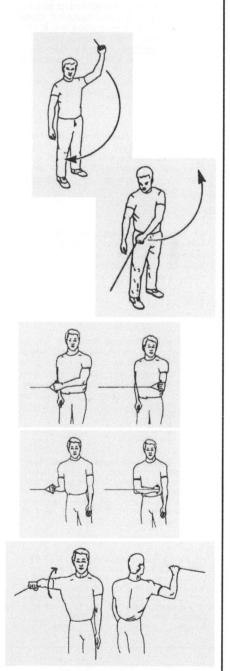

(continued on next page)

Appendix 2
(continued)

2D. (Optional) **Internal Rotation at 90°
Abduction:** Stand with shoulder abducted
to 90°, externally rotated 90° and elbow bent
to 90°. Keeping shoulder abducted, rotate
shoulder forward, keeping elbow bent at 90°.
Return tubing and hand to start position.
I. <u>Slow Speed Sets:</u> (Slow and Controlled)
Perform _____ sets of _____ repetitions
_____ times daily.
II. <u>Fast Speed Sets:</u> Perform _____ sets of
_____ repetitions _____ times daily.

3. **Shoulder Abduction to 90°:** Stand with
arm at side, elbow straight, and palm
against side. Raise arm to the side, palm
down, until arm reaches 90° (shoulder level).
Perform _____ sets of _____ repetitions
_____ times daily.

4. **Scaption, External Rotation:** Stand
with elbow straight and thumb up. Raise
arm to shoulder level at 30° angle in front of
body. Do not go above shoulder height.
Hold 2 seconds and lower slowly. Perform
_____ sets of _____ repetitions _____ times
daily.

5. **Sidelying External Rotation:** Lie on
uninvolved side, with involved arm at side of
body and elbow bent to 90°. Keeping the
elbow of involved arm fixed to side, raise
arm. Hold _____ seconds and lower slowly.
Perform _____ sets of _____ repetitions
_____ times daily.

6A. **Prone Horizontal Abduction
(Neutral):** Lie on table, face down, with
involved arm hanging straight to the floor,
and palm facing down. Raise arm out to the
side, parallel to the floor. Hold 2 seconds
and lower slowly. Perform _____ sets of
_____ repetitions _____ times daily.

6B. **Prone Horizontal Abduction (Full ER,
100° ABD):** Lie on table face down, with
involved arm hanging straight to the floor,
and thumb rotated up (hitchhiker). Raise
arm out to the side with arm slightly in front
of shoulder, parallel to the floor. Hold 2
seconds and lower slowly. Perform _____
sets of _____ repetitions _____ times daily.

(continued on next page)

Appendix 2
(*continued*)

6C. Prone Rowing: Lying on your stomach with your involved arm hanging over the side of the table, dumbbell in hand and elbow straight. Slowly raise arm, bending elbow, and bring dumbbell as high as possible. Hold at the top for 2 seconds, then slowly lower. Perform _____ sets of _____ repetitions _____ times daily.

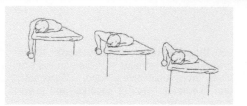

6D.   Prone Rowing into External Rotation: Lying on your stomach with your involved arm hanging over the side of the table, dumbbell in hand and elbow straight. Slowly raise arm, bending elbow, up to the level of the table. Pause one second. Then rotate shoulder upward until dumbbell is even with the table, keeping elbow at 90°. Hold at the top for 2 seconds, then slowly lower taking 2 – 3 seconds. Perform _____ sets of _____ repetitions _____ times daily.

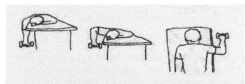

7. Press-ups: Seated on a chair or table, place both hands firmly on the sides of the chair or table, palm down and fingers pointed outward. Hands should be placed equal with shoulders. Slowly push downward through the hands to elevate your body. Hold the elevated position for 2 seconds and lower body slowly. Perform _____ sets of _____ repetitions _____ times daily.

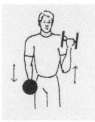

8. Push-ups: Start in the down position with arms in a comfortable position. Place hands no more than shoulder width apart. Push up as high as possible, rolling shoulders forward after elbows are straight. Start with a push-up into wall. Gradually progress to table top and eventually to floor as tolerable. Perform _____ sets of _____ repetitions _____ times daily.

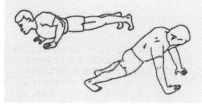

9A.   Elbow Flexion: Standing with arm against side and palm facing inward, bend elbow upward turning palm up as you progress. Hold 2 seconds and lower slowly. Perform _____ sets of _____ repetitions _____ times daily.

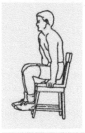

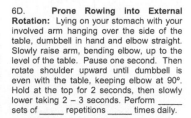

(*continued on next page*)

Appendix 2
(*continued*)

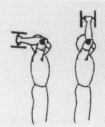

9B. Elbow Extension (Abduction): Raise involved arm overhead. Provide support at elbow from uninvolved hand. Straighten arm overhead. Hold 2 seconds and lower slowly. Perform _____ sets of _____ repetitions _____ times daily.

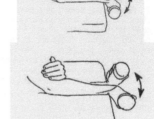

10A. Wrist Extension: Supporting the forearm and with palm facing downward, raise weight in hand as far as possible. Hold 2 seconds and lower slowly. Perform _____ sets of _____ repetitions _____ times daily.

10B. Wrist Flexion: Supporting the forearm and with palm facing upward, lower a weight in hand as far as possible and then curl it up as high as possible. Hold for 2 seconds and lower slowly.

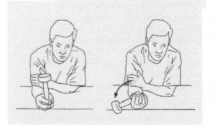

10C. Supination: Forearm supported on table with wrist in neutral position. Using a weight or hammer, roll wrist taking palm up. Hold for a 2 count and return to starting position. Perform _____ sets of _____ repetitions _____ times daily.

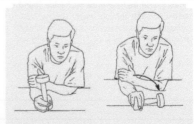

10D. Pronation: Forearm should be supported on a table with wrist in neutral position. Using a weight or hammer, roll wrist taking palm down. Hold for a 2 count and return to starting position. Perform _____ sets of _____ repetitions _____ times daily.

Appendix 3

Advanced Thrower's Ten Program

1A. **External Rotation at 0° Abduction:** Seated on stability ball with elbow at side fixed at 90° and involved arm across front of body. Grip tubing and pull out arm, while keeping elbow at side. Return tubing slowly and controlled. Perform _____ sets of _____ repetitions_____ times daily.

1B. **Internal Rotation at 0° Abduction:** Seated on stability ball with elbow at side fixed to 90° and shoulder rotated out. Grip tubing and pull arm across body keeping elbow at side. Return tubing slowly and controlled. Perform _____ sets of _____ repetitions _____ times daily.

2A. **External Rotation at 0° Abduction with sustained hold:** Seated on stability ball with elbow at side fixed at 90° and involved arm across front of body. With uninvolved arm at side, elbow straight, and palm against side. Raise uninvolved arm to the side, palm down, until arm reaches 90° (shoulder level). Sustain uninvolved arm position while involved arm grips tubing and pulls out keeping elbow at side. Return tubing slowly and controlled. Perform _____ sets of _____ repetitions _____ times daily.

2B. **Internal Rotation at 0° Abduction with sustained hold:** Seated on stability ball with elbow at side fixed at 90° and shoulder rotated out. With uninvolved arm at side, elbow straight, and palm against side. Raise uninvolved arm to the side, palm down, until arm reaches 90° (shoulder level). Sustained uninvolved arm position while involved arms grips tubing and pulls arm across body keeping elbow at side. Return tubing slowly and controlled. Perform _____ sets of _____ repetitions _____ times daily.

3. **Shoulder Abduction to 90° with sustained hold:**
    First Set: Seated on ball with both arms at side, elbows straight, and palms against sides. Raise both arms to the side, palm down, until both arms reach 90° (shoulder level).
    Second Set: Seated on ball with both arms at side, elbows straight, and palms against

(continued on next page)

Appendix 3
(continued)

sides. Raise both arms to the side, palm down, until both arms reach 90°. Return involved arm to side and repeat motion while uninvolved arm sustains position for duration of the set. Repeat for uninvolved side with sustained hold of involved side.

  <u>Third Set:</u> Seated on ball with both arms at side, elbows straight, and palms against sides. Raise both arms to the side, until both arms reach 90°. Alternate returning each arm to side while opposite arm sustains its position at shoulder level.

Perform ____ sets of ____ repetitions ____ times daily.

4. Scaption, External Rotation "Full can":
  <u>First Set:</u> Seated on ball with both arms at side, elbow straight and thumb up. Raise both arms to shoulder level at 30°angle in front of body. Do not go above shoulder height. Hold for 2 seconds and lower slowly.

  <u>Second Set:</u> Seated on ball with both arms at side, elbow straight and thumb up. Raise both arms to shoulder level at 30°angle in front of body. Return involved arm to side and repeat motion while uninvolved arm sustains position for duration of set. Repeat for uninvolved side with sustained hold of involved arm.

  <u>Third Set:</u> Seated on ball with both arms at side, elbow straight and thumb up. Raise both arms to shoulder level at 30°angle in front of body. Alternate returning each arm to side while opposite arm sustains its position at shoulder level.

Perform ____ sets of ____ repetitions ____ times daily.

5. Sidelying External Rotation: Lie on uninvolved side, with involved arm at side of body and elbow bent to 90°. Keeping the elbow of involved arm fixed to side, raise arm with dumbbell in hand. Hold for 2 seconds and lower back to starting position.

Perform ____ sets of ____ repetitions ____ times daily.

6A. Prone Horizontal Abduction:
  <u>First Set:</u> Lie prone on Stability Ball, face down, with both arms hanging straight to floor and palms facing down. Raise both arms out to the side, parallel to the floor, hold for 2 seconds then lower slowly back to starting position.

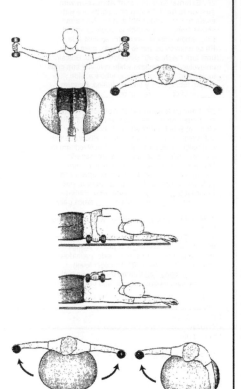

(continued on next page)

Appendix 3
(continued)

  Second Set: Lie prone on Stability Ball, face down, with both arms hanging straight to floor and palms facing down. Raise both arms out to the side, parallel to the floor. Return involved arm to starting position and repeat motion while uninvolved arm sustains hold parallel to floor for duration of set. Repeat for uninvolved arm.

  Third Set: Lie prone on Stability Ball, face down, with both arms hanging straight to floor and palms facing down. Raise both arms out to the side, parallel to the floor. Alternate returning each arm to starting position while opposite arm sustains hold position.
Perform ____ sets of ____ repetitions ____ times daily.

6B. Prone Horizontal Abduction, (Full ER, 100° ABD):

  First Set: Lie on Stability Ball face down, with both arms hanging straight to floor, and thumbs rotated up (hitchhiker). Raise arms out to side with arms slightly in front of shoulders, parallel to the floor. Hold 2 seconds at top and lower slowly.

  Second Set: Lie on Stability Ball, face down, with both arms hanging straight to floor, and thumbs rotated up (hitchhiker). Raise arms out to side with arms slightly in front of shoulders, parallel to the floor. Return involved arm to starting position and repeat motion, while uninvolved arm sustains position parallel to floor. Repeat for uninvolved arm.

  Third Set: Lie on Stability Ball, face down, with both arms hanging straight to floor, and thumbs rotated up (hitchhiker). Raise arms out to side with arms slightly in front of shoulders, parallel to the floor. Alternate returning each arm to starting position while opposite arm sustains hold position.
Perform ____ sets of ____ repetitions ____ times daily.

6C. Prone Row: Lie on Stability Ball face down, with both arms hanging to floor, dumbbells in hand, and elbows straight. Slowly raise each arm, bending elbows, bringing dumbbells as high as possible.
Perform ____ sets of ____ repetitions ____ times daily.

6D. Prone Row into External Rotation:
  First Set: Lying on Stability Ball face with both arms hanging to floor, dumbbells in each hand and elbows straight. Slowly raise both arms, bending elbows, up to the level of the top

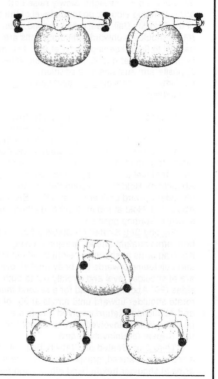

(continued on next page)

Appendix 3
(continued)

of the Stability Ball. Pause one second, then rotate shoulders upward until dumbbells are parallel to floor, keeping elbow at 90°. Hold at top for 2 second then slowly return back to starting position.

Second Set: Lying on Stability Ball face with both arms hanging to floor, dumbbells in each hand and elbows straight. Slowly raise both arms, bending elbows, up to the level of the top of the Stability Ball. Pause one second, then rotate shoulders upward until dumbbells are parallel to floor, keeping elbow at 90°. Return involved arm to starting position and repeat motion while opposite arm sustains position at the top. Repeat for uninvolved arm.

Third Set: Lying on Stability Ball face with both arms hanging to floor, dumbbells in each hand and elbows straight. Slowly raise both arms, bending elbows, up to the level of the top of the Stability Ball. Pause one second, then rotate shoulders upward until dumbbells are parallel to floor, keeping elbow at 90°. Alternate returning each arm to starting position while opposite arm sustains hold position.
Perform _____ sets of _____ repetitions _____ times daily.

7A. Seated Scapular retraction into ER:
First Set: Seated on Stability Ball, with both arms straight ahead, grasping tubing. Keeping arms at shoulder height bend elbows and pull tubing towards the body until elbows are at shoulder level and directly out to both sides (90° Abduction). Hold for a second then rotate shoulder upward until arm is at 90° of ER and Abduction. Hold at top for 2 seconds then return slowly to starting position.

Second Set: Seated on Stability Ball, with both arms straight ahead, grasping tubing. Keeping arms at shoulder height bend elbows and pull tubing towards the body until elbows are at shoulder level and directly out to both sides (90° Abduction). Hold for a second then rotate shoulder upward until arm is at 90° of ER and Abduction. Return involved arm to starting position while uninvolved arm holds position at top. Repeat for uninvolved arm.

Third Set: Seated on Stability Ball, with both arms straight ahead, grasping tubing. Keeping arms at shoulder height bend elbows and pull tubing towards the body until elbows are at shoulder level and directly out to both sides (90° Abduction). Hold for a second then rotate shoulder upward until arm is at 90° of ER and Abduction. Alternate returning each arm to

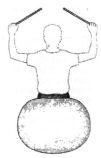

(continued on next page)

Appendix 3
(continued)

starting position while opposite arm sustains hold position at top.
Perform ____ sets of ____ repetitions ____ times daily.

7B. **Seated Low Trap:** Seated on Stability Ball, with both arms fixed at side and elbows bent to 90°, thumbs facing upwards. Grasp tubing with both hands and rotate both shoulders outward (External Rotation), rotating thumbs until parallel with floor. Hold for 2 seconds then return to starting position.
Perform ____ sets of ____ repetitions ____ times daily.

7C. **Seated Neuromuscular Control:** Seated on Stability Ball with involved arm at side, towel roll under involved side, elbow flexed to 90°. Resistance is applied to top of shoulder as shoulder is shrugged up against resistance. Resistance is then applied to bottom of towel roll as shoulder moves downward against resistance. Resistance is next applied to front of shoulder as shoulder moves forward against resistance. Apply resistance to back of shoulder as shoulder moves back against resistance and scapulas are pinched together.
Perform ____ sets of ____ repetitions ____ times daily.

8. **Tilt-board Push-Ups:** Start in down position with arms in comfortable position, both hands no more then shoulder width apart, on tilt-board. Keeping body in straight line, push up as high possible, rolling shoulders forward after elbows are straight. Return slowly to starting position.
Perform ____ sets of ____ repetitions ____ times daily.

9A. **Elbow Flexion (Bicep Curl):** Seated on Stability Ball with both arms facing inward, bend elbow upward turning palm up as you progress. Hold for 2 seconds at top and lower slowly.
Perform ____ sets of ____ repetitions ____ times daily.

9B. **Elbow Extension (Triceps):** Seated on Stability Ball, raise involved arm overhead. Provide support at elbow from uninvolved hand. Straighten arm overhead. Hold for 2 seconds and lower slowly. Repeat for uninvolved arm.
Perform ____ sets of ____ repetitions ____ times daily.

(continued on next page)

Appendix 3
(continued)

10A. **Wrist Extension:** Supporting the forearm and with palm facing downward, raise weight in hand as far as possible. Hold for 2 seconds and lower slowly.
Perform _____ sets of _____ repetitions _____ times daily.

10B. **Wrist Flexion:** Supporting the forearm and with palm facing upward, lower a weight in hand as far as possible and then curl it up as high as possible. Hold for 2 seconds and lower slowly.
Perform _____ sets of _____ repetitions _____ times daily.

10C. **Wrist Supination:** Forearm supported on table with wrist in neutral position. Using a weight, roll wrist taking the palm upward. Hold for 2 seconds and return to starting position.
Perform _____ sets of _____ repetitions _____ times daily.

10D. **Wrist Pronation:** Forearm supported on table with wrist in neutral position. Using a weight, roll wrist taking palm downward. Hold for 2 seconds and return to starting position.
Perform _____ sets of _____ repetitions _____ times daily

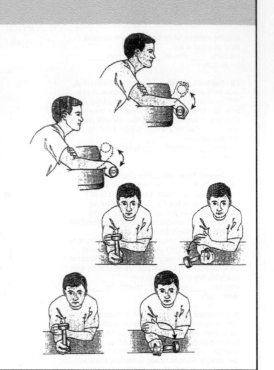

Nonoperative Rehabilitation for
Multi-Directional Instability

This multi-phased program is designed to allow the patient/athlete to return to their previous functional level as quickly and safely as possible. Each phase will vary in length for each individual depending upon the severity of injury, ROM/strength deficits, and the required activity demands of the patient.

I.   PHASE I – ACUTE PHASE

Goals: Decrease pain/inflammation
Re-establish functional range of motion
Establish voluntary muscular activation
Re-establish muscular balance
Improve proprioception

- **Decrease Pain/Inflammation**
  - Therapeutic modalities (ice, electrotherapy, etc.)
  - NSAIDS
  - Gentle joint mobilizations (Grade 1 and II) for neuromodulation of pain

- **Range of Motion Exercises**
  - Gentle ROM exercises – no stretching
  - Pendulum exercises
  - Rope and pulley
    - Elevation to 90 degrees, progressing to 145/150 degrees flexion
  - L-Bar
    - Flexion to 90 degrees, progressing to full ROM
    - Internal rotation with arm in scapular plane at 45 degrees abduction
    - External rotation with arm in scapular plane at 45 degrees abduction
      - Progressing arm to 90 degrees abduction

- **Strengthening Exercises**
  - Isometrics (performed with arm at side)
    - Flexion
    - Abduction
    - Extension
    - External rotation at 0 degrees abduction
    - Internal rotation at 0 degrees abduction
    - Biceps
    - Scapular isometrics
      - Retraction/protraction
      - Elevation/depression
  - Weight shifts with arm in scapular plane (closed chain exercises)
  - Rhythmic stabilizations (supine position)
    - External/internal rotation at 30 degrees abduction
    - Flexion/extension at 45 and 90 degrees flexion

**Note: It is important to refrain from activities and motion in extreme ranges of motion early in the rehabilitation process in order to minimize stress on joint capsule.

- **Proprioception/Kinesthesia**
  - Active joint reposition drills for ER/IR

(continued on next page)

Appendix 4
(*continued*)

II.   **PHASE II – INTERMEDIATE PHASE**

Goals: Normalize arthrokinematics of shoulder complex
Regain and improve muscular strength of glenohumeral and scapular muscle
Improve neuromuscular control of shoulder complex
Enhance proprioception and kinesthesia

Criteria to Progress to Phase II:
-   Full functional ROM
-   Minimal pain or tenderness
-   "Good" MMT

- **Initiate Isotonic Strengthening**
  - Internal rotation (sidelying dumbbell)
  - External rotation (sidelying dumbbell)
  - Scaption to 90 degrees
  - Abduction to 90 degrees
  - Prone horizontal abduction
  - Prone rows
  - Prone extensions
  - Biceps
  - Lower trapezius strengthening

- **Initiate Eccentric (surgical tubing) Exercises at Zero Degrees Abduction**
  - Internal rotation
  - External rotation

- **Improve Neuromuscular Control of Shoulder Complex**

- Rhythmic stabilization drills at inner, mid, and outer ranges of motion (ER/IR, and Flex/Ext)
- Initiate proprioceptive neuromuscular facilitation
  - Scapulothoracic musculature
  - Glenohumeral musculature
    - Open kinetic chain at beginning and mid ranges of motion
      - PNF
      - Manual resistance
        - External rotation
          - Begin in supine position progress to sidelying
          - Prone rows
      - ER/IR tubing with rhythmic stabilization
    - Closed kinetic chain
      - Wall stabilization drills
        - Initiated in scapular plane
        - Progress to stabilization onto ball
        - Weight shifts had on ball
    - Initiate core stabilization drills
      - Abdominal
      - Erect spine
      - Gluteal strengthening

(*continued on next page*)

Appendix 4
(*continued*)

- **Continue Use of Modalities (as needed)**
  - Ice, electrotherapy

III. **PHASE III – ADVANCED STRENGTHENING PHASE**

Goals: Enhance dynamic stabilization
Improve strength/endurance
Improve neuromuscular control
Prepare patient for activity

Criteria to Progress to Phase III:
- Full non-painful ROM
- No pain or tenderness
- Continued progression of resistive exercises
- Good to normal muscle strength

- **Continue Use of Modalities (as needed)**

- **Continue Isotonic Strengthening (PRE's)**
  - Fundamental shoulder exercises II

- **Continue Eccentric Strengthening**

- **Emphasize PNF Exercises (D2 pattern) With Rhythmic Stabilization Hold**

- **Continue to Progress Neuromuscular Control Drills**
  - Open kinetic chain
    - PNF and manual resistance exercises at outer ranges of motion
  - Closed kinetic chain
    - Push-ups with rhythmic stabilization
      - Progress to unsteady surface
        - Medicine ball
        - Rocker board
    - Push-ups with stabilization onto ball
    - Wall stabilization drills onto ball

- **Initiate Isokinetics**
  - Abduction/adduction
  - Internal/external rotation

- **Program Scapular Neuromuscular Control Training**
  - Sidelying manual drills
  - Progress to RS and movements (quadrant)

- **Emphasize Endurance Training**
  - Time bouts of exercise 30-60 sec
  - Increase number of reps
  - Multiple boots bouts during day (TID)

(*continued on next page*)

Appendix 4
(continued)

IV.   **PHASE IV – RETURN TO ACTIVITY PHASE**

Goals: Maintain level of strength/power/endurance
Progress activity level to prepare patient/athlete for full functional return to activity/sport

Criteria to Progress to Phase IV:
- Full non-painful ROM
- No pain or tenderness
- Satisfactory isokinetic test
- Satisfactory clinical exam

- **Continue all exercises as in Phase III**

- **Initiate Internal Sport Program (if appropriate)**

- **Patient Education**

- **Continue Exercise on Fundamental Shoulder Exercise II**

Appendix 5

ARTHROSCOPIC ANTERIOR BANKART REPAIR

I.   **Phase I – Immediate Postoperative Phase "Restrictive Motion" (Weeks 0-6)**

Goals: Protect the anatomic repair
Prevent negative effects of immobilization
Promote dynamic stability and proprioception
Diminish pain and inflammation

Weeks 0-2

- Sling for 2-3 weeks for comfort
- Sleep in immobilizer for 4 weeks
- Elbow/hand ROM
- Hand gripping exercises
- Passive and gentle active assistive ROM exercise
  - Flexion to 70 degrees week 1
  - Flexion to 90 degrees week 2
  - ER/IR with arm 30 degrees abduction
    - ER to 5-10 degrees
    - IR to 45 degrees
    **NO active ER or Extension or Abduction
- Submaximal isometrics for shoulder musculature
- Rhythmic stabilization drills ER/IR
- Proprioception drills
- Cryotherapy, modalities as indicated

Weeks 3-4

- Discontinue use of sling
- Use immobilizer for sleep ** **to be discontinued at 4 weeks unless otherwise directed by physician**
- Continue gentle ROM exercises (PROM and AAROM)
  - Flexion to 90 degrees
  - Abduction to 90 degrees
  - ER/IR at 45 degrees abd in scapular plane
  - ER in scapular plane to 15-20 degrees
  - IR in scapular plane to 55-60 degrees
  **NOTE: Rate of progression based on evaluation of the patient
- No excessive ER, extension or elevation
- Continue isometrics and rhythmic stabilization (submax)
- Core stabilization program
- Initiate scapular strengthening program
- Continue use of cryotherapy

(continued on next page)

Appendix 5
(continued)

Weeks 5-6

- Gradually improve ROM
  - Flexion to 145 degrees
  - ER at 45 degrees abduction: 55-50 degrees
  - IR at 45 degrees abduction: 55-60 degrees
- May initiate stretching exercises
- Initiate exercise tubing ER/IR (arm at side)
- Scapular strengthening
- PNF manual resistance

II.   **Phase II – Intermediate Phase: Moderate Protection Phase (Weeks 7-14)**

Goals: Gradually restore full ROM (week 10)
         Preserve the integrity of the surgical repair
         Restore muscular strength and balance
         Enhance neuromuscular control

Weeks 7-9

- Gradually progress ROM;
  - Flexion to 160 degrees
  - Initiate ER/IR at 90 degrees abd
  - ER at 90 degrees abduction: 70-80 degrees at week 7
  - ER to 90 degrees at weeks 8-9
  - IR at 90 degrees abduction: 70-75 degrees
- Continue to progress isotonic strengthening program
- Continue PNF strengthening

Weeks 10-14

- May initiate slightly more aggressive strengthening
- Progress isotonic strengthening exercises
- Continue all stretching exercises
  **Progress ROM to functional demands (i.e. overhead athlete)
- Progress to isotonic strengthening (light and restricted ROM)

III.   **Phase III – Minimal Protection Phase (Week 15-20)**

Goals: Maintain full ROM
         Improve muscular strength, power and endurance
         Gradually initiate functional activities

Criteria to Enter Phase III

1)   Full non-painful ROM
2)   Satisfactory stability
3)   Muscular strength (good grade or better)
4)   No pain or tenderness

(continued on next page)

Appendix 5
(continued)

Weeks 15-18

- Continue all stretching exercises (capsular stretches)

- Continue strengthening exercises:
  - Throwers ten program or fundamental exercises
  - PNF manual resistance
  - Endurance training
  - Restricted sport activities (light swimming, half golf swings)
- Initiate interval sport program week 16-18

Weeks 18-20

- Continue all exercise listed above
- Process interval sport program (throwing, etc.)

IV.   **Phase IV – Advanced Strengthening Phase (Weeks 21-24)**

    Goals: Enhance muscular strength, power and endurance
             Progress functional activities
             Maintain shoulder mobility

    Criteria to Enter Phase IV

    1)   Full non-painful ROM
    2)   Satisfactory static stability
    3)   Muscular strength 75-80% of contralateral side
    4)   No pain or tenderness

    Weeks 21-24
- Continue flexibility exercises
- Continue isotonic strengthening program
- NM control drills
- Plyometric strengthening
- Progress interval sport programs

V.   **Phase V – Return to Activity Phase (Months 7-9)**
    Goals: Gradual return to sport activities
             Maintain strength, mobility and stability
    Criteria to Enter Phase V
    1)   Full functional ROM
    2)   Satisfactory isokinetic test that fulfills criteria
    3)   Satisfactory shoulder stability
    4)   No pain or tenderness
    Exercises
- Gradually progress sport activities to unrestrictive participation
- Continue stretching and strengthening program

Appendix 6

Interval Throwing Program for Baseball Players – Phase I

The Interval Throwing Program (ITP) is designed to gradually return motion, strength and confidence in the throwing arm after injury or surgery by slowly progressing through graduated throwing distances. The ITP is initiated upon clearance by the athlete's physician to resume throwing, and performed under the supervision of the rehabilitation team, (physician, physical therapist and athletic trainer).

The program is set up to minimize the chance of re-injury and emphasize pre-throwing warm-up and stretching. In development of the interval throwing program, the following factors are considered most important.

1. The act of throwing the baseball involves the transfer of energy from the feet through the legs, pelvis, trunk, and out the shoulder through the elbow and hand. Therefore, any return to throwing after injury must include attention to the entire body.
2. The chance for re-injury is lessened by a graduated progression of interval throwing.
3. Proper warm-up is essential.
4. Most injuries occur as the result of fatigue.
5. Proper throwing mechanics lessen the incidence of re-injury.
6. Baseline requirements for throwing include:
   - Pain-free range of motion
   - Adequate muscle power
   - Adequate muscle resistance to fatigue

Because there is individual variability in all throwing athletes, there is no set timetable for completion of the program. Most athletes, by nature, are highly competitive individuals and wish to return to competition at the earliest possible moment. While this is a necessary quality of all athletes, the proper channeling of the athlete's energies into a rigidly controlled throwing program is essential to lessen the chance of re-injury during the rehabilitation process. The athlete may have the tendency to want to increase the intensity of the throwing program. This will increase the incidence of re-injury and may greatly retard the rehabilitation process. It is recommended to follow the program rigidly as this will be the safest route to return to competition.

During the recovery process the athlete will probably experience soreness and a dull, diffuse aching sensation in the muscles and tendons. If the athlete experiences sharp pain, particularly in the joint, stop all throwing activity until this pain ceases. If continued pain, contact your physician.

Weight Training: The athlete should supplement the ITP with a high repetition, low weight exercise program. Strengthening should address a good balance between anterior and posterior musculature so that the shoulder will not be predisposed to injury. Special emphasis must be given to posterior rotator cuff musculature for any strengthening program. Weight training will not increase throwing velocity, but will increase the resistance of the arm to fatigue and injury. Weight training should be done the same day as you throw; however, it should be after your throwing is completed, using the day in between for flexibility exercises and a recovery period. A weight training pattern or routine should be stressed at this point as a "maintenance program." This pattern can and should accompany the athlete into and throughout the season as a deterrent to further injury. It must be stressed that weight training is of no benefit unless accompanied by a sound flexibility program.

Individual Variability: The ITP is designed so that each level is achieved without pain or complications before the next level is initiated. This sets up a progression in which a goal is achieved prior to advancement rather than advancing to a specific timeframe. Because of this design, the ITP may be used for different levels of skills and abilities from those in high school to professional levels. Progression will vary from person to person throughout the ITP. Example: One athlete may wish to use alternate days throwing with or without using weights in between; another athlete may have to throw every third or fourth day due to pain or swelling. "Listen to your body – it will tell you when to slow down." Again, completion of the steps of the ITP will vary from person to person. There is no set timetable in terms of days to completion.

Warm-up: We recommend 1 set of 10 repititions of RTC be performed prior to ITP. Jogging may also assist in warm-up. Jogging increases blood flow to the muscles and joints thus increasing their flexibility and decreasing the chance of re-injury. Since the amount of warm-up will vary from person to person, the athlete should jog until developing a light sweat, then progress to the stretching phase.

Stretching: Since throwing involves all muscles in the body, all muscle groups should be stretched prior to throwing. This should be done in a systematic fashion beginning with the legs and including the trunk, back, neck and arms. Continue with capsular stretches and L-bar range of motion exercises.

Throwing Mechanics: A critical aspect of the ITP is maintenance of proper throwing mechanics throughout the advancement. The use of the Crow-Hop method simulates the throwing act, allowing emphasis of the proper body mechanics. This throwing method should be adopted from the set of the ITP. Throwing flat footed encourages improper body mechanics, placing increases tress on the throwing arm and, therefore, predisposing the arm to re-injury. The pitching coach and sports biomechanicalist (if available) may be valuable allies to the rehabilitation team with their knowledge of throwing mechanics.

Components of the Crow-Hop method are first a hop, then a skip, followed by the throw. The velocity of the throw is determined by the distance, whereas the ball should have only enough momentum to travel each designed distance. Again, emphasis should be placed

---

(continued on next page)

Appendix 6
(continued)

upon proper throwing mechanics when the athlete beings phase two: "Throwing Off the Mound" or from the athlete's respective position, to decrease the chance of re-injury.

Throwing: Using the Crow-Hop method, the athlete should begin warm-up throws at a comfortable distance (approximately 30-45 ft.) and then progress to the distance indicated for that phase (refer to Table 1). The program consists of throwing at each step 2 to 3 times without pain or symptoms before progressing to the next step. The object of each phase is for the athlete to be able to throw the ball without pain the specified number of feet (45 ft., 60 ft., 90 ft., 120 ft., 150 ft., 180 ft.), 75 times at each distance. After the athlete can throw at the prescribed distance without pain they will be ready for throwing from flat ground 60ft, 6 in. in the normal pitching mechanics or return to their respective position (step 14). At this point, full strength and confidence should be restored in the athlete's arm. It is important to stress the Crow-Hop method and proper mechanics with each throw. Just as the advancement to this point has been gradual and progressive, the return to unrestricted throwing must follow the same principles. A pitcher should first throw only fast balls at 50%, progressing to 75% and 100%. At this time, he may start more stressful pitches such as breaking balls. The position player should simulate a game situation, again progressing at 50-75 –100%. Once again, if an athlete has increased pain, particularly at the joint, the throwing program should be backed off and re-advanced as tolerated, under the direction of the rehabilitation team.

Batting: Depending on the type of injury that the athlete has, the time of return to batting should be determined by the physician. It should be noted that stress placed upon the arm and should in the batting motion are very different from the throwing motion. Return to unrestricted use of the bat should also follow the same progression guidelines as seen in the training program. Begin with dry swings progressing to hitting off the tee, then soft toss and finally live pitching.

Summary: In using the Interval Throwing Program (ITP) in conjunction with a structured rehabilitation program, the athlete should be able to return to full competition status, minimizing any chance of re-injury. The program and its progression should be modified to meet the specific needs of each individual athlete. A comprehensive program consisting of a maintenance strength and flexibility program, appropriate warm-up and cool down procedures, proper pitching mechanics, and progressive throwing and batting will assist the baseball player in returning safely to competition.

Phase I for pitchers

45' Phase	60' Phase	90' Phase	120' Phase
Step 1: A) Warm-up Throwing B) 45' (25 Throws) C) Rest 3-5 min. D) Warm-up Throwing E) 45' (25 Throws) Step 2: A) Warm-up Throwing B) 45' (25 Throws) C) Rest 3-5 min. D) Warm-up Throwing E) 45' (25 Throws) F) Rest 3-5 min. G) Warm-up Throwing H) 45' (25 Throws)	Step 3: A) Warm-up Throwing B) 60'(25 Throws) C) Rest 3-5 min. D) Warm-up Throwing E) 60' (25Throws) Step 4: A) Warm-up Throwing B) 60' (25 Throws) C) Rest 3-5 min. D) Warm-up Throwing E) 60' (25 Throws) F) Rest 3-5 min G) Warm-up Throwing H) 60' (25 Throws)	Step 5: A) 60' (10 throws) B) 90' (20 throws) C) Rest 3-5 min. D) 60' (10 throws) E) 90' (20 Throws) Step 6: A) 60' (7 throws) B) 90' (18Throws) C) Rest 3-5 min. D) 60' (7 throws) E) 90' (18 throws) F) Rest 3-5 min. G) 60' (7 throws) H) 90' (18 Throws)	Step 7: A) 60' (5-7 throws) B) 90' (5-7 throws) C) 120' (15 Throws) D) Rest 3-5 min. E) 60' (5-7 throws) F) 90' (5-7 throwe) G) 120' (15 Throws) Step 8: A) 60' (5 throws) B) 90' (10 throws) C) 120' (15 Throws) D) Rest 3-5 min. E) 60' (5 throwe) F) 90' (10 throws) G) 120' (15 Throws) H) Rest 3-5 min. I) 60' (5 throws) J) 90' (10 throws) K) 120' (15 Throws)

Flat Throwing

A) Throw 60 ft. (10-15 throws) B) Throw 90 ft. (10 throws) C) Throw 120 ft. (10 throws) D) Throw 60 ft. (flat ground) using pitching mechanics 　(20-30 throws)	A) Throw 60 ft. (10-15 throws) B) Throw 90 ft. (10 throws) C) Throw 120 ft. (10 throws) D) Throw 60 ft. (flat ground) using pitching 　mechanics (20-30 throws) E) Rest 3-5 min. F) Throw 60-90 ft. (10-15 throws) G) Throw 80 ft. (flat ground) using pitching 　mechanics (20 throws)

Throwing program should be performed every other day, with one day of rest between steps, unless otherwise specified by your physician

Perform each step 2 times before progressing to the next step.

(continued on next page)

Appendix 6
(*continued*)

Interval Throwing Program – Throwing Off the Mound – Phase II

After the completion of Phase I of the Interval Throwing Program (ITP) and the athlete can throw to the prescribed distance without pain the athlete will be ready for throwing off the mound or return to their respective position. At this point, full strength and confidence should be restored in the athlete's arm. Just as the advancement to this point has been gradual and progressive, the return to unrestricted throwing must follow the same principles. A pitcher should first throw only fast ball at 50%, progressing to 75% and 100%. At this time, the athlete may start more stressful pitches such as breaking balls. The position player should simulate a game situation, again progressing at 50-75-100%. Once again, if an athlete has increased pain, particularly at the joint, the throwing program should be backed off and re-advanced as tolerated, under the direction of the rehabilitation team.

Summary: In using the Interval Throwing Program (ITP) in conjunction with a structured rehabilitation program, the athlete should be able to return to full competition status, minimizing any chance of re-injury. The program and its progression should be modified to meet the specific needs of each individual athlete. A comprehensive program consisting of a maintenance strength and flexibility program, appropriate warm-up and cool-down procedures, proper pitching mechanics, and progressive throwing and batting will assist the baseball player in returning safely to competition.

STAGE ONE: FASTBALLS ONLY

Step 1:	Interval Throwing 15 Throws off mound 50%	(Use Interval Throwing 120' Phase as warm-up except Step 12, 13, 14)
Step 2:	Interval Throwing 30 Throws off mound 50%	
Step 3:	Interval Throwing 45 Throws off mound 50%	ALL THROWING OFF THE MOUND SHOULD BE DONE IN THE PRESENCE OF YOUR PITCHING COACH TO STRESS PROPER THROWING
Step 4:	Interval Throwing 60 Throws off mound 50%	MECHANICS
Step 5:	Interval Throwing 70 Throws off mound 50%	(Use speed gun to aid in effort control)
Step 6:	45 Throws off mound 50% 30 Throws off mound 75%	
Step 7:	30 Throws off mound 50% 45 Throws off mound 75%	
Step 8:	65 Throws off mound 75% 10 Throws off mound 50%	

STAGE TWO: FASTBALLS ONLY

Step 9:   60 Throws off mound 75%
           15 Throws in Batting Practice

Step 10: 50-60 Throws off mound 75%
           30 Throws in Batting Practice

Step 11: 45-50 Throws off mound 75%
           45 Throws in Batting Practice

STAGE THREE

Step 12: 30 Throws off mound 75% (warm-up)
           15 Throws off mound 50% BREAKING BALLS
           45-60 Throws in Batting Practice (fastball only)

Step 13: 30 Throws off mound 75% (warm-up)
           30 Breaking Balls 75%
           30 Throws in Batting Practice

Step 14: 30 throws off mound 75% (warm-up)
           60-90 Throws in Batting Practice (Gradually increase breaking balls)

Step 15: SIMULATED GAME: PROGRESSING BY 15 THROWS PER WORKOUT (Pitch Count)

Index

Note: Page numbers of article titles are in **boldface** type.

Clin Sports Med 32 (2013) 915–921
http://dx.doi.org/10.1016/S0278-5919(13)00085-9
0278-5919/13/$ – see front matter © 2013 Elsevier Inc. All rights reserved.

sportsmed.theclinics.com

Glenoid bone loss, noninvasive evaluation of, 672–678

  prevalance/morphology/classification of, 670–672, 673

Glenoid defects, 626, 627

  glenoid bone grafting in, 628

  nonanatomic procedures in, 628–630

  posterior, repair of, 790, 791

  prognosis in, 627

Glenolabral articular disruption, 658–659, 660

H

Hill-Sachs defects (lesions), 626–627, 631, 665–666, 670–671, 712–713, 789, 790, 808, 810, 845

  engaging, 742–743

  management of, 854

Hill-Sachs impression fracture, 617

  reverse, 619

Hockey players, shoulder instability in, **803–813**

Humeral bone loss, noninvasive evaluation of, 666–670, 671

  prevalence/morphology/classification of, 665

Humeral defects, 630–634

  anatomic procedures in, 630

  coracoid transfer in, 632

  humeral head bone augmentation in, 630

  nonanatomic procedures in, 630–634

  remplissage in, 631–632, 755–756, 854

  rotational humeral osteotomy in, 633

  shoulder arthroplasty in, 633–634

  soft tissue transfer in, 630–631

Humeral head bone grafting, in bone loss, 754–755

Humeral head defects, 626–627

I

Impingement, internal, 698

Instability, anterior, 656–661

    arthroscopic stabilization of, 827–828

    bony block procedures in, 828–829

    epidemiology of, 686–687

    open stabilization of, 826

    preferred management of, 691

    recurrent, in contact athletes, Latarjet-Patte procedure for, **731–739**

    surgical treatment of, in athlete, 826–829

  definition of, 608

  glenohumeral. See *Glenohumeral instability*.

  in athlete, imaging of, **653–684**

  in contact athlete, arthroscopic management of, **709–730**, 718–723

      outcomes of, 723–726

    classification of, 716

    incidence of, 713–714

United States Postal Service
Statement of Ownership, Management, and Circulation
(All Periodicals Publications Except Requestor Publications)

1. Publication Title	2. Publication Number	3. Filing Date
Clinics in Sports Medicine	0 0 0 - 7 0 2	9/4/13

4. Issue Frequency	5. Number of Issues Published Annually	6. Annual Subscription Price
Jan, Apr, Jul, Oct	4	$324.00

7. Complete Mailing Address of Known Office of Publication (*Not printer*) (*Street, city, county, state, and ZIP+4®*)

Elsevier Inc.
360 Park Avenue South
New York, NY 10010-1710

Contact Person
Stephen Bushing
Telephone (Include area code)
215-239-3688

8. Complete Mailing Address of Headquarters or General Business Office of Publisher (*Not printer*)

Elsevier Inc., 360 Park Avenue South, New York, NY 10010-1710

9. Full Names and Complete Mailing Addresses of Publisher, Editor, and Managing Editor (*Do not leave blank*)

Publisher (*Name and complete mailing address*)

Linda Belfus, Elsevier, Inc., 1600 John F. Kennedy Blvd. Suite 1800, Philadelphia, PA 19103-2899

Editor (*Name and complete mailing address*)

Jennifer Flynn-Briggs, Elsevier, Inc., 1600 John F. Kennedy Blvd. Suite 1800, Philadelphia, PA 19103-2899

Managing Editor (*Name and complete mailing address*)

Adrianne Brigido, Elsevier, Inc., 1600 John F. Kennedy Blvd. Suite 1800, Philadelphia, PA 19103-2899

10. Owner (*Do not leave blank. If the publication is owned by a corporation, give the name and address of the corporation immediately followed by the names and addresses of all stockholders owning or holding 1 percent or more of the total amount of stock. If not owned by a corporation, give the names and addresses of the individual owners. If owned by a partnership or other unincorporated firm, give its name and address as well as those of each individual owner. If the publication is published by a nonprofit organization, give its name and address.*)

Full Name	Complete Mailing Address
Wholly owned subsidiary of	1600 John F. Kennedy Blvd, Ste. 1800
Reed/Elsevier, US holdings	Philadelphia, PA 19103-2899

11. Known Bondholders, Mortgagees, and Other Security Holders Owning or Holding 1 Percent or More of Total Amount of Bonds, Mortgages, or Other Securities. If none, check box ☐ None

Full Name	Complete Mailing Address
N/A	

12. Tax Status (*For completion by nonprofit organizations authorized to mail at nonprofit rates*) (Check one)
The purpose, function, and nonprofit status of this organization and the exempt status for federal income tax purposes:
☐ Has Not Changed During Preceding 12 Months
☐ Has Changed During Preceding 12 Months (*Publisher must submit explanation of change with this statement*)

PS Form 3526, September 2007 (Page 1 of 3 (Instructions Page 3)) PSN 7530-01-000-9931 PRIVACY NOTICE: See our Privacy policy in www.usps.com

---

13. Publication Title	14. Issue Date for Circulation Data Below
Clinics in Sports Medicine	July 2013

15. Extent and Nature of Circulation		Average No. Copies Each Issue During Preceding 12 Months	No. Copies of Single Issue Published Nearest to Filing Date
a. Total Number of Copies (*Net press run*)		771	714
b. Paid Circulation (By Mail and Outside the Mail)	(1) Mailed Outside-County Paid Subscriptions Stated on PS Form 3541. (*Include paid distribution above nominal rate, advertiser's proof copies, and exchange copies*)	472	436
	(2) Mailed In-County Paid Subscriptions Stated on PS Form 3541 (*Include paid distribution above nominal rate, advertiser's proof copies, and exchange copies*)		
	(3) Paid Distribution Outside the Mails Including Sales Through Dealers and Carriers, Street Vendors, Counter Sales, and Other Paid Distribution Outside USPS®	90	84
	(4) Paid Distribution by Other Classes Mailed Through the USPS (e.g. First-Class Mail®)		
c. Total Paid Distribution (*Sum of 15b (1), (2), (3), and (4)*)		562	520
d. Free or Nominal Rate Distribution (By Mail and Outside the Mail)	(1) Free or Nominal Rate Outside-County Copies Included on PS Form 3541	75	84
	(2) Free or Nominal Rate In-County Copies Included on PS Form 3541		
	(3) Free or Nominal Rate Copies Mailed at Other Classes Through the USPS (e.g. First-Class Mail)		
	(4) Free or Nominal Rate Distribution Outside the Mail (Carriers or other means)		
e. Total Free or Nominal Rate Distribution (Sum of 15d (1), (2), (3) and (4)		75	84
f. Total Distribution (Sum of 15c and 15e)		637	604
g. Copies not Distributed (See instructions to publishers #4 (page #3))		134	110
h. Total (Sum of 15f and g)		771	714
i. Percent Paid (*15c divided by 15f times 100*)		88.23%	86.09%

16. Publication of Statement of Ownership
☐ If the publication is a general publication, publication of this statement is required. Will be printed ☐ Publication not required
in the **October 2013** issue of this publication.

17. Signature and Title of Editor, Publisher, Business Manager, or Owner

[signature]   Date September 14, 2013

Stephen R. Bushing – Inventory/Distribution Coordinator

I certify that all information furnished on this form is true and complete. I understand that anyone who furnishes false or misleading information on this form or who omits material or information requested on the form may be subject to criminal sanctions (including fines and imprisonment) and/or civil sanctions (including civil penalties).

PS Form 3526, September 2007 (Page 2 of 3)

Printed and bound by CPI Group (UK) Ltd, Croydon, CR0 4YY

19/10/2024

01776488-0002